CONTENTS

List of Figures

THE EPIDEMIOLOGY OF CANCER

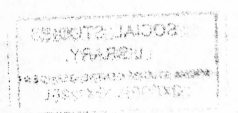

The Epidemiology of Cancer

Edited by Geoffrey J. Bourke

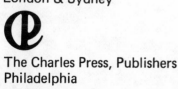

CROOM HELM
London & Sydney

The Charles Press, Publishers
Philadelphia

Croom Helm Ltd; Provident House, Burrell Row,
Beckenham, Kent BR3 1AT

Croom Helm Australia Pty Ltd,
G.P.O. Box 5097, Sydney,
NSW 2001, Australia

and
The Charles Press, Publishers, Suite 14K,
1420 Locust Street, Philadelphia,
Pennsylvania 19102

British Library Cataloguing in Publication Data

The Epidemiology of Cancer.
   1. Cancer   2. Epidemiology
   I. Bourke, Geoffrey J.
   614.5'999   RA645.C3

   ISBN 0-7099-0670-6

Library of Congress Catalog Card Number
84-070185

ISBN 0-914783-03-3

Typeset by Elephant Productions, London SE19
Printed and bound in Great Britain
by Billing & Sons Limited, Worcester.

List of Tables

List of Tables

TO THE MEMORY OF MARESE

PREFACE

Cancer is a condition which accounts for considerable morbidity and an annual toll of approximately 20 per cent of all deaths in developed countries. It thus appears fitting that our current knowledge of the epidemiology of the common cancers should be presented in a single volume for all those interested in this group of diseases including undergraduate and postgraduate students. Each chapter is essentially complete on its own topic. In the first chapter simple epidemiological terms are explained and to those unfamiliar with epidemiology perusal of this chapter is worthwhile prior to reading others.

I am indebted to the many authors from various countries throughout the world who have contributed so generously of their time to assist in the production of this book. Collectively they have made my task as editor an interesting and uncomplicated one.

I am particularly grateful to my secretary, Mrs Christine Delaney, for her meticulous attention to detail and for her endless patience with the typescript. Finally, my thanks are due to Mr T. Hardwick of Croom Helm Ltd for his assistance and encouragement.

Geoffrey J. Bourke

CONTRIBUTORS

Bourke, Geoffrey J., MA, MD, FRCPI, FFCM, FFCMI, Professor and Head, Department of Community Medicine and Epidemiology, University College Dublin; Consultant in Epidemiology and Preventive Medicine, St Vincent's Hospital, Elm Park, Dublin, Ireland

Caldwell, Glyn G., BS, MS, MD, Deputy Director, Chronic Diseases Division, Center for Environmental Control, Centers for Disease Control, Atlanta, Georgia, USA

Cole, Philip, MD, MPH, Dr.PH, Professor and Head, Department of Epidemiology, School of Public Health, University of Alabama in Birmingham, USA

Coulter, John R., MB, BS, MASM, formerly Surgical Research Officer, Institute of Medical and Veterinary Science, Adelaide, Australia; presently, Private Consultant in Occupational and Environmental Hazards

Daly, Leslie, MSc, PhD, Lecturer in Community Medicine and Epidemiology, University College Dublin, Ireland

De Graaff, Jan, MD, PhD, Consultant, Department of Obstetrics and Gynaecology, Vrije Universiteit, Amsterdam, The Netherlands

Fujimoto, Isaburo, MD, Director, Department of Field Research, Center for Adult Diseases, Osaka, Japan

Greenebaum, Ellen, MD, Assistant Professor of Pathology, Albert Einstein College of Medicine at Montefiore Medical Center, New York, USA

Hakama, Matti, ScD, Professor of Epidemiology, Department of Public Health, University of Tampere, Finland

Herity, Bernadette, MB, DPH, FFCMI, Lecturer in Community Medicine and Epidemiology, University College Dublin, Ireland

Koss, Leopold, G., MD, Professor and Chairman, Department of Pathology, Albert Einstein College of Medicine at Montefiore Hospital and Medical Center, New York, USA

Mabuchi, Kiyohiko, MD, Dr.PH, Assistant Professor of Epidemiology and Preventive Medicine, University of Maryland School of Medicine, Baltimore, USA

McMichael, Anthony J., MB, BS, PhD, Senior Principal Research Scientist, Division of Human Nutrition, Commonwealth Scientific and Industrial Research Organization, Adelaide, Australia

Merletti, Franco, MD, MSc, Visiting Scientist, Department of Epidemiology, School of Public Health, University of Alabama in Birmingham, USA; Assistant Professor of Research, Institute of Pathological Anatomy and Histology, University of Turin, Italy

Mettlin, Curtis, PhD, Director of Cancer Control and Epidemiology, Roswell Park Memorial Institute, Buffalo, USA

Miller, Anthony B., MB, MRCP, FRCP (C), FFCM, Director, National Cancer Institute of Canada Epidemiology Unit, University of Toronto, Canada

Muir, Calum S., MB, ChB, PhD, FRC Path., Descriptive Epidemiology Programme, International Agency for Research on Cancer, Lyon, France

Murata, Motoi, PhD, Senior Researcher, Division of Epidemiology, Chiba Cancer Center Research Institute, Chiba, Japan

Oshima, Akira, MD, Chief, Stomach Cancer Epidemiology Section, Department of Field Research, Center for Adult Diseases, Osaka, Japan

Parkin, D. Maxwell, BSc, MB, ChB, MRCP, MFCM, Descriptive Epidemiology Programme, International Agency for Research on Cancer, Lyon, France

Smith, Alwyn, PhD, FRCP, PFCM, FRCGP, Professor of Epidemiology and Social Oncology, University Hospital of South Manchester, England

Stolk, Johannes G., MD, PhD, Professor and Chairman, Department of Obstetrics and Gynaecology, Vrije Universiteit, Amsterdam, The Netherlands

Straus, David, MD, Associate Attending Physician, Sloan Memorial Hospital Cancer Center, New York; Associate Professor of Clinical Medicine, Cornell University Medical College, New York, USA

Tanaka, Noboru, MD, DDS, Director, Chiba Cancer Center Research Institute, Chiba; Professor of Pathology, Nihon University School of

Medicine, Tokyo, Japan

Troop, Patricia A., MSc, MB, ChB, MFCM, Specialist in Community Medicine, Cambridge Health Authority, England

Urbach, Frederick, MD, FACP, Professor and Chairman, Department of Dermatology, Temple University School of Medicine, Philadelphia, USA

Vianna, Nicholas J., MD, MSPH, Director, Division of Health Risk Control, New York State Department of Health, Albany, USA

1 EPIDEMIOLOGY AND CANCER

G.J. Bourke and L. Daly

Introduction

Epidemiology has been defined as the study of the distribution and determinants of disease frequency in man (MacMahon and Pugh, 1970). It is based upon accurate observation and studies of disease in various populations which enable the epidemiologist to obtain a better understanding of disease and how it can be modified or prevented.

Incidence and/or prevalence refer to the frequency of disease. A disease prevalence rate (the number of diseased individuals existing in a population at a specified time per 1,000 of the population) is dependent on the incidence rate (the number of new cases of disease per 1,000 of the population during a specified time), the cure rate and the fatality rate from a particular disease or condition (Alderson, 1976), so incidence and prevalence although quite distinct are closely related to each other.

Epidemiology is by no means the prerogative of specialists in this subject as a method of research and much epidemiological research is undertaken by clinicians. Important contributions in the field have been made by, for example, an ophthalmologist whose observations led to the implication of rubella virus in congenital malformations (Gregg, 1941) and a surgeon (Burkitt, 1962) who studied the epidemiology of the malignant lymphoma now bearing his name.

The origins of epidemiology are deeply rooted in the study of infectious disease and the control of most of these diseases in developed countries has focused attention on prevailing health problems such as heart disease and cancer.

In the following chapters the authors use epidemiological terminology which may not be familiar to every reader and particularly to undergraduates. This short chapter presents an overview for the uninitiated of some of the concepts and techniques frequently encountered.

Mortality

Mortality data are compiled from the diagnoses of the underlying causes

5

of death recorded on death certificates and a review (Bourke, 1969) of the various studies on the accuracy of such statistics demonstrates that many studies using different approaches have shown inaccuracies in death certification which of course indicate errors in mortality statistics. However, mortality statistics in the field of cancer may be more accurate than those in other conditions because in many cancerous conditions surgery and histology are frequently carried out. Mortality statistics have a limited role in cancer and only ever reflect morbidity from a particular malignant neoplasm when mortality from that disease is invariably very high (e.g. lung cancer). Clearly mortality from skin cancer does not in any way represent the morbidity from that condition. This being so the epidemiologist also requires morbidity data on cancer and the common sources of such statistics are cancer registries.

Morbidity

Cancer registries compile morbidity statistics on cancer at either local (e.g. hospital), regional or national level. The subject of cancer registration has been well reviewed by various authors (Doll *et al.*, 1966; Clemmesen, 1978; Donnan, 1982).

Cancer registration is undertaken for a number of reasons and completeness of registration is vital. It is a procedure whereby selected information regarding all patients suffering from cancer occurring in a defined population is brought together centrally as soon as possible after diagnosis (Doll *et al.*, 1966). There are various reasons why cancer registration is considered to be important and these have been outlined (MacLennan *et al.*, 1978; Doll *et al.*, 1966):

(a) The data collected enable the incidence of each type of cancer to be determined by age and sex since such data are used both for planning the development of health services and in aetiological studies. Patients included in the cancer registration scheme should come from a clearly defined population so that morbidity rates can be calculated. Long-established registries are useful for examining time trends which provide information which is again of value for both administrative and research purposes.

(b) The data provide information for research in both epidemiological and clinical areas. Differences in incidence rates in different sections of the population are of interest and follow-up data and calculation of survival rates following various types of treatment in disparate centres are of importance to participating hospitals as a guide to the efficacy of their treatment, and on a national basis for purposes of the control of cancer.

(c) The information provided by registration is also valuable for health education to the public about cancer.

Obviously, there are many difficulties presenting to cancer registries. For example, should one accept histologically verified cases only?; should the responsibility for abstracting the data for the registry be delegated to a medical or non-medical person?; should one concern oneself with patients rather than tumours and ignore further tumours in a patient already in the registry?; what information should be collected, and is it reliable?; should follow-up of patients be maintained to evaluate treatment and if so at what intervals?; and could standardisation of at least basic information be achieved internationally?

The literature is not short of publications on the value of cancer registries and their methods of organisation, many of which have been published by the World Health Organization (1959; 1962; 1964; 1966) and the systematic biases that may occur have been outlined by Doll *et al.* (1966).

Analytical and Experimental Epidemiology

Apart from the study of vital statistics and cancer registry data, much epidemiological research concentrates on the examination of specific subgroups from the general population. Research into the aetiology of a particular cancer may involve examining sets of twins, following up individuals exposed and not exposed to a risk factor, or comparing cancer patients with individuals free of disease. Determination of prognosis and evaluation of treatment requires following up patients with a diagnosed cancer and comparison of treated and untreated groups, or comparison of two different forms of treatment.

Prospective and Retrospective Studies

Two broad methodological categories of research in cancer aetiology can be identified. The prospective (cohort or follow-up) study is the more intuitive of the two approaches and the study of lung cancer in British doctors (Doll and Hill, 1954; Doll and Peto, 1976) is one of the best-known examples. In the early 1950s the smoking habits of nearly 35,000 doctors were determined and it was shown that over the next

20 years mortality from most causes, especially lung cancer, was higher among cigarette smokers. Typically, a prospective study involves the selection of a group which is free from the disease under investigation. Base-line risk factors are then measured and subsequent follow-up over time determines which factors are associated with increased morbidity or mortality. Such studies, however, necessarily involve large numbers of subjects and an extensive period of follow-up.

The retrospective (case-control) study, on the other hand, can provide similar information regarding cancer aetiology but without follow-up and with far fewer subjects. Herity *et al.* (1980), for example, compared a group of 200 patients with cancer of the head and neck with a group of 200 control patients free of such cancer and examined their history of tobacco and alcohol consumption. Both factors were shown to be more common among those with head and neck cancer. The essence of any such study is that the determination of risk factor exposure in groups with and without the cancer (the cases and controls) is retrospective, usually by means of interview or case notes. The retrospective study looks backwards from a disease to the risk factors while the prospective study starts with the risk factors and moves forward to the eventual occurrence of disease.

In a retrospective study the diseased group should ideally be made up of new or incident cases and the control group should comprise individuals free of disease who are representative of the general population. In practice, however, the control group is often formed from hospital patients with diseases unrelated to the risk factor under investigation and is usually chosen to have at least a similar age and sex structure to the cases. Putting it simply the purpose of such matching is to have the two groups resembling each other as closely as possible except for the risk factors under study. There are two possible approaches to matching for a factor such as age. Pair matching requires that each individual case is paired with a control of the same age, whereas frequency matching requires only that the final age distribution (e.g. in five-year age groups) is similar in cases and controls without pairing specific individuals.

Although more commonly employed than the prospective study the retrospective study has many potential sources of bias (Sackett, 1979) and results may be difficult to interpret. Breslow and Day (1980) provide a detailed description of case-control methodology and discuss its limitations and advantages compared to the prospective approach.

Any aetiological study is of course only capable of detecting associations between risk factors and disease, and to demonstrate that such an association is causal is quite a different matter. Criteria for evaluating the causal significance of an association have, however, been proposed (Smoking and Health, 1964) and are widely quoted.

Twin Studies (Gemellology)

Monozygotic (identical) twins have the same genetic make-up while dizygotic (non-identical) twins are genetically like ordinary siblings. If monozygotic twin pairs develop a disease or condition considerably more frequently than dizygotic twin pairs this is accepted as reasonable evidence of an important genetic component in the aetiology of that disease. On the other hand if dizygotic twins have a frequency of a particular disease or condition similar to monozygotic twins then a stronger environmental than genetic influence is accepted. Obviously if a study is made of monozygotic twins separated at birth and living in different environments, genetic influences can be more readily determined.

If malignant tumours are dependent wholly or in large part upon genetic factors then it should be found that monozygotic twins resemble each other with respect to the presence or absence of tumours more often than they differ in this respect, and they should exhibit the same type of tumour more frequently than diverse types of tumours. Furthermore, they should be much more alike in these two respects than dizygotic twins. If monozygotic twins are similarly affected by cancer in greater proportion than are dizygotic twins it may be concluded that the presence of malignancy and the type of tumour are dependent, to a large degree at least, on inherited factors (Macklin, 1940). This author defends well the various criticisms of twin studies.

Twin studies in breast cancer, for example, have provided little useful information with regard to heredity. Hauge *et al.* (1968) recorded concordance (similar occurrence) of breast cancer in 4 (17.4 per cent) of 23 pairs of monozygotic twins and 6 (12.8 per cent) of 47 pairs of dizygotic twins, a result which they concluded suggested a small genetic effect. These studies, however, as pointed out by Knudson *et al.* (1973) were based on the premise that breast cancer is a single homogeneous disease. If the disease is in fact heterogeneous as they suggest the evidence now indicates, the effect would be to diminish or obscure any measure or estimate of a genetic effect.

Randomised Trials

The research strategies outlined above can be broadly classified as observational and no attempt is made to evaluate directly the effect of a planned intervention in terms of treating a particular cancer or in terms of the alteration of risk factors. To determine the value of any such intervention it is necessary to carry out an experimental trial, and the salient points of this approach are best illustrated in the context of cancer therapy.

The biases involved in comparing the results of a particular treatment with previously published or historical data are well known (Peto *et al.*, 1976) and randomised controlled trials (clinical trials) are designed to eliminate these problems. Examples of such trials abound in the literature. For example, Bonadonna *et al.* (1976) showed that recurrence rates after radical mastectomy for breast cancer were lower in 207 patients who received chemotherapy compared to a control group of 179 patients who did not receive this adjuvant treatment.

Essentially, the clinical trial involves dividing a group of patients with a particular cancer into two groups, one of which receives the treatment under investigation while the other acts as a comparison or control group. Selection bias is avoided by randomisation (and by including only new cases). The groups are then followed forward in time and subsequent morbidity or mortality determined. To avoid biases in response the patient may not be informed as to which group he/she is assigned to resulting in what is called a single blind trial. This often necessitates placebo treatment being given to the control group. Double blind trials in which, additionally, the doctor evaluating the treatment response does not know the assigned group of a patient are also used to eliminate observer bias. A detailed description of the design and methodology of clinical trials in cancer is given by Peto *et al.* (1976).

Relative and Attributable Risk

Central to the analysis of any epidemiological study is the quantification of risk. Identification of groups of individuals with a high risk of developing a particular cancer or of experiencing a recurrence, or at high risk of death, has immense practical implications in terms of management and prevention. The notion of risk can be applied to both morbidity and mortality.

In a prospective study or in a clinical trial risks can be calculated directly in the groups of interest and such risks are referred to as absolute risks. In a prospective study, for example, the annual lung cancer mortalities for smokers and non-smokers might be estimated as 1.5 and 0.5 per 1,000, respectively. The risk of a smoker dying from lung cancer relative to that of a non-smoker is calculated as $1.5/0.5 = 3$. Thus smokers have three times the risk of dying from lung cancer compared to non-smokers. A comparative figure formed in this manner is called a relative risk or risk ratio.

In the retrospective study it is not possible to estimate the absolute risks of disease in subgroups of interest but nonetheless a relative risk measure is calculable (Cornfield, 1951). The relative risk in such a study is more correctly referred to as the odds ratio and it is in fact one of the large disadvantages of such studies that all analyses must be performed on the basis of this measure only.

Although the relative risk is a more commonly employed comparative measure the difference between two absolute risks rather than their ratio is also used in prospective studies. In the example given the difference between the lung cancer mortality risk for smokers (1.50) and non-smokers (0.50) is 1.00 per 1,000, which is referred to as the excess or attributable risk in the smokers. The latter term arises from the assumption that all else being equal, the smokers would have had a risk of 0.50 per 1,000 if they did not smoke so that their extra risk of 1.00 per 1,000 is actually attributable to their smoking. In other words smoking accounts for 67 per cent ($1/1.5 \times 100$) of their excess lung cancer mortality risk (the attributable risk per cent).

The relative risk and attributable risk compare risks in different ways. The former is more appropriate for determining the strength of an association and the aetiological importance of a particular risk factor (Cornfield *et al.*, 1959) while the latter is a more direct measure of the actual effect of the risk factor itself. If it is required to measure the impact of a risk factor in the *total* study population (rather than in the exposed group only) the population attributable risk should be calculated. This measures the magnitude of the risk in the exposed and non-exposed groups combined that could be attributed to the risk factor exposure. It is obtained by subtracting the risk in the non-exposed group from the total risk in the study population. Suppose that in the example above the lung cancer mortality risk was 1.25 per 1,000 in the entire population of smokers and non-smokers combined. Had there been no smokers the risk would have been, all else being equal, 0.50 per 1,000. The population attributable risk is therefore estimated as the difference between these two figures which is 0.75 per 1,000. A general discussion of such risk measures is to be found in MacMahon and Pugh (1970).

Proportionate Mortality Studies

In some studies, particularly of occupational mortality, analysis can be in terms of the distribution of the causes of death rather than in terms of the actual mortality rates. Li *et al.* (1969), for example, studied the causes of death of 3,637 chemists in the United States of America (USA) and showed a significantly higher proportion of deaths from cancer as compared to the situation in the general population determined from vital statistics data. Such studies are referred to as proportionate mortality studies.

Synergy and Antagonism

As discussed above the effect of exposure to a single risk factor can be quantified by means of a relative or attributable risk. When the combined effect of two factors is being examined the effects can be illustrated in a 2 × 2 table. Table 1.1 shows the relative risks of cancer of the larynx in groups defined by drinking and smoking habits. Among those who do not drink smoking increases the risk of this cancer by a factor of 6.0, while among the group that do not smoke drinking increases the risk of laryngeal cancer by a factor of 3.0. In those who drink and smoke the risk of cancer is 20 times that of a non-smoker and non-drinker and the relative risk in this latter group is 'assigned' a value of 1.0.

Table 1.1: Hypothetical Data Showing Relative Risks for Cancer of the Larynx

	Non-drinkers	Drinkers
Non-smokers	1.0	3.0
Smokers	6.0	20.0

An important question in relation to such data is whether or not the combined effect of both factors is greater than that expected on the basis of their individual effects in isolation. A synergistic effect is said to be present if the observed effect is greater than expected and an antagonistic effect obtains if the effect is less than expected (Rothman, 1974).

In the example the observed effect of drinking and smoking is given by a relative risk of 20.0 and the main question is how to calculate the expected effect. There are at least two methods of doing this. Among the non-smokers, drinkers have three times the relative risk of non-drinkers and one could expect the same to hold among the smokers. In this group the non-drinkers have a relative risk of 6.0 so that the expected relative risk would be three times this, or 18.0.

The approach outlined above is for obvious reasons referred to as the multiplicative model for the expected risk but there is an alternative model for estimating the expected value. Among non-smokers the *difference* between the relative risk for drinkers (3.0) and that for non-drinkers (1.0) is 2.0. If this difference also held for the smokers one would expect that the relative risk in smokers and drinkers would be 8.0 compared to 6.0 in the smoking non-drinkers. Using the additive model the expected relative risk is 8.0 whereas with the multiplicative model it is 18.0. There is furthermore no definitive answer as to which model is more appropriate (Walter and Holford, 1978), though many favour the additive one (Rothman *et al.*, 1980).

In the example the observed relative risk of 20.0 in the smoking drinkers is greater than that expected on the basis of either the multiplicative or additive models, and a synergistic effect is present no matter which model is chosen. In some situations of course this may not hold and model choice would affect the interpretation of the combined effects of two risk factors.

Survival Rates

In a prospective study or clinical trial the calculation of a mortality rate or risk is straightforward if all individuals are followed for the same length of time (or could have been if they had not died). The five-year mortality rate is the number who died during five years divided by the total number in the study; a five-year survival rate which is often calculated as an alternative would be the number who survived five years divided by the same quantity. Survival rates can also be calculated at annual intervals and the survivorship function (life table, survival curve, cumulative survival) gives the proportion of individuals surviving each year from study commencement, rather than at a fixed time point only (e.g. five years).

In situations, however, when patients enter a study serially over time problems can arise in calculating survival rates. If, for example, patients first entered a study of breast cancer prognosis in 1977 and continued entering as they were diagnosed up to 1982, some patients would have been followed for five years but others who entered the study only recently would have perhaps less than a year's observation. Data collected in such a manner are called censored data since the follow-up on many patients is terminated early; those whose follow-up is terminated in this way are usually called 'withdrawals' to distinguish them from cases actually lost to follow-up. Due to the different lengths of follow-up survival cannot be calculated directly as above but using what are generally called actuarial life table techniques it is still possible to calculate survival curves for such patients. Peto *et al.* (1977) describe this approach in great detail.

The survival rate for a group of cancer patients is necessarily influenced by the mortality that would have been experienced by the group if they had been free of the cancer in question, and it is often worthwhile correcting for this effect. For example, in a follow-up study of breast cancer patients 50 per cent of patients may actually survive five years from diagnosis; if a group free of disease, but similar in terms of age, sex and race, could be expected to have an 80 per cent five-year survival then a five-year relative survival rate is calculated as 50/80 giving 62.5 per cent. The relative survival rate thus adjusts for normal mortality in the population and reflects the real impact of the cancer on survival. Whereas a five-year survival rate gives the actual proportion who survive five years the five-year relative survival gives this as a proportion of the expected survival. A relative survival of 100 per cent suggests no adverse effects of the cancer. The expected survival is calculated on the basis of vital statistics mortality in the population. Pocock *et al.* (1982) discuss this and other techniques for long-term survival analysis in the context of breast cancer.

Comment

This chapter is devoted to an overview of some common techniques in epidemiological research and is aimed primarily at undergraduates or readers who may not be familiar with the epidemiological approach. The remainder of the volume deals with specific topics in cancer epidemiology and it is hoped that this brief and simplified introduction will provide useful background material together with an explanation of some of the terminology in common use.

References

Alderson, M. (1976). *An Introduction to Epidemiology*. Macmillan, Ch. 1, p. 1

Bonadonna, G., Brusamolino, E., Valagussa, P., Rossi, A., Brugnatelli, L., Brambilla, C. *et al.* (1976) Combination chemotherapy as an adjuvant treatment in operable breast cancer. *New England Journal of Medicine*, 294: 405-10

Bourke, G.J. (1969). Accuracy of death certification. *Irish Journal of Medical Science*, 2: 7th series, 35-42

Breslow, N.E. and Day, N.E. (1980). Statistical methods in cancer research. Volume I – The analysis of case-control studies. *International Agency for Research on Cancer. Scientific Publication. No. 32*, IARC, Lyon

Burkitt, D.P. (1962). A tumour syndrome affecting children in tropical Africa. *Postgraduate Medical Journal*, 38: 71-9

Clemmesen, J. (1978). Registration in the study of human cancer. In: Holland, W.W., Karhausen, L. and Wainwright, A.H. (eds.), *Health Care and Epidemiology*, Kimpton, London, Ch. 11, pp. 153-70

Cornfield, J. (1951). A method of estimating comparative rates from clinical data. Applications to cancer of the lung, breast and cervix. *Journal of the National Cancer Institute*, 11: 1269-75

——— Haenszel, W., Hammond, E.C., Lilienfeld, A.M., Shimkin, M.B. and Wynder, E.L. (1959). Smoking and lung cancer: recent evidence and a discussion of some questions. *Journal of the National Cancer Institute*, 22: 173-203

Doll, R. and Hill, B. (1954). The mortality of doctors in relation to their smoking habits. *British Medical Journal*, 1: 1451-55

——— Payne, P. and Waterhouse, J. (eds.) (1966). *Cancer Incidence in Five Continents*. Volume I. International Union against Cancer. Springer-Verlag, Berlin

——— and Peto, R. (1976). Mortality in relation to smoking: 20 years' observations on male British doctors. *British Medical Journal*, 2: 1525-36

Donnan, S. (1982). Cancer registration – Advance or retreat? In: Smith, A. (ed.), *Recent Advances in Community Medicine, No. 2* Churchill Livingstone, Edinburgh, London, Ch. 12, pp. 157-68

Gregg, N.M. (1941). Congenital cataract following German measles in the mother. *Transactions of the Ophthalmological Society of Australia*, 3: 35-46

Hauge, M., Harvald, B., Fischer, M., Gotlieb-Jensen, K., Juel-Nielsen, N., Raebild, I. *et al.* (1968). The Danish twin register. *Acta Geneticae Medicae et Gemellologiae*, 17: 315-31

Herity, B., Moriarty, M., Bourke, G.J. and Daly, L. (1981). A case-control study of head and neck cancer in the Republic of Ireland. *British Journal of Cancer*, 43: 177-82

Knudson, A.G., Jr., Strong, L.C. and Anderson, D.E. (1973). Heredity and cancer in man. *Progress in Medical Genetics*, 9: 113-58

Li, F.P., Fraumeni, J.F., Mantel, N., and Miller, R.W. (1969). Cancer mortality among chemists. *Journal of the National Cancer Institute*, 43: 1159-64

Macklin, M.T. (1940). An analysis of tumors in monozygous and dizygous twins. *Journal of Heredity*, 31: 277-90

MacLennon, R., Muir, C., Steinitz, R. and Winkler, A. (1978). Cancer registration and its techniques. *International Agency for Research on Cancer. Scientific Publication No. 21*, IARC, Lyon

MacMahon, B. and Pugh, T.F. (1970). *Epidemiology: Principles and Methods.* Little Brown, Boston, Ch. 1, p. 1; Ch. 11, pp. 232 ff.

Peto, R., Pike, M.C., Armitage, P., Breslow, N.E., Cox, D.R., Howard, S.V. *et al.* (1976). Design and analysis of randomized clinical trials requiring prolonged observation of each patient. I. Introduction and design. *British Journal of Cancer*, 34: 585-612

——— Pike, M.C., Armitage, P., Breslow, N.E., Cox, D.R., Howard, S.V. *et al.* (1977). Design and analysis of randomized clinical trials requiring prolonged observation of each patient. II. Analysis and examples. *British Journal of Cancer*, 35: 1-39

Pocock, S.J., Gore, S.M. and Kerr, G.R. (1982). Long-term survival analysis: the curability of breast cancer. *Statistics in Medicine*. 1: 93-104

Rothman, K.J. (1974). Synergy and antagonism in cause-effect relationships. *American Journal of Epidemiology*, 99: 385-8

—— Greenland, S. and Walker, A.M. (1980). Concepts of interaction. *American Journal of Epidemiology*, 112: 467-70

Sackett, D.L. (1979). Bias in analytic research. *Journal of Chronic Diseases*, 32: 51-63

Smoking and Health (1964). *Report of the Advisory Committee to the Surgeon General of the Public Health Service*. US Department of Health, Education and Welfare, Washington, DC

Walter, S.D. and Holford, T.R. (1978). Additive, multiplicative and other models for disease risks. *American Journal of Epidemiology*, 108: 341-6

World Health Organization (1959). Third Report of the Subcommittee on Cancer Statistics. In: Sixth Report of the Expert Committee on Health Statistics. *Technical Report Series*, No. 164, WHO, Geneva

—— (1962). Cancer control; Report of an Expert Committee. *Technical Report Series*, No. 251, WHO, Geneva

—— (1964). *The Application of Automatic Data Processing Systems in Health Administration*. WHO, Copenhagen

—— (1966). Cancer treatment; Report of an Expert Committee. *Technical Report Series*, No. 322, WHO, Geneva

2 FAMILIAL ASPECTS OF CANCER

M. Murata and N. Tanaka

Introduction

It is now obvious that human cancer, with few exceptions, shows a certain tendency towards familial aggregation in an exclusively organ-specific manner. Furthermore, the association of at least a hundred different monogenic diseases with cancer has been documented (Mulvihill, 1977). Yet little is known about the true reason for familial clustering of cancer; it is likely to be due to some familial influence either hereditary or environmental, or to their synergistic effect. To unravel this problem, as with that of other chronic diseases, is indeed one of the major current roles of genetic epidemiology (Schull and Weiss, 1980).

Studies are more and more focused on isolating specific dominant types of familial cancer as typical models of inherited susceptibility to cancer. These have resulted from past work using unselected cancer cases which were regarded as being insufficient in terms of revealing the aetiological role of the hereditary factors. However, it is not completely convincing even now if these dominant genes (known or postulated) are wholly responsible for the familial clustering of common cancers. More recently, studies are attempting to elucidate different forms of gene-environment interaction. Although available data are so far insufficient, the resulting evidence is useful for understanding both genetic and environmental carcinogenesis.

To cover the whole familial or genetic aspect of human cancer would be far beyond the scope of this chapter, but a number of outstanding reviews are now available (Anderson, 1970; Knudson *et al.*, 1973; Lynch, 1976; Schimke, 1978; Purtilo *et al.*, 1978). Therefore, it is intended, after giving a general outline of family studies, to discuss how to evaluate their results in terms of gene-environment interaction in carcinogenesis.

Family Studies

Voluminous literature on the retrospective family study of cancer bears

17

consistent evidence of a two- to threefold risk of the same cancer occurring among family members of patients (Clemmesen, 1965; Post, 1966; Knudson *et al.*, 1973; McConnell, 1976; Thomas, 1980). Perhaps breast cancer is the most extensively studied, the next being colon cancer, followed by stomach and uterine cancer. For instance, by simply averaging the values observed in most published studies (Thomas, 1980), the relative risk for breast cancer is 3.8 in mother or daughter, 2.9 in sister and 2.7 for grandmother or aunt of probands, respectively, whereas for stomach cancer it is 2.1 in parents and 2.2 in siblings. Comparison of site-specific concordance rates for certain cancers occurring in monozygotic and in dizygotic twins, e.g. stomach, colon, breast cancers and leukaemia, shows roughly a doubled rate in the monozygotic twins, thereby indicating evidence of hereditary susceptibility to these cancers (Jarvik and Falek, 1962; Harvald and Hauge, 1963; Nakano, 1967).

The population-based study using genealogical data of a defined population is a newly developed type of family investigation which adopts a form of retrospective cohort study. Studies of Mormons in Utah as well as of the Icelandic Cancer Registry have yielded valuable observations in respect of familial clustering. One of their advantages is that the data include non-genetic as well as genetic characteristics of individuals, thus providing an opportunity for studying their synergistic effect (Martin *et al.*, 1980; Tulinius *et al.*, 1980; Skolnik *et al.*, 1981).

It should be pointed out that, contrary to the general findings, the site-specificity of familial aggregation might not be sustained in some cases. A variety of pedigrees of dominantly inherited cancer family syndrome has been identified, wherein cancer occurs involving multiple organs in either the same or different individuals within a pedigree (Lynch *et al.*, 1976). Furthermore, Skolnik *et al.* (1981) have reported that specific pairs of cancers of different organs tend to aggregate more often than expected among different individuals within the same pedigree.

Causes of Familial Aggregation

As mentioned previously, the familial tendency to cancer could be explained by genetic and/or environmental factors. Changing patterns of certain cancers in migrant populations from low- to high-risk countries or vice versa indicate that environmental factors as carcinogens may already act early in life (Haenszel, 1975). So, an epidemiological study aiming to quantify the relative influences of hereditary and environmental factors may not yield clear-cut results; for example, how could we distinguish a possible carcinogenic effect of passive smoking caused by a smoking father from true hereditary susceptibility?

Genetic Predisposition

There are at least three clues pointing to the importance of genetic predisposition. Firstly, when the familial occurrence and non-genetic risk factors are studied the relative risk of the former does not markedly change even after adjusting for the latter (Tokuhata, 1969; Tulinius *et al.*, 1980).

Secondly, recessively inherited genetic diseases such as xeroderma pigmentosum (XP), ataxia telangiectasia, Fanconi's anaemia and Bloom's syndrome are known to be significantly associated with certain malignancies. Cultured somatic cells from such patients show characteristic sensitivity to the agents which induce gene mutation, chromosomal or chromatid aberration, cell killing, or cell transformation for example (Arlett and Lehmann, 1978). Swift (1976) proposes that heterozygotes of such recessive genes are also, though very slightly, prone to malignancy, and that in fact there may be quite a few such individuals in the total population. Furthermore, dominantly inherited neoplasia such as retinoblastoma (RB) and Wilm's tumour (WT) are also being investigated for such cytological abnormalities (Paterson *et al.*, 1979; Weichselbaum *et al.*, 1980). Searches for a possible high-risk individual are carried out by using these cytological tests (Day, 1974; Chen *et al.*, 1978; Arlett and Harcourt, 1980; Kopelovich, 1981). The mechanism of oncogenic association of either recessive or dominant genetic defects requires further exploration.

Thirdly, although previous works mostly failed to show any critical association of a genetic marker trait with specific cancers, a weak tendency was reported in some cases. The association of ABO blood groups could not be overlooked in various kinds of cancer (King and Petrakis, 1977). Genetic control of aryl-hydrocarbon hydroxylase (AHH) inducibility is also strongly suspected, as will be discussed in a later section. Furthermore, recent evidence on the chromosomal linkage of glutamate pyruvate transaminase locus (GPT-1) with the possible dominant gene for a specific hereditary breast cancer may provide some prospect for future studies (King *et al.*, 1980). Not only single gene but also multifactorial genetic mechanisms may be responsible for genetic predisposition. Other findings on the genetic marker association need further substantiation (Barlow *et al.*, 1981; Petrakis *et al.*, 1981).

Environmental Influences

It is well known that many environmental factors are associated with cancer in a site-specific manner: colon cancer but not stomach cancer may be ascribed to a Western type of dietary habit; cigarette smoking is extremely hazardous for the lung but unrelated to breast cancer. Thus it may be suspected that any environmental risk factors will, if common in a family, result in some familial tendency of disease vulnerability (MacMahon, 1979); this may be exemplified in virus-induced neoplasia such as some hepatic and nasopharyngeal cancers (Miller, 1978; Blumberg and London, 1981).

Studies comparing stomach cancer incidence in husband and wife could not detect any significant correlation between them (Macklin, 1955; Woolf, 1961), whereas Ruff and Scanlon (1980) reported eleven couples with identical cancers of various sites. Recent studies from the Swedish Twin Registry are interesting in this respect, because they are primarily aimed at revealing environmental rather than hereditary effects on disease susceptibility. A significantly higher concordance rate was observed among monozygotic than dizygotic twins for cervical cancer (Cederlöf and Floderus-Myrhed, 1980). This finding suggests a genetic influence on the disease, and is apparently contrary to a previous finding of no real evidence of genetic predisposition (Rotkin, 1966). However, another finding in the Swedish Twin Registry suggested a larger shared environmental influence among monozygotic than dizygotic twin pairs; on the other hand, the idea that life style as such might be genetically controlled must also be considered.

Gene–environment Interaction

Gene–environment interaction in human carcinogenesis is clearly documented with ultra-violet-induced skin cancer in XP patients. Generally, however, it is feasible to predict, but rather hard to prove in epidemiological studies, a synergistic effect of genetic predisposition with any exogenous factors. This is because (1) factors associated with a certain cancer are usually multiple, and none of these, except cigarette smoking, has been recognised as an almost invariably incriminated factor; and (2) genetically predisposing conditions are generally unidentifiable except those of highly cancer-prone genetic disorders. Strong (1981) has challenged this by investigating cancer risks among survivors of childhood hereditary cancer, such as nevoid basal cell carcinoma, RB and WT, by comparing those with radiation therapy and those without. The incidence of the development of a second malignant neoplasm was significantly increased with radiation treatment. But, importantly, it occurred with a short latent period of less than a few years and with tissue specificity for those tissues predisposed by the genes; this finding is contrary to the current concept on radiation effect, that is that cancer could be induced in any exposed tissues only with a quite long latent period (Land and Norman, 1978).

For common cancers, on the other hand, there are but scant published data which point to the synergistic effect of genetic and environmental factors. The best-known example is the work of Tokuhata and Lilienfeld (1963) on lung cancer. They compared lung cancer mortality among relatives of lung cancer patients and controls, according to the history of cigarette smoking. The relative risk of the disease, as compared with the mortality in non-smoking relatives of the control group, was 4.0 in non-smoking relatives of the patient group (family history alone), and was 5.3 in smoking relatives of the control group (smoking habit alone), while with both family history and smoking habit it was elevated to 13.6; the latter figure, while obviously showing a non-additive effect of both factors, is smaller than that (roughly, 20) expected from a multiplicative model. This finding indicates that smoking and the hereditary factor are not independent under either an additive or multiplicative model. On the basis of the additive model the two factors act synergistically in the causation of lung cancer. On the other hand using the multiplicative model an antagonistic effect is apparent and the hereditary factor is more important for the risk of lung cancer in non-smokers. Without firm biological reasons for choosing one or other model the interpretation of these results remains ambiguous. Relevant to accepting a synergistic effect a mortality study on smoking discordant twins by the Swedish Twin Registry has given an interesting finding that the excess mortality among smokers, including lung cancer death, could not be entirely attributable to the effect of smoking *per se*, but to some smoking associated features as well (Friberg *et al.*, 1973), which in turn may be under some genetic control. Supporting the existence of antagonism, on the other hand, are the consistent findings that smoking is a stronger risk factor for the squamous cell carcinoma than for adenocarcinoma; so far the relationship between family history and histological types of lung cancer has scarcely been studied, but there is some evidence indicating greater importance of heritable factors in adenocarcinoma (Schimke, 1978).

A plausible explanation of the synergistic effect observed by Toku-hata and Lilienfeld (1963) was subsequently provided by Kellermann *et al.* (1973a; 1973b). The significant role of AHH in the metabolism of carcinogenic polycyclic hydrocarbons has been well documented in experimental animals (Nebert and Atlas, 1977). Kellermann *et al.* (1973a; 1973b) found suggestive evidence of single gene control for this enzyme inducibility in man and its possible correlation with lung cancer. However, later studies could not fully support this, suggesting a complicated feature of its genetic control (Mulvihill, 1976). Findings obtained by Hopkin and Evans (1980) may indicate another explana-tion of that synergism in lung cancer. The frequency of sister chromatid exchange (SCE) induced by cigarette-smoke-condensate in lymphocyte culture is, compared with non-smoking healthy controls, significantly increased in heavy smoking healthy controls, and when compared with the latter it is much more elevated in heavy smoking lung cancer patients. Rüdiger *et al.* (1981) added more evidence, again with SCE. A common familial tendency for lung cancer and chronic obstructive pulmonary disease has been demonstrated by Cohen *et al.* (1977). They observed a higher rate of impaired forced-expiration in family members of both diseases, compared with control groups, after the smoking factor was adjusted for. A multifactorial genetic mechanism seems to be involved in both diseases. More such studies are required, but particularly with reference to histological classification.

Among all common cancers, breast cancer is exclusively noted for its genetic predisposition, but to date no marked evidence has been exhibited regarding the gene–environment interaction. Boice and Stone (1978) demonstrated that the radiation effect in breast carcinogenesis among cohorts of women treated for pneumothorax was about twofold larger if they had a positive family history of the disease than if they did not; but they were not convinced of the result because of the small size of the study population. Use of oral contraceptives has been suggested to be a synergistic risk factor with family history (Matthews *et al.*, 1981; Pike *et al.*, 1981), and has been statistically examined in a number of studies (Brinton *et al.*, 1979; Hoover *et al.*, 1981; Black *et al.*, 1981).

There is accumulating evidence that the hereditary factor in breast cancer may be associated with endogenous (perhaps ovarian) hormone levels, which thus enhance tissue susceptibility to exogenous carcino-gens (Henderson *et al.*, 1975; Fishman *et al.*, 1979; Siiteri *et al.*, 1981). Murata *et al.* (1982) provided supportive evidence for this by showing a significantly younger age at menarche and taller stature of patients with a positive family history compared with non-familial patients; these traits are both known to be, at least in part, genetically controlled. On the other hand, these two groups of patients were quite concordant with regard to age at marriage, which is unlikely to be under any genetic control. Earlier age at menarche and older age at marriage (or more precisely at first pregnancy) are both well-known risk factors for breast cancer (Thomas, 1980).

The younger age at menarche or taller stature observed in the familial breast cancer patients (Murata *et al.*, 1982) may also be interpreted as resulting from a synergistic effect of these traits with some entirely independent hereditary factors. The authors could not solve this problem, because of the lack of a well-matched control population. Bain *et al.* (1980) have shown, by using multivariate analysis, that the relative risk of a positive maternal history of breast cancer is greater the younger the age at menarche or as the total number of years of menstruation increases. It seems that their findings point to a probable synergistic effect. They suggest that the maternal influence on disease susceptibility acts via a predisposition to a prolonged menstrual life. It is as yet rather unclear if any hereditary factors in breast cancer act via, or interact with, some hormonal factors. Furthermore, it should be pointed out that even normal women show different characteristics according to their family history of cancer. By using a participant group of a cervical cancer screening programme we confirmed that a positive family history of breast cancer is associated with earlier age at menarche and older age at marriage among normal women, and that these associations are stronger when they are residents of urban areas. It is suggested that some environmental influence must be involved in these associations.

Colon cancer is distinguishable from other cancers with the infrequent but strong association with familial polyposis coli (FPC), a well-defined, entirely tumourigenic genetic disease (Reed and Neel, 1955). Exceptionally early age at onset and multiple occurrence are the characteristics of colon cancer in FPC patients. Cultured fibroblasts from the patients show a variety of cytological abnormalities in response to various chemical and viral agents (Lipkin, 1978; Danes, 1978; Hori *et al.*, 1980; Kopelovich *et al.*, 1979; Rasheed and Gardner, 1981). These findings, though as yet inconsistent, suggest post-zygotic influence of some exogenous factors in addition to the probable inherited genetic defect for developing the malignancy. However, a comparative epidemiological study on the age-specific incidence rate of colon cancer in English (Veale, 1965) and Japanese FPC patients (Utsunomia *et al.*, 1980) could not detect any difference between them. Their median ages at diagnosis of adenoma without cancer (25.9 *vs.* 26.3 years) and colo-rectal cancer (41.2 *vs.* 40.9 years) are respectively very similar. Thus the effect of a Western-type nutritional condition as a proposed risk factor for colon cancer (Wynder and Reddy, 1975) seems not important for FPC patients.

Caucasian and Japanese colon cancers are individually characterised by their sub-site distribution, with a relatively larger proportion of the distal colon involved in the former, suggesting the influence of nutrition (Correa and Haenszel, 1978). According to Anderson and Romsdahl (1977), in the USA the percentage of proximal colon cancer among all colo-rectal cancers is approximately 51 per cent in familial patients, which is 2.3 times larger than that (22 per cent) of non-familial patients. In Japan, moreover, a preliminary analysis of the cases in the Cancer Institute Hospital, Tokyo, reveals almost the same ratio between familial and non-familial cases, despite the fact that the incidence of colon cancer is generally much lower. Thus, again, the effect of the hereditary factor seems independent from that of the Western-type dietary factor in colon carcinogenesis.

These facts mentioned above do not imply that the influence of a genetic predisposition is completely independent of any exogenous factors for colon cancer; the effect of the Western-type diet is suspected to be active in the promotional phase. Of course, other initiating factors should also be investigated for their relationship with a possible genetic predisposition.

No markedly predisposing genetic condition has been identified for stomach cancer, except for the A blood group and also pernicious anaemia (McConnell, 1976). Genetic predisposition to chronic gastritis in common with stomach cancer has been substantiated especially in Finland (Varis, 1971). Lehtola (1978) observed that the relative risk of stomach cancer was much larger when probands were affected with diffuse type than with intestinal-type stomach cancer, according to Laurén's classification (Laurén, 1965). Chronic gastritis is detected more often in relatives of the former type of stomach cancer patients (Kekki *et al.*, 1975). These results indicate that histological diagnosis is important for investigating the hereditary factor. We are presently conducting an analysis on the relationship between the histological type of tumour, family history and ABO blood groups. The frequency of A blood group is 0.421 in stomach cancer patients, significantly higher than that (0.366) of the Japanese general population. There appears to be no difference either between the patient groups with and without a positive family history of stomach cancer (0.426 *vs.* 0.420), or between those with diffuse type and the other types of tumour (0.430 *vs.* 0.414). Nevertheless, the frequency becomes extremely high when the patients with a positive family history are either younger than 50 years of age (0.571) or with diffuse type of tumour (0.463). Although the number of cases (402 in total) is too small to be considered conclusive, a similar finding has already been reported by another author (Kurita, 1976). Furthermore, the frequency of A blood group is also increased in stomach cancer patients with pernicious anaemia (Hoskins *et al.*, 1965). Development of stomach cancer may be enhanced by these hereditary factors, though their mechanisms are as yet wholly obscured.

Summary and Conclusion

We have reviewed both genetic and environmental aspects of the familial tendency of cancer susceptibility. It appears probable that the environmental factor is by no means irrelevant to the family history of the disease, as has been indicated by those studies from the Swedish Twin Registry as well as our own data on breast cancer. The important role of the genetic factor is also progressively clarified, especially with dominantly inherited neoplasia. Knudson (1981) has proposed that these dominant genes must be a mutation on the locus that controls cell differentiation; this idea may explain the site-specificity of the hereditary factor generally observed. Although presently we are not sure to what extent these mutant genes are responsible for the whole genetic predisposition, the important thing is to distinguish and define these highly predisposed individuals by epidemiological study.

With respect to the synergistic effect of the genetic and environmental factors, most epidemiological data observed for four major cancers seem to have resulted in some confusion. Suggestive evidence of this effect may not necessarily be regarded as conclusive, as observed for lung cancer. Thus, when we consider the genetic and environmental effects on certain cancers, we are driven to the question whether the cancer of an organ is a single disease or not. If rectal cancer is classified as a different entity from colon cancer, then why not the same for proximal and distal colon cancers? As indicated by Strong (1981), if gene-environment interaction should be tissue specific, it is of major importance to discern precisely whether tissues and cell types are associated with an hereditary factor. Finally, the genetic and environmental contribution to cancer aetiology must be more satisfactorily elucidated.

Acknowledgement

The authors are very much indebted to the Cancer Institute Hospital in Tokyo, the Association for Cancer Prevention in Chiba Prefecture, Chiba Cancer Center Hospital, and the Second Department of Surgery of Tokyo Medical and Dental University for generously allowing us to use their data and files.

References

Anderson, D.E. (1970). Genetic varieties of neoplasia. In: M.D. Anderson Hospital and Tumor Institute (ed.), *Genetic Concepts and Neoplasia*, Williams and Wilkins, Baltimore, p. 85
—— and Romsdahl, M.M. (1977). Family history: A criteria for selective screening. In: Mulvihill, J.J., Miller, R.W. and Fraumeni, J.F. (eds.), *Genetics of Human Cancer*, Raven Press, New York, Ch. 21, p. 257
Arlett, C.F. and Lehmann, A.R. (1978). Human disorders showing increased sensitivity to the induction of genetic damage. *Annual Review of Genetics*, 12: 95-115
—— and Harcourt, S.A. (1980). Survey study of radiosensitivity in a variety of human cell strains. *Cancer Research*, 40: 926-32
Bain, C., Speizer, F.E., Rosner, B., Belanger, C. and Hennekens, C.H. (1980). Family history of breast cancer as a risk indicator for the disease. *American Journal of Epidemiology*, 111: 301-8
Barlow, J.J., Diciocco, R.A., Dillard, P.H., Blumenson, L.E. and Matta, K.L. (1981). Frequency of an allele for low activity of α-L-fucosidase in sera: Possible increase in epithelial ovarian cancer patients. *Journal of the National Cancer Institute*, 67: 1005-9
Black, M.M., Kwon, C.S., Leis, H.P. and Barclay, T.H.C. (1981). Family history and oral contraceptives. Unique relationships in breast cancer patients. *Cancer*, 46: 2747-51
Blumberg, B.S. and London, W.T. (1981). Hepatitis B virus and the prevention of primary hepatocellular carcinoma. *New England Journal of Medicine*, 304: 782-3
Boice, J.D. and Stone, B.J. (1978). Interaction between radiation and other breast cancer risk factors. In: *Late Biological Effects of Ionizing Radiation*, Vol. I., IAEA, Vienna, p. 231
Brinton, L.A., Williams, R.R., Hoover, R.N., Stegens, N.L., Feinleib, M. and Fraumeni, J.F. (1979). Breast cancer risk factors among screening program participants. *Journal of the National Cancer Institute*, 62: 37-44
Cederlöf, R. and Floderus-Myrhed, B. (1980). Cancer mortality and morbidity among 23,000 unselected twin pairs. In: Gelboin, H.V., MacMahon, B., Matsushima, T., Sugimura, T., Takayama, S. and Takebe, H. (eds.), *Genetic and Environmental Factors in Experimental and Human Cancer*, Japan Scientific Society Press, Tokyo, p. 151
Chen, P.C., Lavin, M.F., Kidson, C. and Moss, D. (1978). Identification of AT heterozygotes: a cancer prone population. *Nature*, 274: 484-6
Clemmesen, J. (1965). Statistical studies in the aetiology of malignant neoplasms, I. Review and results. *Acta Pathologica et Microbiologica Scandinavica* (Suppl.), 174: 1-543

Cohen, B.H., Diamond, E.L., Graves, C.G., Kreiss, P., Levy, D.A., Menkes, H.A. *et al.* (1977). A common familial component in lung cancer and chronic obstructive pulmonary disease. *Lancet*, 2: 523-6

Correa, P. and Haenszel, W. (1978). The epidemiology of large-bowel cancer. *Advances in Cancer Research*, 26: 1-141

Danes, B.S. (1978). Increased in vitro tetraploidy: tissue specific within the heritable colo-rectal cancer syndromes with polyposis. *Cancer*, 41: 2330-4

Day, R.S. (1974). Studies on repair of adenovirus 2 by human fibroblasts using normal, xeroderma pigmentosum, and xeroderma pigmentosum heterozygous strains. *Cancer Research*, 34: 1965-70

Fishman, J., Fukushima, D.K. and O'Conner, J. (1979). Low urinary estrogen glucuronides in women at risk for familial breast cancer. *Science*, 204: 1089-91

Friberg, L., Cederlöf, R., Lorich, U., Lundman, T. and deFaire, U. (1973). Mortality in twins in relation to smoking habits and alcohol problems. *Archives of Environmental Health*, 27: 294-304

Haenszel, W. (1975). Migrant studies. In: Fraumeni, J.F. (ed.), *Persons at High Risk of Cancer*, Academic Press, New York, Ch. 21, p. 361

Harvald, B. and Hauge, M. (1963). Heredity of cancer elucidated by a study of unselected twins. *Journal of the American Medical Association*, 23: 749-53

Henderson, B.E., Gerkins, V., Rosario, I., Casagrande, J. and Pike, M.C. (1975). Elevated serum levels of estrogen and prolactin in daughters of patients with breast cancer. *New England Journal of Medicine*, 293: 790-5

Hoover, R., Glass, A., Finkle, W.D., Azenvedo, D. and Milne, K. (1981). Conjugated estrogens and breast cancer risk in women. *Journal of the National Cancer Institute*, 67: 815-20

Hopkin, J.M. and Evans, H.J. (1980). Cigarette smoke-induced DNA damage and lung cancer risks. *Nature*, 283: 388-90

Hori, T., Murata, M. and Utsunomiya, J. (1980). Chromosome aberrations induced by N-Methyl-N'-nitro-N-nitrosoguanidine in cultured skin fibroblasts from patients with adenomatosis coli. *Gann: Japanese Journal of Cancer Research*, 71: 628-36

Hoskins, L.C., Loux, H.A., Britten, A. and Zamcheck, N. (1965). Distribution of ABO blood groups in patients with pernicious anemia, gastric carcinoma and gastric carcinoma associated with pernicious anemia. *New England Journal of Medicine*, 273: 633-7

Jarvik, L.F. and Falek, A. (1962). Comparative data on cancer in aging twins. *Cancer*, 15: 1009-18

Kekki, M., Ihamäki, T., Sipponen, P. and Hovinen, E. (1975). Heterogeneity in susceptibility to chronic gastritis in relatives of gastric cancer patients with different histology of carcinoma. *Scandinavian Journal of Gastroenterology*, 10: 737-45

Kellermann, G., Luyten-Kellermann, M. and Shaw, C.R. (1973a). Genetic variation of aryl hydrocarbon hydroxylase in human lymphocytes. *American Journal of Human Genetics*, 25: 327-31

—— Shaw, C.R. and Luyten-Kellermann, M. (1973b). Aryl hydrocarbon hydroxylase inducibility and bronchogenic carcinoma. *New England Journal of Medicine*, 289: 934-7

King, M.C. and Petrakis, N.L. (1977). Genetic markers and cancer. In: Mulvihill, J.J., Miller, R.W. and Fraumeni, J.F. (eds.), *Genetics of Human Cancer*, Raven Press, New York, Ch. 24, p. 281

—— Petrakis, N.L., Go, R.C.P., Elston, R.C. and Lynch, H.T. (1980). An allele increasing susceptibility to human breast cancer may be linked to the GPT locus. *Science*, 208: 406-8

Knudson, A.G. (1981). Human cancer genes. In: Arrighi, F.E., Rao, P.N. and

Stubblefield, E. (eds.), *Genes, Chromosomes, and Neoplasia*, Raven Press, New York, p. 453
———— Strong, L.C. and Anderson, D.E. (1973). Heredity and cancer in man. *Progress in Medical Genetics*, 9: 113-58
Kopelovich, L. (1981). The use of a tumor promoter as a single parameter approach for the detection of individuals genetically predisposed to colo-rectal cancer. *Cancer Research*, 12: 67-74
———— Pfeffer, L. and Bias, N. (1979). Growth characteristics of human skin fibroblasts *in vitro*. A simple experimental approach for the identification of hereditary adenomatosis of the colon and rectum. *Cancer*, 43: 218-23
Kurita, H. (1976). ABO blood groups and cancer family history factors in gastric cancer patients, approached from sex, age and clinical feature. *Nagoya Medical Journal*, 21: 213-27
Land, C.E. and Norman, J.E. (1978). Latent period of radiogenic cancers occurring among Japanese A-bomb survivors. In: *Late Biological Effects of Ionizing Radiation*, IAEA, Vienna, p. 29
Laurén, P. (1965). The two histological main types of gastric carcinoma: Diffuse and so-called intestinal type carcinoma. *Acta Pathologica et Microbiologica Scandinavica*, 64: 31-49
Lehtola, J. (1978). Family study of gastric carcinoma. *Scandinavian Journal of Gastroenterology*, 13 (suppl. 50): 1-54
Lipkin, M. (1978). Susceptibility of human population groups to colon cancer. *Advances in Cancer Research*, 27: 281-304
Lynch, H.T. (1976). Introduction to cancer genetics. In: Lynch, H.T. (ed.), *Cancer Genetics*, Thomas, Springfield, Ch. 1, p. 3
———— Krush, A.J., Thomas, R.J. and Lynch, J. (1976). Cancer family syndrome. In: Lynch, H.T. (ed.), *Cancer Genetics*, Thomas, Springfield, Ch. 19, p. 355
Macklin, M. (1955). The role of heredity in gastric and intestinal cancer. *Gastroenterology*, 29: 507-11
MacMahon, B. (1979). Epidemiological approaches to family resemblance. In: Morton, N.E. and Chung, C.S. (eds.), *Genetic Epidemiology*, Academic Press, New York, p. 3
Martin, A.O., Dunn, J.K., Simpson, J.L., Olsen, C.L., Kemel, S., Grace, M. *et al.* (1980). Cancer mortality in a human isolate. *Journal of the National Cancer Institute*, 65: 1109-13
Matthews, P.N., Millis, R.R. and Hayward, J.L. (1981). Breast cancer in women who have taken contraceptive steroids. *British Medical Journal*, 282: 774-6
McConnell, R.B. (1976). Genetic aspects of gastrointestinal cancer. *Clinics in Gastroenterology*, 5: 483-503
Miller, R.W. (1978). Cancer epidemics in the People's Republic of China. *Journal of the National Cancer Institute*, 60: 1195-203
Mulvihill, J.J. (1976). Host factors in human lung tumors: an example of ecogenetics in oncology. *Journal of the National Cancer Institute*, 57: 3-7
———— (1977). Genetic repertory of human neoplasia. In: Mulvihill, J.J., Miller, R.W. and Fraumeni, J.F. (eds.), *Genetics of Human Cancer*, Raven Press, New York, Ch. 11, p. 137
Murata, M., Kuno, K., Fukami, A. and Sakamoto, G. (1982). Epidemiology of familial predisposition for breast cancer in Japan. *Journal of the National Cancer Institute*, 69: 1229-34
Nakano, K. (1967). Genetical studies of malignant tumor. II. Twin study of malignant tumor. *Kumamoto Medical Journal*, 20: 1051-6
Nebert, D.W. and Atlas, S.A. (1977). Aryl hydrocarbon hydroxylase induction (Ah locus) as a possible genetic marker for cancer. In: Mulvihill, J.J., Miller, R.W. and Fraumeni, J.F. (eds.), *Genetics of Human Cancer*, Raven Press,

New York, Ch. 27, p. 301

Paterson, M.C., Smith, P.J., Bech-Hansen, N.T., Smith, B.P. and Sell, B.M. (1979). γ-ray hypersensitivity and faulty DNA repair in cultured cells from human exhibiting familial cancer proneness. In: Okada, S., Imamura, T., Terashima, T. and Yamaguchi, H. (eds.), *Proceedings of the Sixth International Congress of Radiation Research*, Toppan Printing Co., Tokyo, p. 484

Petrakis, N.L., Emster, V.L., Sacks, S.T., King, E.B., Schweitzer, R.J., Hunt, T.K. *et al*. (1981). Epidemiology of breast fluid secretion: Association with breast cancer risk factors and cerumen type. *Journal of the National Cancer Institute*, 67: 277-84

Pike, M.C., Henderson, B.E., Casagrande, J.T., Rosario, I. and Gray, G.E. (1981). Oral contraceptive use and early abortion as risk factors for breast cancer in young women. *British Journal of Cancer*, 43: 72-6

Post, R.H. (1966). Breast cancer, lactation, and genetics. *Eugenics Quarterly*, 13: 1-29

Purtilo, D.T., Paquin, L. and Gindhart, T. (1978). Genetics of neoplasia – Impact of econogenetics on oncogenesis. *American Journal of Pathology*, 91: 609-87

Rasheed, S. and Gardner, M.B. (1981). Growth properties and susceptibility to viral transformation of skin fibroblasts from individuals at high genetic risk for colorectal cancer. *Journal of the National Cancer Institute*, 66: 43-9

Reed, T.E. and Neel, J.V. (1955). A genetic study of multiple polyposis of the colon. *American Journal of Human Genetics*, 7: 236-63

Rotkin, I.E. (1966). Further studies in cervical cancer inheritance. *Cancer*, 19: 1251-68

Rüdiger, H.W., Harder, W., Maack, P., Kohl, F.V. and Schmidt-Preuss, U. (1981). Decreased rate of Benzo(a)pyrene-induced sister chromatid exchange in fibroblast cultures from patients with lung cancer. *Journal of Cancer Research and Clinical Oncology*, 102: 169-75

Russ, F.E. and Scanlon, E.F. (1980). Identical cancers in husband and wife. *Surgery, Gynecology and Obstetrics*, 150: 664-6

Schimke, R.N. (1978). *Genetics and Cancer in Man*. Churchill Livingstone, Edinburgh, Ch. 9, p. 98

Schull, W.J. and Weiss, K.M. (1980). Genetic epidemiology: Four strategies. *Epidemiological Reviews*, 2: 1-18

Siiteri, P.K., Hammond, G.L. and Nisker, J.A. (1981). Increased availability of serum estrogens in breast cancer: A new hypothesis. In: Pike, M.C., Siiteri, P.K. and Welsch, C.W. (eds.), *Hormones and Breast Cancer*, Cold Spring Harbor Laboratory, New York, p. 87

Skolnik, M., Bishop, D.T., Carmelli, D., Gardner, E., Hadley, R., Hasstedt, S. *et al*. (1981). A population-based assessment of familial cancer risk in Utah Mormon genealogies. In: Arrighi, F.E., Rao, P.N. and Stubblefield, E. (eds.), *Genes, Chromosomes, and Neoplasia*, Raven Press, New York, p. 477

Strong, L.C. (1981). Genetic-environmental interactions in human cancer. In: Arrighi, F.E., Rao, P.N. and Stubblefield, E. (eds.), *Genes, Chromosomes, and Neoplasia*, Raven Press, New York, p. 463

Swift, M. (1976). Malignant disease in heterozygous carriers. In: Bergsma, D. (ed.), *Cancer and Genetics*, Liss, New York, p. 133

Thomas, D.B. (1980). Epidemiologic and related studies of breast cancer etiology. In: Lilienfeld, A.M. (ed.), *Reviews in Cancer Epidemiology*, Elsevier/North Holland, New York/Amsterdam, p. 153

Tokuhata, G.K. (1969). Morbidity and mortality among offspring of breast cancer mothers. *American Journal of Epidemiology*, 89: 139-53

—— and Lilienfeld, A.M. (1963). Familial aggregation of lung cancer in humans. *Journal of the National Cancer Institute*, 30: 289-312

Tulinius, H., Day, N.E., Sigvaldason, H., Bjarnason, O., Johannesson, G., de Ganzalez, M.A.L. *et al.* (1980). A population-based study on familial aggregation of breast cancer in Iceland, taking some other risk factors into account. In: Gelboin, H.V., MacMahon, B., Matsushima, T., Sugimura, T., Takayama, S., and Takebe, H. (eds.), *Genetic and Environmental Factors in Experimental and Human Cancer*, Japan Scientific Societies Press, Tokyo, p. 303

Utsunomiya, J., Murata, M. and Tanimura, M. (1980). An analysis of the age distribution of colon cancer in adenomatosis coli. *Cancer*, 45: 198-205

Varis, K. (1971). A familial study of chronic gastritis: histological, immunological and functional aspects. *Scandinavian Journal of Gastroenterology*, 6 (suppl. 13): pp. 1-50

Veale, A.M.O. (1965). Intestinal polyposis. In: *Eugenics Laboratory Memoirs*, Vol. XL, Cambridge University Press, London, pp. 1-104

Weichselbaum, R.R., Nove, J. and Little, J.B. (1980). X-ray sensitivity of fifty-three human diploid fibroblast cell strains from patients with characterized genetic disorders. *Cancer Research*, 40: 920-5

Woolf, C.M. (1961). The incidence of cancer in the spouses of stomach cancer patients. *Cancer*, 14: 199-200

Wynder, E.L. and Reddy, B.S. (1975). Dietary fat and colon cancer. *Journal of the National Cancer Institute*, 54: 7-10

3 PRECANCEROUS LESIONS

L.G. Koss and E. Greenebaum

Introduction

Within the last 30 years major conceptual changes in reference to human cancer have taken place. From the point of view of pathogenesis perhaps the most significant series of observations pertains to the existence of precursor lesions that can be recognised morphologically by the studies of tissues or cells derived therefrom. Nearly all of our knowledge in this regard comes from the study of events in the epithelial lining of various organs, hence of precursor lesions of carcinomas. Little is known about the precursors of tumours of mesenchymal origin or sarcomas and this group of diseases will not be discussed here.

The sequence of biological events leading to the formation of the precursor lesions of the epithelium is still enigmatic and may vary from organ to organ and from tissue to tissue. Nonetheless, at this time, it appears reasonably certain that human cancer does not originate *ab initio* in healthy tissues but that it follows a number of transformations at the molecular level. It is also likely that most of the initial events in human cancer do not produce obvious morphological modifications. Thus, the precancerous lesions that can be identified microscopically must be construed as early clinical but late biological events. Human cancer has been compared to an iceberg; the obvious clinical disease is its tip while 8/9 of its bulk remains submerged. The morphologically identifiable precancerous events are probably close to the surface although their exact position in reference to obvious clinical disease remains uncertain.

There are several very important but often poorly understood differences that separate precancerous lesions from clinical cancer. Precancerous lesions generally do not cause any clinical symptoms and thus their discovery is either the result of a fortuitous accident or deliberate search by a system of cancer detection, usually based on cytological techniques. Furthermore, not all of the morphological precursor lesions will progress to clinical cancer within the lifespan of the patient. In fact, for some organs such as the uterine cervix, the majority of the precancerous lesions is *not* likely to progress to clinical cancer. For other organs, such as the urinary bladder, there may be two types of precancerous events, each with a different natural history and prognosis. The same may well be true of the endometrium, the breast, and perhaps of the colon as well. Unfortunately, from the epidemiological point of view some of these morphological events of unequal clinical value may occur simultaneously, and the unravelling of their natural history may prove extremely difficult in man.

Definitions

It is a common misconception that the diagnosis and classification of precancerous lesions in man is an exact science. For example, it is particularly unfortunate that some epidemiologists may assume that designations such as 'dysplasia' or 'carcinoma *in situ*' represent objective and scientifically documented differences in the categories of diseases. Nothing could be further from the truth. As has been repeatedly shown, major inter- and intra-observer variations exist in the classification and assessment of the precancerous events (Siegler, 1956; Cocker *et al.*, 1968; Koss, 1978; Klionsky *et al.*, 1969). It has been further noted that the ability of the observer to prognosticate on the outcome of precancerous lesions is limited. It is probably fair to state that precancerous epithelial lesions in man form a spectrum of morphological abnormalities, the outcome of which can never be predicted, except on the basis of statistical analysis. Each one of these lesions if untreated, may either disappear, remain the same, or progress to invasive carcinoma. For some organs fairly accurate statistical predictions can be made. For other organs the data are not available either because of the rarity of the lesions or absence of controlled followup studies.

The type of precancerous lesion that is relatively easy to define is known as carcinoma *in situ*. In these lesions cells with morphological characteristics of cancer have completely replaced the normal epithelium (Koss, 1979a). Unfortunately, the morphological configuration of precancerous lesions does not always follow the preconceived definitions. Thus, lesions with less ominous morphology may behave in identical unpredictable fashion and may also progress to invasive cancer. For such lesions, terms such as dysplasia, atypia, atypical hyperplasia, intraepithelial neoplasia, etc., have been coined. The subclassification of precancerous epithelial lesions may vary from organ to organ and depends to a significant degree on the training, experience and even emotional preferences of the observers.

It may be stated that epithelial lesions in which some or all cells display nuclear abnormalities of cancer, such as nuclear enlargement, hyperchromasia, or abnormal mitotic activity, must be considered as potential precursor lesions of invasive carcinoma. There are, however, some notable but relatively rare exceptions to this rule, including drug-induced or regenerative abnormalities which will not be considered further.

Epidemiological Considerations of Precancerous Lesions

Epidemiology of human cancer has for its purpose the determination by prospective or retrospective studies of the factors that by statistical analysis have shown a consistent and firm association with a specific form of disease. The classical example of a successful documentation is the association of cigarette smoking and lung cancer, based on retrospective and prospective studies (Auerbach *et al.*, 1961; Hammond and Horn, 1958). For other organs and other cancers, the documentation is unfortunately less secure. Much of what is known is based on interviews with patients with obvious and treated clinical disease, compared with a matched group of patients with other diseases. It must be recognised that the acquisition of epidemiological data on precancerous states is much more difficult. Those with precancerous lesions, as a general rule, are not sick and their disease state does not cause any alarm or discomfort. Setting up control groups is difficult indeed. Age and sex alone are obviously not enough. Thus, the controls may be set up according to race, religion, social stratum, occupation, education, geographical location, and perhaps most importantly, life style – which is very difficult to determine. Thus, the epidemiological studies of precancerous lesions are often based on assessment of factors that have been elicited in the studies of obvious clinical disease. It is evident that such studies have limited validity and may give a slanted view of the factors associated with a given precancerous lesion. This caveat appears essential prior to the discussion of the various organ systems.

Buccal Cavity and the Respiratory Tract

There is a great diversity of cancers of the upper digestive and respiratory tracts, but by far the most common site of origin is the epithelial lining of these organs.

Buccal Cavity and the Oropharynx

The most common malignant tumour of the buccal cavity is squamous carcinoma. It has been shown that this tumour originates in altered squamous epithelium that falls into two broad categories: a heavily keratinised variant that appears white on clinical examination and, therefore, is referred to as leukoplakia, and the non-keratinising variant that appears clinically as a red or pink patch and is readily mistaken for an inflammatory lesion.

Sandler (1962) and Stahl *et al.* (1967) have shown that by deliberate cytological screening of visible but not necessarily suspect lesions of the buccal cavity a significant proportion of carcinomas *in situ* may be detected.

Sandler's study clearly documented the existence of detectable precancerous changes in the buccal epithelium, often masquerading as benign lesions. In order of frequency such lesions occur in the floor of the mouth, tongue and soft palate. Many of the American veterans included in this survey were heavy smokers and drinkers of alcoholic beverages. Many had poor oral hygiene and poor dentition. It is unfortunate that a complete epidemiological survey was not conducted on this population to calculate the risk associated with these various factors. Nonetheless, the common denominator of oral carcinoma appears to be chronic irritation (Decker and Goldstein, 1982) and exposure to tobacco either in the form of smoking or chewing (Malaowalla *et al.*, 1976; Wynder and Hoffman, 1976). Jussawalla and Deshpande (1971) have shown that the distribution of cancers in the oropharynx varies with the form of addiction: in betel leaf chewers the cancers usually develop at a point of contact with the bolus; in smokers the anatomical distribution of cancers corresponds to areas of deposition of particulate matter contained in tobacco smoke. Silverman *et al.* (1977) surveyed 57,518 Indian workers at risk for oral cancer by cytological techniques and failed to observe a single precancerous lesion. The may be, at least in part, explained by the high prevalence of leukoplakias in the mouth of betel leaf chewers. Such lesions do not lend themselves to cytological detection because of the heavy layers of keratin on their surface.

Other conditions that have been epidemiologically linked to oral precancerous lesions are Plummer-Vinson syndrome, perhaps associated with iron and riboflavin deficiency (Suzman, 1933; Ahlbom, 1936; McCoy *et al.*, 1980; Decker and Goldstein, 1982). The assessment of poor oral hygiene as an epidemiological factor is difficult. Using edentia as an objective criterion, Wynder *et al.* (1957) have found it in 44 per cent of patients with oral cancer and in 28 per cent of controls, which is not a particularly persuasive result.

The Larynx

Precancerous epithelial lesions (carcinoma *in situ*) have been recognised in the larynx for many years (Altmann *et al.*, 1952). As in the buccal cavity, such lesions are either keratin-forming or not and may be recognised either on laryngoscopic examination or with the use of cytological techniques (Koss, 1979a).

Epidemiological factors implicated in carcinoma *in situ* of the larynx are probably similar to those observed in invasive cancer of this organ, e.g. tobacco smoking. The occurrence of laryngeal carcinoma appears to be in proportion to the number of cigarettes smoked and is enhanced by alcohol intake (Rothman *et al.*, 1980). Experimental evidence in support of the carcinogenic role of tobacco has been provided in inbred Syrian hamsters; a progressive transformation of the laryngeal epithelium leading to carcinoma *in situ* and invasive cancer has been observed after exposure to tobacco smoke (Homburger *et al.*, 1979).

Alcohol has also been identified as a risk factor in oral, laryngeal and oesophageal cancers; however, there is neither epidemiological nor experimental evidence that alcohol *per se* is carcinogenic; yet in combination with cigarette smoking, excessive alcohol intake significantly increases the risk for these cancers (Wynder *et al.*, 1977). Occupational exposure to asbestos is also believed to be a risk factor for laryngeal carcinoma (Rothman *et al.*, 1980).

Laryngeal Papillomatosis. Laryngeal papillomatosis is a chronic recurrent disease beginning in early childhood. An infrequent 'adult' form is also known. The recent major interest in papillomatosis of childhood is due to the fact that this tumour is induced by papillomaviruses and may progress to squamous cancer (zur Hausen, 1977). A possible link between laryngeal papillomatosis and the papillomavirus infection of the female genital tract has been provided by the casual observations that mothers of some of the children with the laryngeal disease may have suffered from condylomata acuminata prior to or during pregnancy (Duff, 1971).

The Trachea

Carcinomas of the trachea, either of squamous type or originating in the minor salivary (mucous) glands, are extremly uncommon in contradistinction to bronchogenic carcinoma. There is virtually nothing known about their epidemiology.

The Lung

With the exception of relatively uncommon tumours of pulmonary parenchyma, nearly all cancers of the lung originate in the bronchi. They are broadly divided into three types: carcinomas forming solid sheets with or without keratin formation (epidermoid or squamous carcinomas), gland-forming cancers (adenocarcinomas), and the highly aggressive small cell cancers (oat cell carcinomas).

The exact sequence of precancerous events is best known for the squamous carcinomas. In man the studies of Auerbach *et al.* (1961) have documented the following sequence of events: the earliest morphological changes have been loss of cilia, followed by an increase in the number of cell layers and an increase in the proportion of atypical cells. Carcinoma *in situ*, defined as bronchial epithelial lesions composed entirely of atypical cells and lacking cilia, was found only in heavy cigarette smokers. Many of the carcinoma *in situ* lesions and small occult primary carcinomas occurred as multiple lesions in patients dying of lung cancer.

The studies by Auerbach *et al.* (1961) have provided solid morphological support to several retrospective and prospective epidemiological surveys implicating cigarette smoking as the key factor in the genesis of epidermoid carcinoma of the lung. Experimental evidence in dogs, rats and hamsters (Schreiber *et al.*, 1974; Schreiber and Nettesheim, 1972; Saffiotti *et al.*, 1967; Rockey *et al.*, 1962) has confirmed this sequence of events in the trachea and the main bronchi after exposure to tobacco smoke, tobacco distillate or chemical carcinogens.

The sequence of events is much less clear in reference to adenocarcinomas of the lung, a type of lesion that is seen with increasing frequency. It is generally assumed that focal transformation of terminal bronchioles or even alveolar cells (so called tumourlets) takes place most often in peripheral areas of the lung, sometimes around scars from previous diseases such as tuberculosis.

The linkage of adenocarcinomas to tobacco smoking is less solid than for squamous carcinoma, the typical smoker's cancer. It is generally assumed that, in smokers, tobacco-related compounds that accumulate in the areas of the scars act as a local carcinogen (Limas *et al.*, 1971; Meyer and Liebow, 1965). The smoking–cancer link is again very well established for oat cell carcinoma, which is seldom observed in non-smokers (Kreyberg, 1968).

The Mayo Clinic study, which was part of the National Lung Cancer Project in the United States of America (USA), casts an interesting light on the nature of 'smokers lung cancer' in the 1970s and 1980s. Instead of the expected predominance of squamous carcinoma of the main bronchi, the classical lesion of smokers, most lung cancers occurred at the periphery of the lung (Woolner, 1981). This observation is in keeping with the data from Auerbach *et al.* (1979), who reported a marked reduction in the frequency of carcinoma *in situ* in the lungs of cigarette smokers in the 1970s, when compared with the 1950s, and attributed the change to the widespread use of filtered cigarettes. Thus the epidemiological profile of patients with lung cancer may be undergoing a significant modification due to changing smoking habits.

Exposure to asbestos fibres (especially chrysotile and amosite) has also been shown to be epidemiologically linked to lung cancer (Lemen *et al.*, 1980). There appears to be a synergy between tobacco smoking and asbestos exposure (Selikoff *et al.*, 1968). Uranium workers (Saccomanno, 1974) also appear to be at risk for lung cancer.

It has been suggested that human papilloma virus (HPV), which may play a role in carcinogenesis in the larynx and female genital tract, may also be of interest in the bronchial tree. Condylomatous lesions have been found in association with invasive bronchial squamous carcinomas (Syrjänen, 1980).

The Gastrointestinal Tract

The Oesophagus

For reasons still unknown but perhaps related to dietary factors, cancer of the oesophagus is found with high frequency in several parts of the world such as the southern littoral of the Caspian Sea, parts of Southern Africa (in the black population), the Brittany region of France, and in Central and Northern China. Because of the extremely high rate of oesophageal cancer in parts of China, a mass cytological screening programme for people over 40 years old has been instituted. The results suggest that there is a sequence of mucosal events strongly resembling that in the uterine cervix; changes range from mild to severe dysplasia that may lead to carcinoma *in situ* and to invasive carcinoma (Shu, 1982). Shu demonstrated that the degree of morphological abnormality of the epithelium is related to the likelihood of progression to carcinoma. Thus, the progression to carcinoma of the slight abnormalities of the epithelium, classified as mild dysplasia, was uncommon; on the other hand, the severe changes, classified as severe dysplasia, had a very high probability of progression to carcinoma: 15 per cent within 4 years, and over 50 per cent within 12 years. It would thus appear that the slight and moderate neoplastic changes in the oesophageal epithelium are at least in part reversible, as is also the case in the uterine cervix. Although the risk of oesophageal carcinoma is minuscule in the USA relative to China, the value of cytological screening of high-risk populations is being currently evaluated (Greenebaum *et al.*, 1982).

There has been an awareness of some of the risk factors associated with oesophageal carcinoma in China for over 2,000 years: excess alcohol, hot beverages and an inadequate diet. More recently, additional factors have been implicated in the genesis of oesophageal carcinoma: tobacco, fermented and mouldy foods, pickled vegetables, many of which contain various fungi including *Geotrichum candidum* and *Aspergillus* species, nitrosamines, deficiencies of molybdenum and ascorbic acid (Li, 1982). A fascinating finding is the high prevalence of gullet cancer in chickens raised by the human populations who are at high risk for oesophagus cancer (Shu, 1982).

The Stomach

Over the last 25 years, the rate of gastric cancer has been dropping very sharply in the USA but it has remained very high in certain areas of the world, notably Japan, Korea, parts of Colombia, South America and Finland.

The sequence of neoplastic events leading to gastric cancer is not fully understood. Chronic atrophic gastritis is the one common denominator that has emerged from the major Japanese effort at gastric cancer detection (Kawachi *et al.*, 1976) and the remarkable studies by Correa *et al.* (1976) in Colombia.

The precursor lesions probably represent a continuum: chronic atrophic gastritis (CAG), intestinal metaplasia, gastric gland atypia, carcinoma *in situ*. Of the two main epidemiological types of gastric carcinoma only the intestinal or 'epidemic' type has been found to be associated with precursor lesions identifiable by the usual histopathological procedures (Correa, 1982); the endemic or diffuse type has not.

The sporadic association of gastric cancer with atrophic gastritis in folate deficiency anemia has been known for many years. Current epidemiological evidence points to environmental rather than genetic determinants. Correa *et al.* (1976) studied two Colombian populations and determined that the population at high risk for gastric carcinoma also had a high prevalence of CAG and that the subgroup with CAG can be identified as early as age 20 in both populations. Second generation migrants to a low-risk environment acquire the low risk of the host country, as is also the case with Japanese migrating to Hawaii (Haenszel *et al.*, 1972).

The sex ratio for CAG is nearly 1:1 in Finland and Colombia, although clinical cancer shows a male predominance, and this would suggest that the initiating factors are equally active in both sexes but that the promoting events are more common or effective in males (Correa, 1982). In fact, atypical precancerous gland changes in intestinal metaplasia are more frequent and more advanced in males (Cuello *et al.*, 1979).

Environmental factors associated with precursor lesions have been investigated; however, dietary surveys of populations with precursor lesions are only available from Colombia. The dietary pattern of precursor populations is similar to that of gastric cancer populations (Correa, 1982). The diet associated with precursor lesions is starchy, low in fat, low in protein, low in fresh vegetables and high in salt and nitrates. The high intake of salt is due to the salting to preserve meat (Haenszel *et al.*, 1976), and the nitrate content of the well water is 10 times greater in high-risk areas of Colombia than in low-risk areas, while urinary and salivary nitrate concentrations are significantly higher in individuals of high-risk areas (Cuello *et al.*, 1976).

Gastric juice nitrites have been further investigated in high-risk individuals in order to gain a clinical tool to study patients with suspected precancerous lesions. Subjects with precursor lesions tend to have less acidic gastric juices and the abnormal presence of nitrite and bacteria (Tannenbaum, 1979).

Disregarding the epidemiological factors, a major effort at gastric cancer detection in Japan has significantly reduced mortality from this disease in very high-risk populations. The gastric cancer detection centres are based in hospitals, clinics and mobile units which offer the asymptomatic population a combination of roentgenological and cytological examination. As a consequence of this major national effort, the majority of gastric cancers in Japan are nowadays uncovered at an early stage, while the lesion is either still confined to the gastric mucosa, or has not infiltrated beyond the submucosa. The five-year survival of patients with such lesions treated by surgery is close to 90 per cent (Murakami, 1979), representing a nearly total reversal of survival patterns of 15 or 20 years ago when only a tiny proportion of patients with symptomatic gastric cancer lived for five years (Muto, 1968).

Colon

Carcinoma of the colon is now the most frequent internal cancer in adults of both sexes in the USA. As Burkitt (1972) has pointed out, this form of cancer is very rare among Africans whose diet is rich in fibre and who normally have several bowel movements a day. It still remains to be seen if, in fact, the dietary factors fully account for the observed geographic differences, if a change in the dietary habits in the Western countries is possible, and if it will contribute to a reduction of colon cancer in the future. In the West, the key factors showing clear epidemiological association with colon cancer are: family history of colon cancer, proliferative changes in colonic epithelium (polyps and polyposis) and chronic ulcerative colitis.

Positive statistical associations are found between polyps and colon carcinoma with respect to interpopulation comparisons of frequency, time trends and socioeconomic gradients (Correa, 1982). There are two types of polyps: the adenomatous polyps leading to carcinoma in a rather small proportion of cases, and the villous adenomas, about 40 per cent of which lead to carcinoma (Morson, 1974). The so-called hyperplastic and juvenile polyps have no proven premalignant role (Correa, 1982).

There is a strong positive correlation between carcinoma and the multiplicity, size and atypia of polyps. In the autosomal dominant genetic disorders with multiplicity of colonic polyps (familial polyposis, Gardner's syndrome, Peutz-Jeghers syndrome), the development of colon cancer is an almost fully predictable event (McKusick, 1975). Gilbertsen (1974) reported on the value of periodic protosigmoidoscopy with removal of lower bowel polyps. In a 25-year study of more than 18,000 patients, 85 per cent of the statistically anticipated adenocarcinomas of the rectosigmoid did not develop. The cancers that did appear were found while still sharply localised to the bowel wall.

In spite of the statistical evidence associating adenomatous polyps with colon cancer, there are no case-control studies of polyp-bearers to determine if the risk factors for polyps correspond to the risk factors for carcinoma (Haenszel and Correa, 1971; Correa, 1982).

Chronic Ulcerative Colitis.   In patients with chronic ulcerative colitis of long duration, premalignant changes have been identified in the flat mucosa of the colon (Yardley and Keren, 1974; Nugent *et al.*, 1979). These changes show architectural distortion of glands, loss of stratification of goblet cells and nuclear abnormalities. Severe abnormalities in colonic mucosa frequently signal the presence of colonic carcinoma elsewhere. Thus rectal biopsies and brush cytological examination are warranted to monitor the mucosal condition in patients with chronic ulcerative colitis.

Anus

There have been several cases reported of the malignant transformation of condylomata acuminata to squamous carcinoma of the anus (Friedberg and Serlin, 1963; Sturm *et al.*, 1975; Prasad and Abcarian, 1980; Choo and Morely, 1980). In fact, there are cases where it is difficult to distinguish morphologically between an atypical condyloma and a squamous carcinoma. This suggests that at least some anal condylomata are premalignant lesions. Carcinoma of the anus is likely to become more common in males as the prevalence of anal condylomata increases with the increasing promiscuity of male homosexuals.

The Female Genital Tract

The Uterine Cervix

Precancerous events in the epithelium of the uterine cervix are the best-known and explored target of epidemiological studies. It has been repeatedly documented that the risk factors are generally related to sexual events. Young age at first sexual encounter and multiplicity of sexual partners have been shown to be of particular significance. All other epidemiological factors, such as economic and social status, number of pregnancies, etc., can be related to these two key events (Koss, 1981).

The geographical distribution of precancerous lesions is known only in the Western world. Cytological screening programmes have not as yet been instituted on a large scale in most of the countries where mortality from carcinoma of the uterine cervix remains alarmingly high, such as many areas of Africa, Asia and Central and South America. In general, it must be assumed that the rate of discovery of precancerous lesions should be in proportion to the rate of invasive cancer in the same population.

It has been repeatedly documented that screening and eradication of precancerous lesions lead to a statistically significant drop in morbidity and mortality from cervix cancer (Christopherson and Scott, 1977; Boyes and Worth, 1976; Miller, 1978). The converse, i.e. follow-up of precancerous lesions until they become invasive, has been sporadically documented either in deliberate follow-up studies (Koss *et al.*,

1963; Richart and Barron, 1969) or in incidental observations as a consequence of faulty screening technique (Rylander, 1977). The nomenclature of precancerous lesions of the uterine cervix has been the subject of considerable controversy.

The Nomenclature. Quite contrary to the belief of many, including highly trained clinical professionals, terms such as dysplasia, carcinoma *in situ*, anaplasia, atypical metaplasia, have never been adequately and objectively defined and are the expression of a subjective microscopical assessment of these lesions by pathologists. Repeatedly, the same lesions have been differently classified by several otherwise equally competent observers (Siegler, 1956; Cocker *et al.*, 1968; Koss, 1978; Klionsky *et al.*, 1969). The concept of cervical intra-epithelial neoplasia (CIN) proposed by Richart (1967) has the benefit of relative simplicity; it encompasses the entire spectrum of neoplastic changes and can be graded from I to III to satisfy the need of pathologists to express the degree of morphological abnormality.

Objective assessment of these lesions in reference to DNA content and behaviour has shown that the lesions can be divided into two groups: the diploid-tetraploid group with relatively good prognosis and high probability of spontaneous disappearance, and the aneuploid group with a tendency to persist and progress (Fu *et al.*, 1981). The DNA content studies have cut across the entire spectrum of morphological abnormalities and have documented that relatively slight modification of epithelial structure (mild or moderate dysplasia, CIN I and II) can be aneuploid whereas some of the severe abnormalities (severe dysplasia, carcinoma *in situ*) may belong to the diploid-tetraploid, hence relatively favourable group.

Behaviour. Regardless of the problems with the nomenclature, the behaviour of precancerous lesions of the uterine cervix is insecure. It has been repeatedly documented that the prevalence of precancerous lesions is much higher than the calculated incidence of invasive carcinoma. In follow-up studies (Koss *et al.*, 1963; Richart and Barron, 1969) three different behavioural options have been documented: the lesions can either disappear, remain confined to the epithelium, or in a relatively small proportion of cases, progress to invasive cancer. The reasons for this behaviour pattern are not known. While the DNA studies (Fu, 1981) may offer a prognostic handle, the morphological diagnosis is not reliable in assessing future behaviour of any given lesion.

Pathogenesis. The epidemiological studies of women with precancerous lesions (or, for that matter, invasive carcinoma) of the uterine cervix have suggested significant similarities between carcinoma of the uterine cervix and a venereal disease. The search for a sexually transmissible agent started in the 1940s and included gonorrheal infection, syphilis and even the common parasite, trichomonas vaginalis (Meisels, 1969; Koss, 1975a).

Within more recent times the search for a viral agent has found two major targets: herpes simplex virus Type II and papilloma virus.

Herpes Simplex Virus Type II (HSV-2). This virus produces significant microscopic changes in the affected epithelial cells such as nuclear inclusions (Koss, 1979a), and this is readily detected in ordinary cervical smears. The evidence linking HSV-2 to cancerous events in the uterine cervix was initially based on the linkage between these morphological changes and precancerous cell changes (Melnick, 1976; Naib, 1969). Subsequent studies of antibodies to HSV-2 provided the information that women with neoplastic events had a consistently higher level than matched controls, although the differences depended on the techniques used (Kessler, 1974).

More substantial evidence of linkage has been provided by newer techniques of immunology and molecular biology. Aurelian (1981) has documented seroepidemiologically the presence of HSV-2 encoded antigens in 72 per cent of patients with invasive cervical carcinoma and 11 per cent of controls. More recently still, McDougall *et al.* (1981) have shown by DNA hybridisation, small fragments of viral DNA may be present in cells from carcinoma of the cervix.

Papilloma Viruses (PV). Viruses of the human papilloma family have had a long documented association with condylomata acuminata, a well-known, sexually transmitted disease. Condylomata acuminata have clinically visible manifestations in the form of wart-like, pedunculated lesions affecting the skin of the male and female genital tract (zur Hausen, 1977). Within recent years the concept of a different form of this disorder has been described affecting the mucous membranes of the vagina, cervix (Meisels and Fortin, 1976) and, in at least some instances, the epithelium of the male urethra (personal observations).

The mucosal condylomata form flat lesions that usually cannot be seen by the naked eye and require colposcopy for their identification. The lesions have been known since their detailed description as koilocytotic atypia (Koss and Durfee, 1956), although their viral aetiology has only come to light recently by demonstration of viral particles in the nuclei of the affected cells (Laverty *et al.*, 1978; Della Torre *et al.*, 1978; Meisels *et al.*, 1981).

The cytotoxic effects of the PV result in the formation of a broad zone of perinuclear cytoplasmic destruction that appears as a 'hollow' or 'cavity' in the affected squamous cells, hence the name 'koilocytosis'. Other, less characteristic cell abnormalities have been described by Koss (1979a) and by Meisels and Fortin (1976).

Because of the characteristic cytoxic changes, the diagnosis of PV infection of the cervix or vagina can be established by an ordinary cervical smear. This simple procedure also allows follow-up of women with this disorder.

The current information, derived from several sources, suggests that flat condylomata are the most common form of initial neoplastic events, particularly in young women (Purola and Savia, 1977; Meisels *et al.*, 1977; Syrjänen *et al.*, 1981). Evidence has also been provided that there is a common association of flat condylomata with other forms of cervical intraepithelial neoplasia and even with invasive carcinoma (Koss and Durfee, 1956; Syrjänen, 1981; Meisels *et al.*, 1977). This association has been recently tested in a controlled study by Reid *et al.* (1982), who concluded that there is a statistically valid, consistent and specific association of PV infection with precancerous events and cancer of the uterine cervix. Supportive evidence has also been provided in a study of four immunodeficient women in whom the presence of the virus could be documented in association with treatment-resistant condylomata and carcinoma *in situ* which, in one of them, progressed to invasive cancer (Shokri-Tabibzadeh *et al.*, 1981).

Still further evidence suggestive of a possible carcinogenic role of PV comes from studies of carcinoma of the vulva (Woodruff *et al.*, 1980). Approximately half of women with this disease had a history of condylomata acuminata. A rare skin disorder associated with a subtype of PV, epidermodysplasia verruciformis, has also been known to progress to invasive carcinoma in a small proportion of cases (Jablonska *et al.*, 1972; Ruiter, 1973).

In spite of all this evidence, the key question in reference to the viral aetiology of carcinomas of the cervix, vulva and vagina, possibly also of the anus, has not been resolved. This question succinctly stated several years ago is 'Passenger or Driver?' (*British Medical Journal*, 1964). Notwithstanding the tremendous recent progress in molecular biology, it may be some time yet until this question is resolved.

The Vulva

The association of precancerous lesions of the vulva (carcinoma *in situ*, Bowen's disease) with PV infection has already been discussed. An interesting disease, Bowenoid papulosis, that may yet prove to be a precancerous event, has also been linked to PV infection (Wade *et al.*, 1978; Zelickson and Prawer, 1980; Steffen, 1982).

Vagina

The precursors of the squamous and adenocarcinomas of the vagina share many epidemiological features with those of the cervix and the vulva.

A clear link has been established between adenocarcinoma of the vagina and maternal ingestion of diethylstilboesterol (DES) during pregnancy. The precursor lesion is vaginal adenosis which is a replacement of the normal squamous epithelium of portions of the vagina and the cervix by glandular epithelium, usually of endocervical type. Maternal ingestion of DES induces adenosis by mechanisms not well understood at this time. Adenosis had been reported in association with vaginal adenocarcinoma in children of DES mothers (Herbst *et al.*, 1971; Herbst *et al.*, 1974), but occasionally also in older women (Plaut and Dreyfuss, 1940; Studdiford, 1957).

Both vaginal adenosis and adenocarcinoma occur most commonly on the anterior vaginal wall. Other DES-induced abnormalities, such as transverse vaginal and cervical ridges, are found frequently in DES-exposed offspring but they are not believed to present any danger to the patient. Current evidence suggests that the association of adenosis with adenocarcinoma occurs very rarely. There are perhaps several million young women with adenosis in the USA but only a few hundred cases of adenocarcinoma of the vagina (Stafl and Mattingly, 1974). The reasons for the transition of anomalous vaginal epithelial development to neoplasia is not yet understood.

Although the issue is somewhat controversial, an increased incidence of CIN of epidermoid type is now being reported in the cervices and vaginas of DES-exposed offspring (Fowler *et al.*, 1981). The women with adenosis have a significantly enlarged transformation zone, the area affected in the development of precancerous lesions of epidermoid type.

The Endometrium – Adenocarcinoma

It is generally assumed that morphological abnormalities of endometrial glands classified as endometrial hyperplasia constitute precursor lesions of endometrial adenocarcinoma. The evidence for this is based mainly on retrospective studies such as the review of prior endometrial biopsies in women with overt endometrial carcinoma (Hertig and Sommers, 1949; Beutler *et al.*, 1963). A specific form of endometrial abnormality known as endometrial carcinoma *in situ* has been singled out in one such study by Hertig and Sommers (1949) as an important precursor lesion.

Prospective studies of patients with endometrial hyperplasia followed without treatment are very few and are generally poorly documented. The study by Gusberg and Kaplan (1963) is most frequently cited; in it 12 per cent of women with atypical endometrial hyperplasia developed endometrial carcinoma. An important aspect of retrospective and prospective studies is the bias in the selection of subjects, all of whom are women who required an initial endometrial sampling because of bleeding. A further complicating factor is the treatment of endometrial hyperplasia by hormonal manipulation which obviously alters the natural history of these lesions.

Ultrastructural studies by Ferenczy (1981) documented some important differences between various forms of hyperplasia and endometrial carcinoma: hyperplastic lesions showed evidence of oestrogen dependence which carcinomas did not.

A further observation of note in this regard was a study of detection of endometrial carcinoma in approximately 2,500 asymptomatic women, age 45 and above (Koss *et al.*, 1981; 1982). The prevalence rate of occult carcinomas, with the addition of two carcinomas missed on screening, was approximately 6.9/1,000; the incidence rate obtained on second screening was approximately 2/1,000. It was of note that the prevalence rate of hyperplasia (including polyps) was only 8/1,000; hence only slightly higher than the rate for carcinomas. If hyperplasia were the precancerous lesions in this group of women, one would have expected a ratio of hyperplasia to carcinomas of 7 or 8 to 1, as calculated from Gusberg and Kaplan's data (1963).

Thus, it is likely that there are two pathways of endometrial carcinoma: one associated with symptomatic hyperplasia and one in which endometrial carcinoma appears *de novo* in non-hyperplastic endometrium. A recent study of occult endometrial carcinomas in necropsy material (Horwitz *et al.*, 1981) confirms that such occult carcinomas do occur with the frequency of 22 to 31 per 10,000 women, age 45 or older, with intact uteri.

The epidemiological studies of endometrial carcinoma have been repeatedly carried out on patients with clinically overt symptomatic disease. Wynder *et al.* (1966) and Elwood *et al.* (1977) have emphasised the increased risk associated with nulliparity, late onset of menopause and obesity. This last factor only applied to extremely obese women in the Elwood study. The use of unopposed exogenous oestrogens has been repeatedly considered as a major risk factor in endometrial carcinoma (Ziel and Finkle, 1975; Smith *et al.*, 1975; Mack *et al.*, 1976), although specific objections of selection bias were raised by Horwitz and Feinstein (1978).

In the studies of asymptomatic women with occult carcinoma, age at onset of menopause, parity, and use of exogenous oestrogens were evaluated with essentially negative results (Koss *et al.*, 1982). It may well be that the proposed two pathways of endometrial carcinoma account for these differences. In the endometrial hyperplasia pathway, the epidemiological factors play a role as discussed by Wynder *et al.* (1966) and Elwood *et al.* (1977). In the carcinomas not preceded by hyperplasia, the one epidemiological factor of significance appears to be age.

Mammary Carcinoma

There are two important groups of precancerous lesions of the female breast: those affecting the primary ducts and secondary larger ducts, and those affecting the terminal portions of the secretory apparatus of the breast, namely the acini or lobules and the adjacent terminal ducts. The malignant changes affecting the larger ducts are well defined morphologically as they are usually made up of clearly malignant, large cells. Rarely is there any diagnostic debate about the nature of the duct lesions except for the so-called minimal carcinomas. To the best of our knowledge no one has ever deliberately followed up women with intraductal malignant disease without treatment. It is generally assumed that intraductal carcinomas, if untreated, will kill the patient (Koss, 1982). The lesions of acini or lobules are much less obvious; the affected area of the breast may be very small. The affected cells are also small and therein the morphological changes are subtle. It takes a practised eye to identify lobular carcinoma *in situ*, particularly if only one or two acini are affected.

Lobular carcinoma *in situ* or lobular neoplasia is not a clinical disease; it is strictly a microscopic abnormality. It may or may not occur simultaneously with other forms of breast cancer. When seen alone it occurs mainly in premenopausal women; it is often multicentric and bilateral. Occult invasive carcinoma occurs simultaneously in about 5 per cent of cases in the same or in the contralateral breast. Occasionally axillary lymph node metastases (Rosen, 1980) and Paget's disease of the nipple (Ashikari *et al.*, 1970) have been observed in the absence of documented invasive growth. It is generally assumed that these events indicated inadequate sampling of the breast, but in at least some cases known to us the sampling of the breast was complete or at least adequate.

There is a strong genetic component to lobular carcinoma *in situ*. The disease appears to occur more often in families with history of breast cancer in close female relatives such as the mother or sister. In such women the probability of developing invasive breast cancer has been calculated by Lattes as about 14 times higher than the expected rate (Anderson, 1974; Lattes, 1980; Rosen, 1980).

The controversy surrounding lobular carcinoma *in situ* is based on the clinical significance of the lesion. Which is more important in a precancerous state, the fact that some patients who harbour it may develop future cancer or the fact that many of the patients with this disorder will remain well and live a normal lifespan without additional treatment? Thus the question of clinical handling and treatment is actively debated (Koss, 1982).

There are some significant differences between the ductal and lobular lesions *in situ*. Because intraductal carcinoma is readily identified as breast cancer, prospective follow-up information is very scarce and based mainly on either diagnostic or patient failure. Rosen (1980) cited 78 such patients collected from his own experience or reported by others. In 41 of them (53 per cent) subsequent invasive cancers were documented, sometimes many years later, and always in the same breast. This modest experience cannot be considered conclusive but it does point out some fundamental differences with lobular carcinoma *in situ*; the bilaterality of the lesion is absent and the rate of progression in the ipsilateral breast is much higher. In the absence of meaningful prospective studies of intraductal carcinoma, which probably cannot and should not be conducted, any comparison with the lobular lesions must be based on circumstantial evidence. It appears rather certain, however, that precancerous changes in the ducts play a much more important, direct role in the genesis of mammary carcinoma than the changes in the lobules, although the two are often associated.

Thus, not unlike the observations recorded above for the endometrium and below for the urinary bladder, one finds in the breast two types of precancerous events of unequal value; the highly aggressive ductal changes which are at the origin of about 90 per cent of breast cancers and the lobular changes which are a major warning sign that cancerous transformation of the excretory apparatus of the breast may occur with a much higher degree of probability than in the population at large. This probability increases significantly if the patient's genetic background is unfavourable.

From the epidemiological point of view, the only factor that has been shown to be significantly associated with the lobular carcinoma *in situ* is the history of cancer in close female relatives, mothers or sisters (Anderson, 1974; Rose, 1980; Lattes, 1980). In spite of very extensive studies, risk factors for intraductal carcinoma have not been identified.

The Urinary Tract

Urothelial Carcinoma of the Urinary Bladder

Epidemiological studies of cancer of the urinary bladder began in the year 1895 when Rehn published his first observations on excessive occurrence of bladder tumours among aniline workers. Since that time massive evidence has accumulated documenting the relationship of bladder cancer to industrial exposure, notably aromatic amines (Koss, 1975b). Another line of inquiry has been the high rate of carcinoma of the bladder in people exposed to bilharzia (*Schistosoma haematobium*) infestation (Goebel, 1905; Ferguson, 1911).

Carcinoma of the urinary bladder has two separate but often overlapping pathways: the papillary and the non-papillary (Koss, 1979b). The more common first pathway is characterised by occurrence of papillary tumours, which usually cause symptoms such as haematuria that bring the patient to the urologist. The natural history of the papillary tumours is usually protracted and stretching over a period of many years. The tumours are treated, recur, are treated again, until in some patients at least, invasive carcinoma develops.

The non-papillary pathway begins as a flat carcinoma *in situ* which may remain completely asymptomatic until invasive carcinoma develops. Because of the insidious onset, the initial diagnosis of non-papillary carcinoma *in situ* is often either based on a fortuitous biopsy or is the result of screening by cytological examination of the sediment of voided urine. For this reason, the exact duration of non-papillary carcinoma remains conjectural. On the other hand, evidence has been presented that about 60 to 70 per cent of patients with flat carcinoma *in situ* will develop invasive bladder cancer within five years (Koss, 1975b).

Current evidence strongly suggests that in the majority of patients with invasive cancer of the bladder there is little or no evidence of previous papillary disease. Thus one must assume that these patients' illness started with occult non-papillary carcinomas *in situ* (Brawn, 1982). It has also been shown by mapping studies of bladders that in patients with papillary disease who develop invasive carcinoma the invasion usually occurs from areas of non-papillary neoplastic disease adjacent to the papillary tumours (Koss, 1975b; Althausen *et al.*, 1976).

The epidemiological studies of bladder cancer do not address the issue of precursor lesions and of the two different pathways of disease. Personal observations on workers exposed to the potent bladder carcinogen, paraaminodiphenyl, strongly suggest that the epidemiological factors may be the same for all precancerous events (Koss *et al.*, 1969). The difference in the pathway of the disease may well reside in the individual patient's response to injury.

Evidence exists that atypical and keratinising squamous metaplasia of the bladder epithelium in patients infested with *Schistosoma haematobium* is the precursor lesion for bladder cancer of the squamous cell type. Hicks *et al.* (1977) propose that low doses of carcinogenic nitrosamine produced in the urine as a result of chronic or recurrent bacterial infections may induce preneoplastic urothelial changes. These may then be promoted to tumour growth either by exposure to other urine-borne carcinogens or by other factors including mechanical irritation from urinary calculi or repeated ulceration as occurs in the bilharzial bladder.

The alkylating agent, cyclophosphamide, has been shown to be a causative factor in carcinoma of the bladder (Pearson and Soloway, 1978; Wall and Clausen, 1975; Fairchild *et al.*, 1979; Plotz *et al.*, 1979), and the bracken fern *Pteridium aquilinum* has been shown to induce bladder tumours in cattle (Evans and Mason, 1965).

Urothelial Carcinoma of the Renal Pelvis

Recent studies by mapping of the renal pelvis have shown that the two tumour pathways, the papillary and the non-papillary, operative in carcinoma of the urinary bladder are also operative in the epithelium of the renal pelves (Mahadevia *et al.*, 1982; Chasko *et al.*, 1981; Kakizoe *et al.*, 1980). Flat carcinoma *in situ* has been identified.

The frequency with which renal pelvic carcinoma either follows or is followed by carcinomas of other portions of the lower urinary tract, such as the bladder or the ureter, clearly documents that the same carcinogenic events that govern the occurrence of bladder cancer are also operative in the renal pelvis. In addition, specific causes of renal pelvic cancer have been identified.

Retrospective studies of patients with urothelial tumours of the renal pelvis revealed a strong association with abuse of phenacetin-containing analgesics (Johansson *et al.*, 1974). Phenacetin is metabolised in man to 2-hydroxy-phenetidin which has an ortho-aminophenol configuration, as does paraaminodiphenyl. This metabolite is excreted in the urine, and probably represents a local carcinogenic hazard. Most of the patients affected showed varying degrees of renal papillary necrosis, some showed focal tubular hyperplasia, and in many the tumours were multiple. In mapping studies of renal pelves and ureters of such patients, the presence of non-papillary carcinoma *in situ* as the source of invasive cancer has been demonstrated (Mahadevia *et al.*, 1983; Chasko *et al.*, 1981).

Interstitial nephritis has been proposed as a premalignant lesion predisposing to upper urinary tract tumours. As many as 20-40 per cent of patients in the Balkans suffering from endemic nephropathy subsequently develop an upper urinary tract tumour (Sorrentino and DeMartino, 1979).

The most impressive figures come from Yugoslavia, the only country in Europe in which renal pelvic tumours are more common than those of the renal parenchyma (the average proportion in Europe is 1:3). Sorrentino and DeMartino (1979) propose that patients with Balkan nephropathy, phenacetin nephropathy and infected pelvic calculi may be more susceptible to the action of carcinogens. They propose that interstitial nephritis, by impeding the reabsorption from the pelvis by pyelolymphatic reflux and by making more difficult the lymphatic drainage of the pelvic and ureter walls, leads to a condition favouring carcinogenesis (even if the carcinogens are weak, e.g. phenacetin metabolites). Thus, interstitial nephritic damage would be the initiated state while phenacetin exposure, infected pelvic calculi and unknown Balkan environmental stimuli would act as promoters in the two-stage carcinogenesis model.

The aetiology of Balkan nephropathy is not known; however, viral-like particles have frequently been detected ultrastructurally in affected kidneys (Georgescu and Diosi, 1981).

Summary and Conclusions

This review of precancerous events in several organ systems brought into focus some striking similarities and some notable differences. In general, the genesis of carcinomas derived from the squamous epithelium appears to progress through a series of identifiable morphological changes of uncertain prognosis prior to the development of invasive cancer. This appears to be true for the buccal cavity, the larynx, the oesophagus and the uterine cervix and must be explored for other organs as well.

In reference to bronchogenic carcinoma, which is derived from the respiratory epithelium, again by a series of changes, the information on the biological behaviour of carcinoma *in situ* and related lesions is not reliable. Auerbach *et al.* (1961) have observed many more areas of carcinoma *in situ* than invasive cancers. Woolner *et al.* (1981) have also noted in the lung cancer detection study that carcinomas *in situ* may be multifocal in a synchronous or metachronous manner. Thus, in the lung we are also confronted with the possibility that not all precancerous events will necessarily progress to invasive cancer within the lifetime of the patient. Furthermore, as already discussed, the pattern of morphological events in lung cancer may be changing, perhaps because of the use of filtered cigarettes.

Studies of organs such as the breast, the endometrium and the urinary bladder, suggest that there are two pathways of precancerous events, one of which is exceedingly slow and of insecure outcome, the other more aggressive, more rapid and leading to invasive cancer in a high percentage of patients.

Future studies of epidemiology of human cancer must take these observations into account. The possibility should be explored that the neoplastic events preceding clinically obvious cancer may be governed by a totally different set of epidemiological parameters than invasive cancer of the same origin.

References

Ahlbom, H.E. (1936). Simple achlorhydric anemia, Plummer-Vinson syndrome, and carcinoma of the mouth, pharynx and oesophagus in women. Observations at Radiumhemmet, Stockholm. *British Medical Journal*, 2: 331-3
Althausen, A., Prout, G.R., Jr., and Daly, J. (1976). Non-invasive papillary carcinoma of the bladder associated with carcinoma *in situ*. *Journal of Urology*, 116: 575-80

Altmann, F., Ginsberg, I. and Stout, A.P. (1952). Intraepithelial carcinoma (cancer *in situ*) of larynx. *Archives of Otolaryngology*, 56: 121-33

Anderson, D.E. (1974). Genetic study of breast cancer: Identification of a high risk group. *Cancer*, 34: 1090-7

Ashikari, R., Park, K., Huvos, A.G. and Urban, J.A. (1970). Paget's disease of the nipple. *Cancer*, 26: 680-5

Auerbach, O., Stout, A.P., Hammond, E.C. and Garfinkel, L. (1961). Changes in bronchial epithelium in relation to cigarette smoking and in relation to lung cancer. *New England Journal of Medicine*, 265: 253-67

——— Hammond, E.C. and Garfinkel, L. (1979). Changes in bronchial epithelium in relation to cigarette smoking, 1955-1960 vs. 1970-1977. *New England Journal of Medicine*, 300: 381-6

Aurelian, L., Kessler, I., Rosenshein, N.B. and Barbour, G. (1981). Viruses and gynecologic cancers: Herpesvirus protein (ICP 10/AG-4), a cervical tumor antigen that fulfils the criteria for a marker of carcinogenicity. *Cancer*, 48: 455-71

Beutler, H.K., Dockerty, M.B. and Randall, L.M. (1963). Precancerous lesions of the endometrium. *American Journal of Obstetrics and Gynecology*, 86: 433-43

Boyes, D.A. and Worth, A.J. (1976). Cytologic screening for cervical carcinoma. In: Jordan, J.A. and Singer, A. (eds.), *The Cervix*, Saunders, London/Philadelphia, ch. 35, p. 404

Brawn, P.N. (1982). The origin of invasive carcinoma of the bladder. *Cancer*, 50: 515-19

British Medical Journal (editorial) (1964). A virus in Burkitt's tumour, 1: 1197-8

Burkitt, D.P. (1972). Epidemiology of cancer of the colon and rectum. *Cancer*, 28: 3-13

Chasko, S.B., Gray, G.F. and McCarron, J.P. (1981). Urothelial neoplasia of the upper urinary tract. In: Sommers, S.C. and Rosen, P.P. (eds.), *Pathology Annual*, Appleton-Century-Crofts, New York, vol. 2, p. 127

Choo, Y-C. and Morley, G.W. (1980). Multiple primary neoplasms of the ano-genital region. *Obstetrics and Gynecology*, 56: 365-9

Christopherson, W.M. and Scott, M.A. (1977). Trends in mortality from uterine cancer in relation to mass screening. *Acta Cytologica*, 21: 5-9

Cocker, J., Fox, H. and Langley, F.A. (1968). Consistency in the histological diagnosis of epithelial abnormalities of the cervix uteri. *Journal of Clinical Pathology*, 21: 67-70

Correa, P. (1982). Morphology and natural history of precursor lesions. In: Schottenfeld, D. and Fraumeni, J.F., Jr. (eds.), *Cancer Epidemiology and Prevention*, Saunders, Philadelphia, ch. 6, p. 90

——— Cuello, C., Duque, E., Burbano, L.C., Garcia, F.T., Bolanos, O. *et al.* (1976). Gastric cancer in Colombia, III. Natural history of precursor lesions. *Journal of the National Cancer Institute*, 57: 1027-35

Cuello, C., Correa, P., Haenszel, W., Gordillo, G., Brown, C., Archer, M. *et al.* (1976). Gastric cancer in Columbia. I. Cancer risk and suspect environmental agents. *Journal of the National Cancer Institute*, 57: 1015-20

——— Lopez, J., Correa, P., Murray, J., Zarama, G. and Gordillo, G. (1979). Histopathology of gastric dysplasias. Correlations with gastric juice chemistry. *American Journal of Surgical Pathology*, 3: 491-500

Decker, J. and Goldstein, J.C. (1982). Current concepts in otolaryngology. Risk factors in head and neck cancer. *New England Journal of Medicine*, 306: 1151-5

Della Torre, G., Pilotti, S., dePalo, G. and Rilke, F. (1978). Viral particles in cervical condylomatous lesions. *Tumori*, 64: 549-53

Duff, T.B. (1971). Laryngeal papillomatosis. *Journal of Laryngology and Otology*, 85: 947-56

Elwood, J.M., Cole, P., Rothman, K.J. and Kaplan, S.D. (1977). Epidemiology of endometrial cancer. *Journal of the National Cancer Institute*, 59: 1055-60

Evans, I.A. and Mason, J. (1965). Carcinogenic activity of bracken. *Nature*, 208: 913-14

Fairchild, W.V., Spence, C.R., Solomon, H.D. and Gangai, M.P. (1979). The incidence of bladder cancer after cyclophosphamide therapy. *Journal of Urology*, 122: 163-4

Ferenczy, A. (1981). The ultrastructural dynamics of endometrial hyperplasia and neoplasia. In: Koss, L.G. and Coleman, D.V. (eds.), *Advances in Clinical Cytology*, Butterworths, London, ch. 1, p. 1

Ferguson, A.R. (1911). Associated bilharziosis and primary malignant disease of the urinary bladder, with observations on a series of forty cases. *Journal of Pathology*, 16: 76-94

Fowler, W.C., Schmidt, G., Edelman, D.A., Kaufman, D.G. and Fenoglio, C.M. (1981). Risks of cervical intraepithelial neoplasia among DES-exposed women. *Obstetrics and Gynecology*, 58: 720-4

Friedberg, M.J. and Serlin, O. (1963). Condyloma acuminatum: Its association with malignancy. *Diseases of the Colon and Rectum*, 6: 352-5

Fu, Y.S., Reagan, J.W. and Richart, R.M. (1981). Definition of precursors. *Gynecologic Oncology*, 12: S220-S231

Georgescu, L. and Diosi, P. (1981). Virus-like particles in the kidneys of three patients with endemic Balkan nephropathy. *Revue Roumaine de Médicine-Virologie*, 32: 305-6

Gilbertsen, V.A. (1974). Proctosigmoidoscopy and polypectomy in reducing the incidence of rectal cancer. *Cancer*, 34 (Suppl.): 936-9

Goebel, C. (1905). Ueber die bei Bilharziakrankheit vorkommenden Blastentumoren mit besonderer Berucksichtigung des Carcinoms. *Zeitschrift Für Krebsforschung*, 3: 369-513

Greenebaum, E., Schreiber, K., Shu, Y.J. and Koss, L.G. (1983). Use of the esophageal balloon in the diagnosis of carcinoma of the head, neck and upper gastro-intestinal tract. (In Press) *Acta Cytologica*

Gusberg, S.B. and Kaplan, A.L. (1963). Precursors of corpus cancer. IV. Adenomatous hyperplasia as stage 0 carcinoma of the endometrium. *American Journal of Obstetrics and Gynecology*, 87: 662-76

Haenszel, W. and Correa, P. (1971). Cancer of the colon and rectum and adenomatous polyps. A review of the epidemiologic findings. *Cancer*, 28: 14-24

―――― Correa, P., Cuello, C., Guzman, N., Burbano, L.C., Lores, H. *et al.* (1976). Gastric cancer in Colombia. II. Case-control epidemiologic study of precursor lesions. *Journal of the National Cancer Institute*, 57: 1021-6

―――― Kurihara, M., Segi, M. and Lee, R.K.C. (1972). Stomach cancer among Japanese in Hawaii. *Journal of the National Cancer Institute*, 49: 969-88

Hammond, E.C. and Horn, D. (1958). Smoking and death rates – report on forty-four months of follow-up of 187,783 men. Part II. Death rates by cause. *Journal of the American Medical Association*, 166: 1294-308

Herbst, A.L., Robboy, S.J., Scully, R.E. and Poskanzer, D.C. (1974). Clear-cell adenocarcinoma of the vagina and cervix in girls: Analysis of 170 registry cases. *American Journal of Obstetrics and Gynecology*, 119: 713-24

―――― Ulfelder, H. and Poskanzer, D.C. (1971). Adenocarcinoma of the vagina. Association of maternal stilbestrol therapy with tumor appearance in young women. *New England Journal of Medicine*, 284: 878-81

Hertig, A.T. and Sommers, S.C. (1949). Genesis of endometrial carcinoma. I. Study of prior biopsies. *Cancer*, 2: 946-56

Hicks, R.M., Walters, C.L., Elsebai, I., El Aasser, A-B., El Merzabani, M. and Gough, T.A. (1977). Demonstration of nitrosamines in human urine: Preliminary observations on a possible aetiology for bladder cancer in association with chronic urinary tract infections. *Proceedings of the Royal Society of Medicine*, 70: 413-16

Homburger, F., Soto, H., Althoff, J., Dalquen, P. and Heitz, P. (1979). Animal model of human disease: carcinoma of the larynx in hamsters exposed to cigarette smoke. *American Journal of Pathology*, 95: 845-8

Horwitz, R.I. and Feinstein, A.R. (1978). Alternative analytic methods for case control studies of estrogen and endometrial cancer. *New England Journal of Medicine*, 299: 1089-94

—— Feinstein, A.R., Horwitz, S.M. and Robboy, S.J. (1981). Necropsy diagnosis of endometrial cancer and detection-bias in case/control studies. *Lancet*, 2: 66-8

Jablonska, S., Dabrowski, J., Jakubowicz, K. (1972). Epidermodysplasia verruciformis as a model in studies of the role of papovaviruses in oncogenesis. *Cancer Research*, 32: 583-9

Johansson, S., Angervall, L., Bengtsson, U. and Wahlquist, L. (1974). Urothelial tumors of the renal pelvis associated with abuse of Phenacetin-containing analgesics. *Cancer*, 33: 743-53

Jussawalla, D.J. and Deshpande, V.A. (1971). Evaluation of cancer risk in tobacco chewers and smokers: an epidemiologic assessment. *Cancer*, 28: 244-52

Kakizoe, T., Fujita, J., Tatsuro, M., Matsumoto, K. and Kishi, I. (1980). Transitional cell carcinoma of the bladder in patients with renal pelvic and ureteral cancer. *Journal of Urology*, 124: 17-19

Kawachi, T., Kurisu, M., Numanyu, N., Sasajima, K., Sano, T. and Sugimura, T. (1976). Precancerous changes in the stomach. *Cancer Research*, 36: 2673-7

Kessler, I.I. (1974). Perspectives on the epidemiology of cervical cancer with special reference to the herpes virus hypothesis. *Cancer Research*, 34: 1091-110

Klionsky, B., Anderson, W.A.D., Bennington, J.L., Carnes, W., Carvalho, G., Cendana, G.E. *et al.* (1969). Joint position statement by the cancer control program. Committee on Reproducibility of Histopathologic Diagnosis. *Acta Cytologica*, 13: 309-11

Koss, L.G. (1975a). Epidemiology of carcinoma of the uterine cervix. In: Proceedings of the XI International Cancer Congress. *Excerpta Medica Congress Series*, 3: 307-13

—— (1975b). *Tumors of the Urinary Bladder*, Second Series, Fascicle 11. Atlas of Tumor Pathology. Armed Forces Institute of Pathology, Washington, DC

—— (1978). Nomenclature of precancerous and early cancerous lesions of the uterine cervix. *Contemporary Ob/Gyn*, 11: 119-26

—— (1979a). *Diagnostic Cytology and its Histopathologic Bases*, 3rd edn., Lippincott, Philadelphia

—— (1979b). Mapping of the urinary bladder: Its impact on the concepts of bladder cancer. *Human Pathology*, 10: 533-48

—— (1981). Pathogenesis of carcinoma of the uterine cervix. In: Dallenbach-Hellweg, G. (ed.), *Current Topics in Pathology*, Springer Verlag, Berlin, Heidelberg, vol. 70, p. 112

—— (1982). Precancerous lesions of the breast – Theoretical and practical considerations. In: *Proceedings of the Second Symposium on Mammary Pathology*. Plenum Publishing Corporation, New York (in press)

—— and Durfee, G.R. (1956). Unusual patterns of squamous epithelium of the uterine cervix: cytologic and pathologic study of koilocytotic atypia. *Annals of the New York Academy of Sciences*, 63: 1245-61

—— Melamed, M.R. and Kelly, R.E. (1969). Further cytologic and histologic studies of bladder lesions in workers exposed to paraaminodiphenyl: Progress report. *Journal of the National Cancer Institute*, 43: 233-43

—— Schreiber, K., Oberlander, S.G., Moukhtar, M., Levine, H.S. and Moussouris, H.F. (1981). Screening of asymptomatic women for endometrial cancer. *Obstetrics and Gynecology*, 57: 681-91

—— Schreiber, K., Oberlander, S.G., Moukhtar, M., Levine, H.S. and Moussouris, H.F. (1982). Unpublished data

—— Stewart, F.W., Foote, F.W., Jordan, M.J., Bader, G.M. and Day, E. (1963). Some histological aspects of behavior of epidermoid carcinoma in situ and related lesions of the uterine cervix. A long term prospective study. *Cancer*, 16: 1160-211

Kreyberg, L. (1968). Nonsmokers and the geographic pathology of lung cancer. In: Liebow, A.A. and Smith, D.E. (eds.), *The Lung*, Williams & Wilkins, Baltimore, ch. 18, p. 273

Lattes, R. (1980). Lobular neoplasia (lobular carcinoma *in situ*) of the breast – a histological entity of controversial clinical significance. *Pathology: Research and Practice*, 166: 415-29

Laverty, C.R., Russell, M.B., Hills, E. and Booth, N. (1978). The significance of noncondylomatous wart virus infection of the cervical transformation zone. A review with discussion of two illustrative cases. *Acta Cytologica*, 22: 195-201

Lemen, R.A., Dement, J.M. and Wagoner, J.K. (1980). Epidemiology of asbestos related diseases. *Environmental Health Perspectives*, 34: 1-11

Li, Jun-Yao (1982). The Epidemiology of Esophageal Cancer in China. NCI Monograph (in press)

Limas, C., Hugo, J. and Garcia-Bunuel, R. (1971). 'Scar' carcinoma of the lung. *Chest*, 59: 219-22

Mack, T.M., Pike, M.C., Henderson, B.E., Pfeffer, R.I., Gerkins, V.R. and Arthur, M. (1976). Estrogens and endometrial cancer in a retirement community. *New England Journal of Medicine*, 294: 1262-7

Mahadevia, P.S., Karwa, G.L. and Koss, L.G. (1983). Mapping of urothelium in carcinomas of renal pelvis and ureter. A report of nine cases. *Cancer*, 51: 890-7

Malaowalla, A.M., Silverman, S., Jr., Mani, N.J., Bilimoria, K.F. and Smith, L.W. (1976). Oral cancer in 57,518 industrial workers of Gujarat, India. A prevalence and follow-up study. *Cancer*, 37: 1882-6

McCoy, G.D., Hecht, S.S. and Wynder, E.L. (1980). The roles of tobacco, alcohol and diet in the etiology of upper alimentary and respiratory tract cancers. *Preventive Medicine*, 9: 622-9

McDougall, J.K., Galloway, D.A., Crum, C., Levine, R., Richart, R. and Fenoglio, C.M. (1981). Detection of nucleic acid sequences in cervical tumors. *Gynecologic Oncology*, 12: S42-S55

McKusick, V.A. (1975). *Mendelian Inheritance in Man*, 4th edn., Johns Hopkins University Press, Baltimore, p. 22A

Meisels, A. (1969). Microbiology of the female reproductive tract as determined in a cytologic specimen. III. In the presence of cellular atypias. *Acta Cytologica*, 13: 64-71

—— and Fortin, R. (1976). Condylomatous lesions of the cervix and vagina. I. Cytologic patterns. *Acta Cytologica*, 20: 505-9

—— Fortin, R. and Roy, M. (1977). Condylomatous lesions of cervix. II. Cytologic, colposcopic and histopathologic study. *Acta Cytologica*, 21: 379-90

—— Roy, M., Fortier, M., Morin, C., Casas-Cordero, M., Shah, K.V. *et al.* (1981). Human papillomavirus (HPV) infection of the cervix. The atypical condyloma. *Acta Cytologica*, 25: 7-16

Melnick, J.L., Courtney, R.J., Powell, K.L., Schaffer, P.A., Benyesh-Melnick, M., Dressman, G.R. *et al.* (1976). Studies on herpes simplex virus and cancer. *Cancer Research*, 36: 845-56

Meyer, E.C. and Liebow, A. (1965). Relationship of interstitial pneumonia, honeycombing and atypical epithelial proliferation. *Cancer*, 18: 322-51

Miller, A.B. (1978). Epidemiology of carcinoma of the cervix. In: Burghardt, E., Holzer, E. and Jordan, J.A. (eds.), *Cervical Pathology and Colposcopy*, Thieme, Stuttgart, p. 103

Morson, B.C. (1974). Evolution of cancer of the colon and rectum. *Cancer*, 34: 845-9

Murakami, T. (1979). Early cancer of the stomach. *World Journal of Surgery*, 3: 685-92

Muto, M., Maki, T., Majima, S. and Yamaguchi, I. (1968). Improvement in the end-results of surgical treatment of gastric cancer. *Surgery*, 63: 229-35

Naib, Z.M., Nahmias, A.J., Josey, W.E. and Kramer, J.H. (1969). Genital herpetic infection: Association with cervical dysplasia and carcinoma. *Cancer*, 23: 940-5

Nugent, F.W., Haggitt, R.C., Colcher, H. and Kutteruf, G.C. (1979). Malignant potential of chronic ulcerative colitis. Preliminary report. *Gastroenterology*, 76: 1-5

Pearson, R.M. and Soloway, M.S. (1978). Does cyclophosphamide induce bladder cancer? *Urology*, 11: 437-47

Plaut, A. and Dreyfuss, M.L. (1940). Adenosis of vagina and its relation to primary adenocarcinoma of vagina. *Surgery, Gynecology and Obstetrics*, 71: 756-65

Plotz, P.H., Klippel, J.H., Decker, J.L., Grauman, D., Wolff, B., Brown, B.D. *et al.* (1979). Bladder complications in patients receiving cyclophosphamide for systemic lupus erythematosus or rheumatoid arthritis. *Annals of Internal Medicine*, 91: 221-3

Prasad, M.L. and Abcarian, H. (1980). Malignant potential of perianal condyloma acuminatum. *Diseases of the Colon and Rectum*, 23: 191-7

Purola, E. and Savia, E. (1977). Cytology of gynecologic condyloma acuminatum. *Acta Cytologica*, 21: 26-31

Rehn, L. (1895). Blasengeschwülste bei Fuchsinarbeitern. *Archivs Klinikum Chirurgia*, 50: 588-600

Reid, R., Stanhope, C.R., Herschman, B.R., Booth, E., Phibbs, G.D. and Smith, J.P. (1982). Genitai warts and cervical cancer. 1. Evidence of an association between subclinical papillomavirus infection and cervical malignancy. *Cancer*, 50: 377-87

Richart, R.M. (1967). The natural history of cervical intraepithelial neoplasia. *Clinical Obstetrics and Gynecology*, 10: 748-84

―――― and Barron, B.A. (1969). A follow-up study of patients with cervical dysplasia. *American Journal of Obstetrics and Gynecology*, 105: 386-93

Rockey, E.E., Speer, F.D., Ahn, K.J., Thompson, S.A. and Hirose, T. (1962). The effect of cigarette smoke condensate on the bronchial mucosa of dogs. *Cancer*, 15: 1100-16

Rosen, P.P. (1980). Lobular carcinoma *in situ*: Recent clinicopathologic studies at Memorial Hospital. *Pathology, Research and Practice*, 166: 430-55

Rothman, K.J., Cann, C.I., Flanders, D. and Fried, M.P. (1980). Epidemiology of laryngeal cancer. *Epidemiologic Reviews*, 2: 195-209

Ruiter, M. (1973). On the histomorphology and origin of malignant cutaneous changes in epidermodysplasia verruciformis. *Acta Dermato-Venerologica* (Stockholm), 53: 290-8

Rylander, E. (1977). Negative smears in women developing cervical cancer. *Acta Obstetrica and Gynecologica Scandinavia*, 56: 115-18

Saccomanno, G., Archer, V.E., Auerbach, O., Saunders, R.P. and Brennan, L.M. (1974). Development of carcinoma of the lung as reflected in exfoliated cells. *Cancer*, 33: 256-70

Saffiotti, J., Montasano, R., Sellukamar, A.R. and Borg, S.A. (1967). Experimental cancer of the lung. Inhibition by vitamin A of the induction of tracheobronchial squamous metaplasia and squamous cell tumors. *Cancer*, 20: 857-64

Sandler, H.C. (1962). Cytologic screening for early mouth cancer. Interim report of the Veterans Administration Co-operative study of oral exfoliative cytology. *Cancer*, 15: 1119-24

Schreiber, H. and Nettesheim, P. (1972). A new method for pulmonary cytology in rats and hamsters. *Cancer Research*, 32: 737-45

―――― Saccomanno, G., Martin, D.H. and Brennan, L. (1974). Sequential cytologic changes during development of respiratory tract tumors induced in hamsters by benzo(a)pyrene-ferric oxide. *Cancer Research*, 34: 689-98

Selikoff, I.J., Hammond, E.C. and Churg, J. (1968). Asbestos exposure, smoking and neoplasia. *Journal of the American Medical Association*, 204: 106

Shokri-Tabibzadeh, S., Koss, L.G., Molnar, J. and Romney, S. (1981). Association of human papillomavirus with neoplastic processes in the genital tract of four women with impaired immunity. *Gynecologic Oncology*, 12: S129-S140

Shu, Y.J. (1982). *Cytopathology of Esophageal Cancer*, New York, Masson Publishing (in press)

Siegler, E.E. (1956). Microdiagnosis of carcinoma in situ of the uterine cervix. A comparative study of pathologists' diagnoses. *Cancer*, 9: 463-9

Silverman, S., Jr., Bilimoria, K.F., Bhargava, K., Mani, N.J. and Shah, R.A. (1977). Cytologic, histologic and clinical correlations of precancerous and cancerous oral lesions in 57,518 industrial workers of Gujarat, India. *Acta Cytologica*, 21: 196-8

Smith, D.C., Prentice, R., Thompson, D.J. and Herrmann, W.L. (1975). Association of exogenous estrogen and endometrial carcinoma. *New England Journal of Medicine*, 293: 1164-7

Sorrentino, F. and DeMartino, A.M. (1979). Chronic interstitial nephritis as a cause of tumours of the upper urinary tract. A hypothesis. *Urologia Internationalis*, 34: 393-402

Stafl, A. and Mattingly, R.F. (1974). Vaginal adenosis: A precancerous lesion? *American Journal of Obstetrics and Gynecology*, 120: 666-77

Stahl, S.S., Koss, L.G., Brown, R.C., Jr., and Murray, D. (1967). Oral cytologic screening in a large metropolitan area. *Journal of the American Dental Association*, 75: 1385-8

Steffen, C. (1982). Concurrence of condylomata acuminata and Bowenoid papulosis. Confirmation of the hypothesis that they are related conditions. *American Journal of Dermato-pathology*, 4: 5-8

Studdiford, W.E. (1957). Vaginal lesions of adenomatous origin. *American Journal of Obstetrics and Gynecology*, 73: 641-56

Sturm, J.T., Christenson, C.E., Uecker, J.H. and Perry, J.F., Jr. (1975). Squamous-cell carcinoma of the anus arising in a giant condyloma acuminatum. Report of a case. *Diseases of the Colon and Rectum*, 18: 147-51

Suzman, M.M. (1933). Syndrome of anemia, glossitis and dysphagia. Report of eight cases with special reference to observations at autopsy in one instance. *Archives of Internal Medicine*, 51: 1-21

Syrjänen, K.J. (1980). Epithelial lesions suggestive of a condylomatous origin found closely associated with invasive bronchial squamous cell carcinomas. *Respiration*, 40: 150-60

―――― Heinonen, U.M. and Kauraniemi, T. (1981). Cytologic evidence of the association of condylomatous lesions with dysplastic and neoplastic changes in the uterine cervix. *Acta Cytologica*, 25: 17-22

Tannenbaum, S.R., Moran, D., Rand, W., Cuello, C. and Correa, P. (1979). Gastric cancer in Colombia. IV. Nitrite and other ions in gastric contents of residents from a high-risk region. *Journal of the National Cancer Institute*, 62: 9-12

Wade, T.R., Kopf, A.W. and Ackerman, B. (1978). Bowenoid papulosis of the penis. *Cancer*, 42: 1890-903

Wall, R.L. and Clausen, K.P. (1975). Carcinoma of the urinary bladder in patients receiving cyclophosphamide. *New England Journal of Medicine*, 293: 271-3

Woodruff, J.D., Braun, L., Cavalieri, R., Gupta, R., Pass, R. and Shah, K.V. (1980). Immunological identification of papillomavirus antigen in paraffin-processed condyloma tissues from the female genital tract. *Obstetrics and Gynecology*, 56: 727-32

Woolner, L.B., Fontana, R.S., Sanderson, D.R., Miller, W.E., Muhm, J.R., Taylor, W.F. *et al.* (1981). Mayo Lung Project. Evaluation of lung cancer screening through December 1979. *Mayo Clinic Proceedings*, 56: 544-55

Wynder, E.L., Bross, I.J. and Feldman, R.M. (1957). A study of the etiologic factors in cancer of the mouth. *Cancer*, 10: 1300-23

—— Escher, G.C. and Mantel, N. (1966). An epidemiological investigation of cancer of the endometrium. *Cancer*, 19: 489-520

—— and Hoffman, D. (1976). Tobacco and tobacco smoke. *Seminars in Oncology*, 3: 5-15

—— Mushinski, M.H. and Spivak, J.C. (1977). Tobacco and alcohol consumption in relation to the development of multiple primary cancers. *Cancer*, 40: 1872-8

Yardley, J.H. and Keren, D.F. (1974). 'Precancer' lesions in ulcerative colitis. A retrospective study of rectal biopsy and colectomy specimens. *Cancer*, 34: 835-44

Zeil, H.K. and Finkle, W.D. (1975). Increased risk of endometrial carcinoma among users of conjugated estrogens. *New England Journal of Medicine*, 293: 1167-70

Zelickson, A.S. and Prawer, S.E. (1980). Bowenoid papulosis of the penis. Demonstration of intranuclear viral-like particles. *American Journal of Dermatopathology*, 2: 305-8

zur Hausen, H. (1977). Human papillomaviruses and their possible role in squamous cell carcinomas. *Current Topics in Microbiology and Immunology*, 78: 1-30

4 CANCERS OF THE HEAD AND NECK

A.J. McMichael

Introduction

Anatomical contiguity aside, cancers of the 'head and neck' are a disparate group. Further, while this grouping is commonly understood to comprise cancers of the oral cavity, pharynx, nasopharynx, nasal and paranasal sinuses, and larynx, there is no such formal definition. For the purpose of completeness, cancers of the oesophagus and the thyroid gland are also included in this chapter.

The relative frequency of these various cancers in Western populations is indicated in the age-standardised incidence data from South Australia for the four-year period 1977-80 (Table 4.1). The reported incidence rates of these individual cancers vary internationally by at least 10- to almost 100-fold, depending on site and sex (Table 4.2). In particular, cancers of the mouth, oesophagus and nasopharynx are dominant cancers in certain parts of the non-Western world, such as India, East Africa, Central Asia and China.

Oral Cavity and Pharynx

Introduction

Cancers of the oral cavity and pharynx are much less common in Western countries than elsewhere in the world. For example, in women, these cancers account for less than 2 per cent of all cancers among Caucasians in North America, yet over 10 per cent in India (Waterhouse et al., 1976).

The anatomic sites specified in the International Classification of Diseases (ICD), 9th Revision, are: lip (140), tongue (141), salivary glands (142), gingiva (143), floor of mouth (144), other and unspecified parts of the mouth (145), oropharynx (146), nasopharynx (147), hypopharynx (148), and lip, oral cavity, and pharynx unspecified (149). Within the oral cavity, in Western populations, cancer occurs most frequently in the tongue (especially the ventral and lateral aspects and the posterior one third) and then the lip, the floor of the mouth, buccal mucosa and soft palate.

Table 4.1: Cancers of the Head and Neck, Number, Per Cent Distribution and Age-standardised Incidence Rate (per 100,000), by Anatomic Site, South Australia, 1977-1980

Site (ICD Code) 9th Revision	Male			Female		
	No.	%[a]	Rate[b]	No.	%[a]	Rate[b]
Lip (140)	246	31.0	8.7	39	11.8	1.0
Tongue (141)	47	5.9	1.6	32	9.7	0.9
Salivary glands (142)	44	5.5	1.5	21	6.3	0.6
Mouth (143-145)	50	6.3	1.7	27	8.1	0.7
Oropharynx (146)	46	5.8	1.6	14	4.2	0.4
Mouth and pharynx (140-146)	433	54.5	15.1	133	40.1	3.6
Nasopharynx (147)	14	1.8	0.5	3	0.9	0.1
Hypopharynx (148)	22	2.8	0.8	8	2.4	0.2
Oesophagus (150)	131	16.5	4.6	51	15.4	1.3
Nose, nasal cavity and middle ear (160)	25	3.2	0.9	15	4.5	0.4
Larynx (161)	131	16.5	4.5	14	4.2	0.4
Thyroid (193)	37	4.7	1.3	108	32.5	3.6

Notes: a. Column per cent; total = 100%.
b. Age-standardised to the World Standard Population, Waterhouse *et al.*, 1976.
Source: South Australian Central Cancer Registry (1982).

Oral and pharyngeal cancers are primarily squamous cell (epidermoid) carcinoma, usually well differentiated. Leukoplakia, erythroplasia, lichen planus and submucous fibrosis, each entailing altered tissue morphology, are considered to be precursor conditions (Pindborg, 1980). Indeed, a recent follow-up study in India concluded that 'oral cancer was always preceded by some kind of precancerous lesion' (Gupta *et al.*, 1980).

Survival rates vary considerably by anatomic site, and by the stage at which the tumour is detected, its histopathology, and the type of treatment. From Table 4.3, among cancers of the mouth and pharynx in the United States of America (USA), lip and salivary gland cancers have the highest five-year survival, whereas cancer of the pharynx has the lowest. Overall, little improvement in survival occurred between 1960-63 and 1970-73. The consistently higher survival among women reflects the generally earlier diagnosis among this sex (Myers and Hankey, 1982).

Table 4.2: International Range of Incidence for Major Cancers of the Head and Neck, by Sex, around 1970[a] (annual age-standardised incidence per 100,000 persons)

Site (ICD code) (8th Revision)	Sex	Rate	High (H) Population	Rate	Low (L) Population	Ratio H/L
Lip (140)	M	27.1	Canada, Newfoundland	0.3	Japan, Miyagi	90.3
	F	1.7	Brazil, Sao Paulo	0.1	England, SMCR[b]	17.0
Oral cavity and pharynx (140-146, 148)	M	33.2	India, Bombay	4.2	Nigeria, Ibadan	7.9
	F	25.5	Singapore, Indian	1.3	Israel, Non-Jews	19.6
Nasopharynx (147)	M	19.1	US Bay Area, Chinese	0.3	German Dem. Rep.	63.7
	F	7.1	Singapore, Chinese	0.1	German Dem. Rep.	71.0
Oesophagus (150)	M	63.8	Rhodesia, Bulawayo: African	1.5	Nigeria, Ibadan	42.5
	F	10.8	India, Bombay	0.4	US, Utah	27.0
Larynx (161)	M	14.1	Brazil, Sao Paulo	1.4	Nigeria, Ibadan	10.1
	F	2.6	India, Bombay	0.2	Norway	13.0
Thyroid (193)	M	5.0	Iceland	0.5	England, SMCR	10.0
	F	18.7	Hawaii, Filipino	0.8	Romania, Timis	23.4

Notes: a. Excludes published rates based on less than 10 cases.
b. England, SMCR = South Metropolitan Cancer Registry (London).
Source: Waterhouse *et al.*, 1976.

Incidence and Mortality

Reported incidence rates around the world vary 8- to 20-fold (Table 4.2). The highest rates occur in India, Sri Lanka and other Southeast Asian countries (Waterhouse *et al.*, 1976). The high rate among Canadian males in Newfoundland (29.9 per 100,000) is due to a remarkably high rate of lip cancer (27.1); high rates also occur in other Canadian provinces, Brazil, rural Poland, Utah (USA) and Malta. Lip cancer is rare in females and in dark-skinned and Oriental persons of either sex.

More than 90 per cent of all oral and pharyngeal cancers occur in

patients over 45 years of age, with a sharp rise in incidence occurring
in the seventh age decade in Western populations (Mahboubi and Sayed,
1982). The male to female ratio ranges from 5:1 to 1:1 in diverse
populations, being approximately 4:1 in South Australia (Table 4.1).
A male: female sex ratio of around 2:1 has also been reported for oral
and pharyngeal cancers, but not for other cancers, in dogs (Cohen *et
al.*, 1964; Dorn *et al.*, 1968). Among Indians in Singapore and Natal
(South Africa) oral cavity cancers are about twice as frequent in women
as in men (Waterhouse *et al.*, 1976).

Table 4.3: Trend in Five-year Relative Survival Rates (per cent) for
Cancers of the Head and Neck, United States of America

Site	White males		White females	
	1960-63	1970-73	1960-63	1970-73
Lip	84	87	88	Too few cases
Tongue	23	32	44	46
Salivary gland	55	53	82	85
Mouth	42	40	50	51
Pharynx	21	27	35	31
Oesophagus	4	4	6	4
Nose, nasal cavity, middle ear	39	48	44	50
Larynx	54	63	46	56
Thyroid	75	82	87	87

Source: Myers and Hankey, 1982.

Analysis of age-specific death rates since around 1940 indicates that
in some populations a substantial increase has occurred in males and
females, while in others mortality has either been stable or has declined
(Mahboubi and Sayed, 1982). For example, mortality among males has
increased in France, remained relatively steady in Scandinavia, Canada,
Israel and Japan, and declined in England and New Zealand. Among
women in Canada and England, however, mortality from oral cavity
cancers has increased as it has also, to a lesser extent, among white
females in the USA.

In the USA, the rates are elevated among males in urban areas and
among females in the rural South (Blot and Fraumeni, 1977). Low
socioeconomic groups have a higher risk of oral and pharyngeal cancer
(Wynder and Stellman, 1977). Those engaged in occupations such as

bartending or waiting-on-table are at highest risk, while professional, administrative and clerical groups are at lower risk. These interoccupational differences are correlated with differences in group smoking and drinking behaviour (McMichael and Hartshorne, 1982).

Aetiological Considerations

The factors thought to cause oral and pharyngeal cancer vary both geographically and culturally. In India, tobacco chewing is important, while in Western populations alcohol and tobacco smoking are major factors. Nutritional deficiency is another suspected factor that may vary geographically. Hirayama (1966) collected data from six countries in Southeast Asia which showed a strong association between tobacco chewing and oral cancer. Lesser associations were evident for smoking, alcohol consumption and a vegetarian diet.

The habits of chewing tobacco and smoking cigarettes have long been associated with oral cancer (Sanghvi, 1981). Tobacco chewing is widespread in India, with 'pan' vendor stalls on many street corners in the cities, and the incidence of oral and pharyngeal cancers is very high (Table 4.2). The part of the oral cavity affected by cancer corresponds to the usual location of the chewed quid (Hirayama, 1966).

The predominant aetiological factors vary regionally within India (Sanghvi, 1981). In Bombay, the risk of oropharyngeal cancer (and cancers of the larynx and oesophagus) is also strongly related to the smoking of an inexpensive tobacco-and-dried-leaf cigarette, called 'bidi'. One bidi delivers about twice the amount of carcinogenic hydrocarbons as a single cigarette. Jayant *et al.* (1977) have estimated that, in India, around 75 per cent of cancers of the oral cavity, pharynx and larynx, and 50 per cent of oesophageal cancers, are attributable to the separate and combined habits of 'pan' chewing and tobacco smoking.

Tobacco chewing has also been associated with oral cancers elsewhere in Southeast Asia and certain Central Asian Soviet Republics (Ashby *et al.*, 1979), although these tobacco preparations often include other substances, such as betel, lime, aromatic oils and flavourings. Nevertheless, a recent case-control study of oral cancer among rural Southern women in the USA, which found a strong association with tobacco-snuff usage (particularly for cancers of the contact areas of the gum and buccal mucosa), suggested that the likely carcinogen was the tobacco-derived N'-nitroso-nornicotine (Winn *et al.*, 1981).

In an early case-control study of oral cancer, Wynder *et al.* (1957) showed that 29 per cent of cases were excessive smokers as compared with 17 per cent of controls. In subsequent studies of oral cancer,

Wynder and Stellman (1977) demonstrated a significant dose-response relationship for both cigar and pipe usage; Graham *et al.* (1977) found heavy smokers to have a 6-fold greater risk than individuals who had never smoked; further, this risk increased synergistically when cigarette smoking co-existed with both heavy alcohol consumption and poor dentition. Heavy alcohol consumption has been consistently associated with cancers of the oral cavity and pharynx. However, since heavy drinkers tend also to smoke, separation of the effects of alcohol and tobacco has posed methodological difficulties.

Mortality from oral and pharyngeal cancers in Australia has risen, declined, and then risen again, thereby following closely (with a time lag) the fluctuations in per caput consumption of alcohol (McMichael and Hetzel, 1978). Further, the staggered pattern of fluctuations in age-specific cancer rates reflects differing cancer risks in successive birth cohorts, each with their different lifetime drinking opportunities and habits.

Cohort studies of male alcoholics have shown increased mortality and morbidity from oral and pharyngeal cancer, even when lung cancer mortality (an index of cigarette consumption) has not been elevated (Sundby, 1967; Hakulinen *et al.*, 1974). An early case-control study in the USA showed that persons drinking more than 160 g daily of alcohol have a 10-fold higher risk of developing oral cancer than minimal alcohol drinkers (Wynder *et al.*, 1957). Graham *et al.* (1977) demonstrated a dose-response relationship of oral cancer with alcohol consumption. Herity *et al.* (1981) reported from a case-control study in Ireland, a strong dose-response gradient between alcohol consumption and cancer of the tongue.

Not only do individuals who drink large quantities of alcohol also tend to smoke disproportionately, but there appears to be a synergistic effect between alcohol and tobacco in the production of oral cancer. For persons who drink at least 1.5 oz (42 g) of alcohol and smoke 40 or more cigarettes per day, Rothman and Keller (1972) found the risk of oral cancer to be 15 times greater than in non-smoking, non-drinking persons. However, in the absence of poor dentition, Graham *et al.* (1977) found no synergistic relationship between tobacco and alcohol use and oral cancer. From other studies, the combined alcohol–tobacco exposure appears to reduce the latent period of oral cancer, by comparison with single exposure to one or other agent (Feldman *et al.*, 1975; Bross and Coombs, 1976).

Various nutritional deficiencies have been associated with oral and pharyngeal cancer. The Plummer-Vinson (Paterson-Kelly) syndrome, a condition that results in part from chronic iron and vitamin deficiency and that predisposes to cancers of the hypopharynx and oesophagus, has been implicated, particularly among Swedish women (Smith, 1973). A case-control study in Pakistan found oral cancer cases to be relatively deficient in vitamin A (Ibrahim *et al.*, 1977); however, in the USA Graham *et al.* (1977) found no dietary differences between cases and controls. A study in Bombay found an apparent interactive effect between diet and tobacco, wherein persons with diets low in milk, eggs, meat or fish were at considerably increased risk of oral cancer from tobacco chewing and smoking (Notani and Sanghvi, 1976).

Defective dentition and poor oral hygiene have been implicated inconsistently in oral cancer (Graham *et al.*, 1977), and are often closely related to smoking and drinking habits and to nutritional status. The decline in oral cancer incidence in some population groups may partially reflect improved dental hygiene (Smith, 1973).

Occupational factors appear to play a minor role. An association between sunlight exposure and lip cancer in fair-skinned persons employed in various outdoor occupations is well established (Mahboubi and Sayed, 1982). An increased risk of oral and pharyngeal cancer has also been observed in both British and American textile workers, particularly in certain jobs such as 'carding' (Moss and Lee, 1974).

Preventive Possibilities

Unlike most other cancers of the head and neck, the mouth and pharynx are directly accessible to visual inspection. Screening by clinical examination and, in high-risk groups (tobacco chewers, smokers and heavy drinkers), exfoliative cytology would enhance detection of precancerous lesions and early malignancies. Dentists, as well as clinicians, should routinely and carefully examine the oral cavity of their patients.

Primary prevention depends substantially on abstinence from tobacco consumption and avoidance of heavy alcohol drinking. In established smokers (or chewers), a more realistic goal is a reduction in exposure, by altering the commodity, the behaviour, or both. In the longer term, upper alimentary tract cancers constitute a further reason for the health education of school children emphasising the hazards of tobacco usage and heavy alcohol consumption.

Nasopharynx

Introduction

Nasopharyngeal cancer is rare in most countries, accounting for much less than 1 per cent of all cancers in Western populations. In South Australia, it is the least common cancer of the head and neck (Table 4.1). However, it occurs with high frequency in southern China and Southeast Asia.

Cancers of the nasopharynx (ICD code 147, 9th Revision) comprise nasopharyngeal squamous-cell carcinoma (NPC), and malignant tumours of glandular epithelium and of soft tissue. NPC is by far the most common type, regardless of race or geography. The relative five-year survival rate for all cases of nasopharyngeal cancer during 1965-9 in the USA was 28 per cent and 32 per cent among white males and females, respectively (Shanmugaratnam, 1982). NPC exists in three histologically distinguishable categories — keratinising (differentiated) squamous carcinoma, non-keratinising carcinoma, and undifferentiated carcinoma. Prognosis declines with the degree of undifferentiation.

Incidence and Mortality

Nasopharyngeal carcinoma is distinguished by a marked geographic and ethnic variation in incidence. The highest rates (10 to 20 cases per 100,000) occur in the southern Chinese (Kwangtung, Kwangsi and Fukien) provinces, both in China and after migration to Southeast Asia and the United States (Clifford, 1970; Ho, 1972). Lower rates are observed among northern Chinese populations. Elsewhere in Asia, NPC is common among non-Chinese in Vietnam, Thailand, Indonesia, Singapore and the Philippines. However, it is no more common among Japanese and Asian Indians than among whites in Europe and North America (Muir, 1971).

In both Chinese and non-Chinese populations around the world, the incidence of NPC is consistently twice as high in males as females. Balakrishnan and Gangadharan (1982) have pointed out that, while the age-incidence peaks at 50-59 years, in males a smaller, earlier peak occurs at ages 15-19, in both Chinese and non-Chinese. This peak comprises predominantly poorly differentiated NPC. These authors also note that, whereas among Chinese the excessive incidence of NPC is most apparent in middle age, in the region stretching from India to northeast Africa there is a relatively high incidence at young ages, while in Europe and North America, where more well-differentiated NPC occurs, the rates tend to increase most sharply at older ages.

Aetiological Considerations

The causes of NPC remain elusive, despite intensive epidemiological investigations focusing on geographical clustering, ethnic-racial differences and close association with Epstein-Barr virus (EBV). Measurement of nitrosamine ingestion, HLA typing and seroepidemiological surveys of EBV have been conducted in endemic areas (Hirayama and Ito, 1981). Domestic, dietary, medical and occupational factors have also been considered, particularly in case-control studies, within various Chinese and non-Chinese communities.

Henderson and Louie (1978), reviewing case-control studies of NPC among southern Chinese, noted increased risks associated with the traditional life style, a prior history of ear and nose disease, use of traditional Chinese nasal medication, and domestic or occupational exposure to smoke and fumes. While these data could indicate an aetiological role for inhaled carcinogens, perhaps potentiated by altered intranasal air currents resulting from preceding disease, Ho (1972) has pointed out that women, who are more exposed to cooking fires, have a lower risk than men and that the 'boat people' of Hong Kong, who cook in the open air, nevertheless have high rates of NPC. Ho has subsequently posited a three-factor aetiology for NPC in southern Chinese, comprising a genetic susceptibility, EBV infection and carcinogens derived from certain foods (particularly Cantonese salted and fried fish) traditionally consumed in early childhood. The plausibility of this hypothesis has been well discussed by Yu *et al.* (1981), including reference to recent experimental induction of nasal and paranasal carcinomas in rats fed Cantonese salted fish.

Cigarette smoking has generally not been implicated in NPC aetiology (Henderson and Louie, 1978). However, subdivision of NPC by histological type may be important. Balakrishnan and Gangadharan (1982) consider that the major aetiological factor in well-differentiated NPC may be inhalation of carcinogens. The similarity of the age-incidence pattern for cancer of the bronchus and for well-differentiated NPC, and the widespread male preponderance, suggest that cigarette smoking may be a risk factor. These authors report a recent case-control study in which the relative risks associated with cigarette smoking were 2.18 for well-differentiated NPC, and 1.19 for undifferentiated NPC.

A strong genetic influence is suggested by the high rates in southern Chinese, at home and abroad, and the intermediate rates in populations admixed with Chinese. Genetic marker studies have demonstrated a clear association of the HLA system (particularly the HLA-A2 and

B-sin 2 alleles) with high risk in the Chinese (Simons *et al.*, 1978). Less strong associations with B locus antigens have been reported in Malays (Simons *et al.*, 1978) and in Tunisians (Betuel *et al.*, 1975). Balakrishnan and Gangadharan (1982) have further suggested that any such genetic factor influences not only predisposition to NPC, but also promotes faster growth. However, if indeed a race-related genetic susceptibility exists, the fact that the reduced rates in Chinese migrants to the USA cannot be accounted for by genetic admixture, suggests that an environmental 'trigger' must also operate (Henderson and Louie, 1978).

Observations of Caucasian cases of undifferentiated NPC indicate that Epstein-Barr viral DNA is regularly present in the tumour cells, whether the cases occur in high-, medium- or low-frequency populations (Andersson-Anvret *et al.*, 1979). Seroepidemiological surveys in Chinese populations, and in Tunisia, East Africa, France and the USA, have clearly established an association between NPC and EBV. Nevertheless, the likelihood that the EBV is aetiologically involved in NPC remains uncertain — is the virus 'driver' or 'passenger'?

A new aetiological possibility, recently proposed by Hirayama and Ito (1981) on the basis of both epidemiological and experimental evidence, entails an interaction between EBV, bacterial fatty acids with EBV activation effect, and ingested plant-derived, promoter substances — particularly croton oil. The geographic distribution of *Croton tiglium* and other related plants, commonly used as Chinese herbal drugs, coincides almost exactly with the regions of high and intermediate risk, for NPC in China.

Preventive Possibilities

Early detection depends primarily upon early recognition of enlarged cervical lymph nodes and symptoms such as earache and nasal discharge. Although cytological screening of healthy populations has not been evaluated, its use in proven cases of NPC indicates that it has a sensitivity of approximately 50 per cent and a specificity of 100 per cent (Shanmugaratnam, 1982).

In view of the uncertain environmental aetiology of NPC, primary preventive measures are debatable. The EBV hypothesis has prompted suggestions that vaccines could be used in high-risk populations — if a demonstrably safe vaccine were developed. The exclusion of nitrosamine-containing foods, especially salted fish, and perhaps particularly in childhood, should also be recommended in high-risk populations; such measures could then be evaluated, in either a controlled or uncontrolled context.

Oesophagus

Introduction

In Western countries, cancer of the oesophagus accounts, like laryngeal cancer, for approximately 1-2 per cent of cancer deaths. Elsewhere in the world, such as Central Asia, parts of China, and eastern and southern Africa, it is a leading cause of cancer death, accounting, for example, for 21.8 per cent of cancer deaths in China (Li *et al.*, 1980). The descriptive epidemiology of oesophageal cancer, characterised by marked differences in incidence within confined geographical regions, between sexes and over time, suggests the aetiological importance of environmental factors.

Only a minority of oesophageal cancers (ICD code 150, 9th Revision) occur within the upper third of the oesophagus (i.e. within the 'head and neck'). Squamous cell carcinomas predominate. Survival from cancer of the oesophagus is universally poor, with only about 4 per cent of cases in USA whites surviving for five years (Table 4.3).

Incidence and Mortality

The data in Table 4.2, restricted to populations with formal cancer registration, understate the remarkable, approximately 500-fold, variation in incidence of oesophageal cancer around the world. The incidence levels around the eastern shores of the Caspian Sea, in both northern Iran and Kazakhstan, are the highest observed anywhere in the world for any individual type of cancer (Cook-Mozaffari, 1979). The estimated annual incidence rates reach as high as 500 per 100,000 in men, and, unusually, the rates in women are sometimes even higher. The lifetime risk of oesophageal cancer is around 25 per cent in this region.

Black males in Bulawayo, Zimbabwe (Rhodesia), have an incidence of 63.8 per 100,000, while in Ibadan, Nigeria, the reported rate is 1.5 (Table 4.2). Fifty-fold or greater variations in incidence between communities living less than 500 miles apart are common (Cook-Mozaffari, 1979). Similarly, between Normandy and Brittany, in northwest France, and other parts of Western Europe there is a 15-fold gradient.

Within China, approximately 30-fold variations in oesophageal cancer mortality exist both between the provinces and between the various ethnic groups (Li *et al.*, 1980). In relation to the latter observation, it is of interest that within the Central Asian 'Oesophageal Cancer Belt' the highest rates are always found among people of Turkic or Mongol origin (Day and Muñoz, 1982).

While male rates generally predominate, the sex ratio (M: F) tends to be lowest where the absolute incidence rates are highest. The ratio varies from near unity in Central Asia, to around 5:1 in eastern and southern Africa, to 25:1 in Normandy and Brittany.

Similar variations characterise the time trends in oesophageal cancer. In both southern and eastern Africa, incidence has increased markedly in recent decades. However, in the exceptionally high incidence areas of Central Asia, the epidemic-like frequency of oesophageal cancer appears to have been longstanding (Cook-Mozaffari, 1979). In Europe, mortality rates have continued to increase in France, Italy, Portugal and Spain, while rates have been stable or are declining elsewhere. In the USA, oesophageal cancer mortality has tripled in 35 years among black males, while declining slightly among white males.

Increases have recently occurred in Britain and Australia, in both sexes, especially at younger ages (McMichael, 1978). Analysis of these data by birth cohort indicates a strong correlation with the prevailing level of alcohol consumption during young adulthood, over an era of marked fluctuations in alcohol consumption (McMichael and Hetzel, 1978). In England and Wales, the rates of oesophageal cancer mortality are high in the service, sport and recreation occupational grouping (which includes barmen and publicans), in labourers, and in farmers, foresters and fishermen (Registrar-General, 1978); elevations occur in similar occupational groups in Australia, along with other low socio-economic status occupations (McMichael and Hartshorne, 1982). Low socioeconomic status and low educational attainment have been associated with heightened risk of oesophageal cancer in various cultural settings (Day and Muñoz, 1982).

Aetiological Considerations

The search for causes of oesophageal cancer has proceeded in two somewhat distinct contexts. In Western populations, chronic exposure to alcoholic drinks and tobacco smoking, particularly in combination, are the major established risk factors. In Asian and African populations, nutritional deficiencies, mucosal irritation, genetic susceptibility and chemical carcinogens are all under continuing investigation (Day and Muñoz, 1982).

The relatively greater effect of alcoholic drinks, compared with tobacco, has been demonstrated consistently in case-control studies in Europe and North America (Tuyns *et al.*, 1977; Pottern *et al.*, 1981). The risk increase is greater for the more concentrated alcoholic drinks (Tuyns *et al.*, 1979; Pottern *et al.*, 1981). A role for nutritional deficiencies, either controlling for the effects of smoking and drinking

(Ziegler *et al.*, 1981), or in the absence of those factors in a study of strict religious orders in England (Kinlen, 1982) has also been suggested.

The mode of action of alcohol is uncertain. It may act as a vehicle for the carcinogen. Kuratsune *et al.* (1965) have shown that benzo(a)-pyrene penetrates more into the rat oesophageal mucosa when in a strong ethanol solution than in a weak one. There is some evidence of experimental mutagenicity or carcinogenicity of non-ethanol fractions present in certain alcoholic drinks. However, van Rensburg (1981) postulates that the specific nutritional deficiencies associated with excessive alcohol intake (e.g. zinc and magnesium depletion) render the oesophageal mucosa more susceptible to malignant transformation.

In contrast to Western countries, and, to a lesser extent, eastern and southern Africa (McGlashan *et al.*, 1982), where male rates of oeso-phageal cancer greatly exceed female rates, and where alcohol and tobacco are the major risk factors, in the Central Asian high-risk regions the similar rates in men and women suggest shared risk factors. Alcohol and tobacco are unimportant factors in either sex within those popula-tions. So far, despite extensive research in the Caspian littoral region, the cause or causes of oesophageal cancer remain uncertain.

Case-control studies in northern Iran have shown that the disease is most frequent among the poorest persons, whose food is deficient in animal protein, vitamins A and C and riboflavin. The consumption of sukteh (opium pipe scrapings, rich in polycyclic aromatic hydrocarbons) has also been suspected. Potentially carcinogenic mycotoxins and natural toxins in dietary staples have been suspected too, as they have been in northern China (Li *et al.*, 1980). A synthesis of this varied evidence has suggested the hypothesis that the eating of opium pyro-lysates, in conjunction with frequent use of very hot tea, acting on an oesophagus rendered susceptible by chronic dietary deficiencies, could explain the high incidence in the Caspian region (Day and Muñoz, 1982).

Analogous models of oesophageal carcinogenesis emerge from studies in China (Li *et al.*, 1980) and Japan (Hirayama, 1979). A recent prevalence survey of precursor lesions of oesophageal cancer in high-risk Linxian County in China, with one-year follow-up of a subsample, suggested that the natural history of oesophageal cancer starts with an oesophagitis which, in a few individuals, progresses to atrophy and dysplasia of the epithelium and finally to cancer (Muñoz *et al.*, 1982). Thermal injury from scalding hot beverages, physical injury caused by ingesting very coarse food, and deficiencies of riboflavin, vitamin A, and zinc were proposed as causes of these precursor lesions.

In an extensive review of the evidence, van Rensburg (1981) points out that, among non-Western populations, low rates of oesophageal cancer occur where the dietary staples are sorghum, millet, cassava, yams or peanuts, whereas high rates occur where corn or wheat are the staples. After reviewing the animal and human evidence of effects upon oesophageal carcinogenesis of deficiencies of specific micronutrients, and their concentrations and bioavailability in various diets, van Rensburg concludes:

> Most evidence suggests that a chronic low status of zinc, magnesium, riboflavin, and nicotinic acid, together with an adequate energy and protein intake, will increase the predisposition of the esophageal epithelium to neoplastic transformation and promote tumor growth. Such a mechanism would apply equally to alcoholics in New York as it does to Iranians, Chinese, or Africans at high risk for esophageal cancer.

Preventive Possibilities

Increased secondary prevention by early detection of oesophageal cancer has not been clearly demonstrated. The early detection programme in China, using abrasive cytology and oesophagoscopy, has not yet been shown conclusively to reduce mortality, although Li *et al.* (1980) report that cases detected and treated while *in situ* have a 90 per cent five-year survival.

The huge geographic variation in oesophageal cancer incidence makes clear the pre-eminent aetiological role of environmental factors. It seems likely that the control of various exogenous factors (alcohol, tobacco, opium tar, thermal injury), and the avoidance of nutritional deficiencies, particularly in non-Western high-risk populations, would reduce the incidence of oesophageal cancer substantially. However, in those same non-Western populations, the constellation of causal factors still awaits clarification.

Nasal Cavity and Paranasal Sinuses

Introduction and Occurrence

Cancers of the nasal cavity and paranasal sinuses (ICD code 160, 9th Revision), like cancers of the nasopharynx and hypopharynx, are relatively uncommon in Western populations (Table 4.1); they are also uncommon in most other countries.

The highest male incidence rates (around 2.5 per 100,000) have been reported in Japan and parts of Africa. The male:female sex ratio is usually about 2:1. Incidence rates rise continuously with increasing age. In England and Wales, rates in males are inversely related to socio-economic class (Registrar-General, 1978).

Data from the USA on histological type (Cutler and Young, 1975) indicate that 70 per cent of these cancers are carcinomas, predominantly squamous cell. The internal nose is the most common site, followed by the maxillary sinus. Melanomas, sarcomas and lymphomas occur rarely. Approximately half the cases in the USA survive for five years (Table 4.3); case survival has improved moderately since 1960-63.

Aetiological Considerations

Whereas the oral cavity is the point of first contact with what is eaten, drunk, or smoked, the nose is much less exposed to behaviourally-determined factors. Not surprisingly, then, occupational contaminants of the inhaled air have been most implicated in nose and paranasal sinus cancers. Because of the rarity of these cancers, any effects of these same (or other) contaminants at lesser, non-occupational, concentrations would be virtually undetectable.

The very high risk of cancers of the nasal cavity and paranasal sinuses in nickel workers, especially furnace operators, has been apparent for 50 years. Both epidemiological and laboratory experimental data particularly implicate nickel subsulphide and nickel carbonyl (Redmond et al., 1982). A high risk in woodworkers, first reported in 1965, has been consistently reported (Cecchi et al., 1980). Acheson (1976), as well as reporting a cluster of these cancers in woodworkers in England, also related the cancer to working in the footwear industry. That relationship has also been reported from Italy (Cecchi et al., 1980).

Other occupational exposures – to organic dusts (e.g. dusts in textile mills, flour mills, bakeries), mustard gas, chromate pigment manufacture, hydrocarbon gas production, radium dial painting and the petroleum and chemical industries – have also been implicated in cancers of the nose and paranasal sinuses. Non-occupational exposures to radioactive thorotrast, used clinically, and to snuff may also increase the risk. Cigarette smoking, however, appears not to be implicated (Redmond et al., 1982).

Preventive Possibilities

Given the rarity of the disease, screening for cancers of the nasal cavity and paranasal sinuses should be confined to high-risk groups, such as nickel workers. Since early diagnosis of these cancers clearly improves prognosis, education of the appropriate medical and dental specialists in their differential diagnosis is desirable, particularly since delay between symptoms and definitive diagnosis has often been unnecessarily long (Redmond *et al.*, 1982).

Primary prevention currently depends largely on the control of occupational exposures, such as has now been largely achieved in various populations of nickel refinery workers. For workers exposed to organic dusts (such as wood and leather) for which, however, excess risks of lung and laryngeal cancers are not apparent, it is likely that the carcinogenic agents are trapped in the nasal passages and sinuses because of their greater particle size (Stokinger, 1977). Industrial hygiene measures, including personal protective devices, ought, therefore, to reduce the risk of cancer of these sites.

Larynx

Introduction

In English-speaking Western countries, cancer of the larynx accounts for approximately 2 per cent of male cancers and 0.5 per cent of female cancers. In South Australia, the incidence rate is approximately ten times higher in males than in females (Table 4.1), accounting for 16.5 and 4.2 per cent, respectively, of all head and neck cancers.

Cancer of the larynx (ICD code 161, 9th Revision) comprises, clinically, three subgroups. Supraglottic tumours, above the true vocal cords, include the epiglottis, false cords and laryngeal ventricles. They arise from ciliated columnar epithelium. Glottic tumours are those of the true vocal cords, and generally arise from stratified squamous epithelium. Subglottic (infraglottic) tumours, much rarer, arise below the true vocal cords.

Cancer of the glottis, accounting for over half of the total, has the most favourable prognosis. Unlike supraglottic cancers, glottic cancer frequently presents with early hoarseness and further, the glottis is less richly supplied with lymphatic drainage. The five-year survival in US whites, during 1970-73 (Table 4.3), was 63 per cent and 56 per cent in men and women, respectively. Indeed, this is the only head and neck cancer for which male survival exceeds female. Between the 1960s and the 1970s, the increase in survival was largely due to an improved prognosis of patients with regional disease (Austin, 1982).

Incidence and Mortality

The incidence of laryngeal cancer, as shown in Table 4.2, varies by a factor of 10 or more around the world, with the highest rates reported in Brazil and India. Further, across the range of incidence rates, male rates exceed female rates by a factor of 5 to 10.

In Europe, the highest incidence rates appear to be in Italy and Spain; high rates are also reported from Colombia, Israel, Finland and Hawaii (Rothman *et al.*, 1980). Dunham and Bailar (1970) produced world maps showing that some areas with very high death rates from lung cancer also have very high rates of laryngeal cancer (e.g. Argentina, Cuba), while in Mediterranean countries and extending east to India, the high rates of laryngeal cancer are not matched by high rates of lung cancer, but instead by high rates of oral and oesophageal cancer. By contrast, Maori females of New Zealand, with the highest reported rate of lung cancer in the world for females, have a near-zero rate of laryngeal cancer (Waterhouse *et al.*, 1976).

In most areas of the world there is evidence that the incidence of laryngeal cancer is currently increasing in males and, in more developed countries, in females also. In Sweden, laryngeal cancer incidence increased about 50 per cent during the 1960s. In both Australia and England and Wales, mortality from laryngeal cancer has declined in each sex since the 1930s, although in Australian males the rates have increased again since around 1960 (McMichael, 1978). Sharp recent increases in mortality have been reported in Italy and Poland (Rothman *et al.*, 1980).

The almost three-fold variation in laryngeal cancer mortality by social class in England and Wales (Registrar-General, 1978) indicates the likely aetiological involvement of class-related factors — smoking, alcohol consumption, dietary habits and occupational exposure.

Aetiological Considerations

As with cancers of the mouth and pharynx, tobacco use and alcohol consumption are the best demonstrated risk factors for laryngeal cancer. In particular, the strong relationship with smoking has been known since the major follow-up studies of smoking in the 1950s. These early studies consistently indicated a risk of laryngeal cancer in heavy smokers 20 to 30 times higher than in non-smokers (Rothman *et al.*, 1980). The dose-response relationship appear linear.

A subsequent large case-control study of Wynder *et al.* (1976), reanalysed by Rothman *et al.* (1980), revealed a similar linear and strong dose-response relationship with cigarette smoking. Data from this and other case-control studies show an intermediate risk increase in smokers of pipes and cigars. In Ireland, Herity *et al.* (1981) reported a nearly 40-fold increase in risk of laryngeal cancer in heavy smokers versus non-smokers. They further observed a significant synergistic effect between smoking and alcohol consumption.

Although ethanol *per se* is not suspected of carcinogenicity, the consumption of alcoholic drinks has been shown in several case-control studies to be associated with a moderate increase in laryngeal cancer risk, after controlling for cigarette smoking (Rothman *et al.*, 1980). Follow-up studies of alcoholics (Sundby, 1967) and Danish brewery workers (Jensen, 1979) have shown excesses of cancer mortality and morbidity largely confined to cancers of the upper alimentary tract and larynx. Further, both McMichael (1978; 1979) and Tuyns and Audigier (1976) have shown that fluctuations in age-specific mortality from laryngeal cancer over time have, like oesophageal cancer, followed the fluctuations in per caput alcohol consumption noticeably more closely than those of per caput tobacco consumption.

Although alcohol consumption appears to have some moderate influence on laryngeal cancer risk independently of its usual association with cigarette smoking, there is evidence of a synergistic carcinogenic effect between those two factors (Rothman *et al.*, 1980). Nevertheless, those authors point to the methodological difficulty in precluding residual confounding between alcohol and smoking.

While there is increasing evidence that dietary factors and nutritional status modify human carcinogenesis, little attention has been paid to these factors in laryngeal cancer. Graham *et al.* (1981), in a large case-control study in the USA, reported a protective effect of vitamins A and C, after controlling for smoking and drinking habits. While this finding accords with other human and experimental data, they recognised the uncertain validity of estimating the usual past dietary intake of micronutrients, by questionnaire.

Among various occupational exposures studied, asbestos has been most consistently related to laryngeal cancer (Rothman *et al.*, 1980; Burch *et al.*, 1981). Exposure to wood dust and nickel may also be implicated (Rothman *et al.*, 1980), although a recent Canadian case-control study found no association with nickel (Burch *et al.*, 1981). Cohorts of workers engaged in the wartime manufacture of mustard gas have shown clear-cut excesses of laryngeal cancer (Manning *et al.*, 1981).

Preventive Possibilities

The early diagnosis of laryngeal cancer is enhanced by laryngoscopic examination and biopsy of suspicious lesions. Simpler tests — involving serology, cytology, or voice spectography — have not yet proven useful for mass screening (Austin, 1982).

The potential for primary prevention is, in principle, great. The major identified risk factors are tobacco and alcohol, with the latter factor acting synergistically — most probably acting directly in supra-glottic laryngeal cancer, but perhaps acting via induced nutritional deficiencies in the production of glottic cancers. The value of ceasing smoking is indicated by Wynder and Stellman (1977), who reported a progressive lowering of the relative risk of laryngeal cancer with increasing duration of continued abstinence.

Nevertheless, reducing or eliminating consumption of tobacco or alcohol is a manifestly difficult public health and individual counselling challenge. The earlier remarks for oral cavity therefore apply here also.

Thyroid Gland

Introduction and Occurrence

Unlike all the other cancers considered in this chapter, thyroid cancer is not a disease of the upper aero-digestive tract. However, in view of its anatomical location, it is included here, albeit briefly.

Thyroid cancer (ICD code 193, 9th Revision) comprises epithelial carcinomas (95 per cent), and occasional sarcomas and lymphomas. Of the carcinomas, the most common is the papillary type, particularly at younger ages, followed by follicular carcinoma.

Although thyroid cancer accounts for less than 2 per cent of cancers in most populations, it occurs relatively often in adolescence and young adulthood (Waterhouse *et al.*, 1976). Some of the reported international variation in incidence (Table 4.2) may reflect the difficulties of differentiating histologically between carcinoma and adenoma. It is much more common in women than men, and, in South Australia, its incidence in women is the same as for all cancers of the mouth and pharynx (Table 4.1). Unlike many other cancer sites, thyroid cancer lacks any systematic variation between developed and underdeveloped, or urban and rural populations (Waterhouse *et al.*, 1976).

The five-year survival in the USA is, except for cancer of the lip, higher for thyroid cancer than for other head and neck cancers (Table 4.3).

Aetiological Considerations

The one clearly established causal factor for thyroid cancer is ionising radiation (Ron and Modan, 1980). A history of repeated childhood irradiation, for conditions such as tinea capitis, tonsillar enlargement, or thymic enlargement, confers a substantial increase in risk. Less extensive data implicate adult X-irradiation and nuclear fallout (Hempelmann and Furth, 1978). Disorders of thyroid function, such as non-toxic goitre, thyrotoxicosis, thyroiditis and thyroid adenoma, have been suspected on the basis of either descriptive epidemiological findings or case reports. However, no case-control studies or follow-up studies appear to have yet been reported in relation to these and other possible aetiological factors, such as diet, iodine status and hormones.

Preventive Possibilities

Screening programmes based on thyroid gland palpation, with or without radio-iodine scanning, while recently popular in the USA in high-risk childhood-irradiated populations, have nevertheless not been shown to enhance prognosis. Indeed, the majority of persons subsequently investigated operatively were false positives (Favus *et al.*, 1976).

In relation to primary prevention, despite the strong evidence of radiation-induced thyroid cancer, other aetiological possibilities have been largely ignored. A programme of analytical epidemiological research is therefore now needed, to investigate the strong predilection for women, and the roles of thyroid stimulating hormone (TSH) and other hormones and exogenous food- and water-borne mutagens and goitrogens.

Summary

Cancers of the head and neck are a disparate group in most respects. With the exception of thyroid cancer, incidence rates are higher in men than women — reflecting the predominant influence of male-oriented exposures (tobacco smoking and chewing, alcohol consumption and occupational exposures). The substantial geographical and other variations in incidence for oesophageal and nasopharyngeal cancers indicate the importance of environmental factors in their aetiology; yet causal mechanisms remain less clear for these two cancers than for oral, pharyngeal and laryngeal cancers. Nevertheless, for each of these five cancers there appears to be a complex of predisposing, initiating, co-initiating and promoting factors involved, each of which may, in turn, derive from nutritional, environmental or genetically determined sources. For cancers of the nasal cavity and paranasal sinuses and of the thyroid gland, fewer causal factors have been identified. The former cancers, universally uncommon, are predominantly related to occupational exposures; the latter to childhood irradiation (and being female). Prognosis varies hugely, from very poor in oesophageal cancer to very good in lip and thyroid cancer.

References

Acheson, E.D. (1976). Nasal cancer in the furniture and boot and shoe manufacturing industries. *Preventive Medicine*, 5: 295-315

Andersson-Anvret, M., Forsby, N., Klein, G., Henle, W. and Biorklund, A. (1979). Relationship between the Epstein-Barr virus genome and nasopharyngeal carcinoma in Caucasian patients. *International Journal of Cancer*, 23: 762-6

Ashby, J., Styles, J.A. and Boyland, E. (1979). Betel nuts, arecaidine, and oral cancer. *Lancet*, 1: 112

Austin, D.F. (1982). Larynx. In: Schottenfeld, D. and Fraumeni, J.F. (eds.), *Cancer Epidemiology and Prevention*, Saunders, Philadelphia, ch. 31, p. 554

Balakrishnan, V. and Gangadharan, P. (1982). Cancer of the nasopharynx in man: Younger age peak and related aspects. In: Reznik, G. (ed.), *Comparative Nasal Cavity Tumors in Animals and Man*, CRC Press, Boca Raton, USA (in press)

Betuel, H., Cammoun, M., Colombani, J., Day, N.E., Ellouz, R. and de-Thé, G. (1975). The relationship between nasopharyngeal carcinoma and the HL-A system among Tunisians. *International Journal of Cancer*, 16: 249-54

Blot, W.J. and Fraumeni, J.F. (1977). Geographic patterns of oral cancer in the United States: Etiologic implications. *Journal of Chronic Diseases*, 30: 745-57

Bross, I.D.J. and Coombs, J. (1976). Early onset of oral cancer among women who drink and smoke. *Oncology*, 33: 135-9

Burch, J.D., Howe, G.R., Miller, A.B. and Semenciw, R. (1981). Tobacco, alcohol, asbestos, and nickel in the etiology of cancer of the larynx: A case-control study. *Journal of the National Cancer Institute*, 67: 1219-24

Cecchi, F., Binatti, E., Kriebel, D., Nastasi, L. and Santucci, M. (1980). Adenocarcinoma of the nose and paranasal sinuses in shoemakers and woodworkers in the province of Florence, Italy (1963-77). *British Journal of Industrial Medicine*, 37: 222-5

Clifford, P. (1970). A review on the epidemiology of nasopharyngeal carcinoma. *International Journal of Cancer*, 5: 287-309

Cohen, D., Brodey, R.S. and Chen, S.M. (1964). Epidemiologic aspects of oral and pharyngeal neoplasms of the dog. *American Journal of Veterinary Research*, 25: 1776-9

Cook-Mozaffari, P. (1979). The epidemiology of cancer of the oesophagus. *Nutrition and Cancer*, 1: 51-60

Cutler, S.J. and Young, J.L. (1975). *Third National Cancer Survey: Incidence Data*. National Cancer Institute Monograph, 41. DHEW Publication No. (NIH) 75-787, Washington, DC, p. 411 (Table 45)

Day, N.E. and Muñoz, N. (1982). Esophagus. In: Schottenfeld, D. and Fraumeni, J.F. (eds.), *Cancer Epidemiology and Prevention*, Saunders, Philadelphia, ch. 34, p. 596

Dorn, C.R., Taylor, D.O.N., Schneider, R., Hibbard, H.H. and Klauber, M.R. (1968). Survey of animal neoplasms in Alameda and Contra Costa Counties, California. II. Cancer morbidity in dogs and cats from Alameda County. *Journal of the National Cancer Institute*, 40: 307-18

Dunham, L.J. and Bailar, J.C. (1970). World maps of cancer mortality rates and frequency ratios. *Industrial Medicine*, 39: 259-75

Favus, M.J., Schneider, A.B., Stachura, M.E., Arnold, J.E., Ryo, U.Y., Pinsky, S.M. *et al.* (1976). Thyroid cancer occurring as a late consequence of head and neck irradiation. Evaluation of 1056 patients. *New England Journal of Medicine*, 294: 1019-25

Feldman, J., Hazan, M., Nagarajan, M. and Kissin, B. (1975). A case-control investigation of alcohol, tobacco and diet in head and neck cancer. *Preventive Medicine*, 4: 444-63

Graham, S., Dayal, H., Rohrer, T., Swanson, M., Sultz, H., Shedd, D. *et al.* (1977). Dentition, diet, tobacco, and alcohol in the epidemiology of oral cancer. *Journal of the National Cancer Institute*, 59: 1611-18

—— Mettlin, C., Marshall, J., Priore, R., Rzepka, T. and Shedd, D. (1981). Dietary factors in the epidemiology of cancer of the larynx. *American Journal of Epidemiology*, 113: 675-80

Gupta, P.C., Mehta, F.S., Daftary, D.K., Pindborg, J.J., Bhonsle, R.B., Jalnawalla, P.N. *et al.* (1980). Incidence rates of oral cancer and natural history of oral precancerous lesions in a 10-year follow-up study of Indian villagers. *Community Dentistry and Oral Epidemiology*. 8: 287-333

Hakulinen, T., Lehtinaki, L. and Lehtonen, M. (1974). Cancer morbidity among two male cohorts with increased alcohol consumption. *Journal of the National Cancer Institute*, 52: 1711-14

Hempelmann, L.H. and Furth, J. (1978). Etiology of thyroid cancer. In: Greenfield, L.D. (ed.), *Thyroid Cancer*, CRC Press, West Palm Beach, Fla., ch. 3, p. 37

Henderson, B.E. and Louie, E. (1978). Discussion of risk factors for nasopharyngeal carcinoma. In: de-Thé, G. and Ito, Y. (eds.), *Nasopharyngeal Carcinoma: Etiology and Control*, International Agency for Research on Cancer, Lyon, ch. 18, p. 251

Herity, B., Moriarty, M., Bourke, G.J. and Daly, L. (1981). A case-control study of head and neck cancer in the Republic of Ireland. *British Journal of Cancer*, 43: 177-82

Hirayama, T. (1966). An epidemiological study of oral and pharyngeal cancer in Central and Southeast Asia. *Bulletin of the World Health Organization*, 34: 41-69

—— (1979). Diet and cancer. *Nutrition and Cancer*, 1: 67-81

—— and Ito, Y. (1981). A new view of the etiology of nasopharyngeal carcinoma. *Preventive Medicine*, 10: 614-22

Ho, J.H.-C. (1972). Nasopharyngeal carcinoma. In: Klein, G. and Weinhouse, S. (eds.), *Advances in Cancer Research*, Vol. 15, Academic Press, New York, ch. 2, p. 57

Ibrahim, K., Jafarey, N.A. and Zuberi, S.J. (1977). Plasma vitamin 'A' and carotene levels in squamous cell carcinoma of oral cavity and oropharynx. *Clinical Oncology*, 3: 203-7

Jayant, K., Balakrishnan, V., Sanghvi, L.D. and Jussawalla, D.J. (1977). Quantification of the role of smoking and chewing tobacco in oral, pharyngeal, and oesophageal cancers. *British Journal of Cancer*, 35: 232-5

Jensen, O.M. (1979). Cancer morbidity and causes of death among Danish brewery workers. *International Journal of Cancer*, 23: 454-63

Kinlen, L.J. (1982). Meat and fat consumption and cancer mortality: A study of strict religious orders in Britain. *Lancet*, 1: 946-9

Kuratsune, M., Kohchi, S. and Horie, A. (1965). Carcinogenesis in the esophagus. 1. Penetration of benzo(a)pyrene and other hydrocarbons into the esophageal mucosa. *Gann*, 56: 177-87

Li, M.H., Li, P. and Li, P.J. (1980). Recent progress in research on oesophageal cancer in China. In: Klein, G. and Weinhouse, S. (eds.), *Advances in Cancer Research*, Vol. 33, Academic Press, New York, ch. 5, pp. 173-249

Mahboubi, E. and Sayed, G.B. (1982). Oral cavity and pharynx. In: Schottenfeld, D. and Fraumeni, J.F. (eds.), *Cancer Epidemiology and Prevention*, Saunders, Philadelphia, ch. 33, p. 583

Manning, K.P., Skegg, D.C.G., Stell, P.M. and Doll, R. (1981). Cancer of the larynx and other occupational hazards of mustard gas workers. *Clinical Otolaryngology*, 6: 165-70

McGlashan, N.D., Bradshaw, E. and Harington, J.S. (1982). Cancer of the oesophagus and the use of tobacco and alcoholic beverages in Transkei, 1975-6. *International Journal of Cancer*, 29: 249-56

McMichael, A.J. (1978). Increases in laryngeal cancer in Britain and Australia in relation to alcohol and tobacco consumption trends. *Lancet*, 1: 1244-7

—— (1979). Laryngeal cancer and alcohol consumption in Australia. *Medical Journal of Australia*, 1: 131-4

—— and Hetzel, B.S. (1978). Time trends in upper alimentary tract cancer mortality and alcohol consumption in Australia. *Community Health Studies*, 1: 43-7

—— and Hartshorne, J.M. (1982). Mortality risks in Australian men in occupational groups, 1968-78. *Medical Journal of Australia*, 1: 253-6

Moss, E. and Lee, W.R. (1974). Occurrence of oral and pharyngeal cancers in textile workers. *British Journal of Industrial Medicine*, 31: 224-32

Muir, C.S. (1971). Nasopharyngeal carcinoma in non-Chinese populations with special reference to southeast Asia and Africa. *International Journal of Cancer*, 8: 351-63

—— (1981). Epidemiology of cancer of the oesophagus in France and in the world, *Gastroenterology and Clinical Biology*, 5: 239-42

Muñoz, N., Crespi, M., Grassi, A., Qing, W.G., Qiong, S. and Cai, L.Z. (1982). Precursor lesions of oesophageal cancer in high-risk populations in Iran and China. *Lancet*, 1: 876-9

Myers, M.H. and Hankey, B.F. (1982). Cancer patient survival in the United States. In: Schottenfeld, D. and Fraumeni, J.F. (eds.), *Cancer Epidemiology and Prevention*, Saunders, Philadelphia, ch. 9, p. 166

Notani, P.N. and Sanghvi, L.D. (1976). Role of diet in the cancers of the oral cavity. *Indian Journal of Cancer*, 13: 156-60

Pindborg, J.J. (1980). *Oral Cancer and Precancer*. John Wright & Sons, Bristol

Pottern, L.M., Morris, L.E., Blot, W.J., Ziegler, R.G. and Fraumeni, J.F. (1981). Esophageal cancer among black men in Washington, DC. 1. Alcohol, tobacco, and other risk factors. *Journal of the National Cancer Institute*, 67: 777-83

Redmond, C.K., Sass, R.E. and Roush, G.C. (1982). Nasal cavity and paranasal sinuses. In: Schottenfeld, D. and Fraumeni, J.F. (eds.), *Cancer Epidemiology and Prevention*, Saunders, Philadelphia, ch. 29, p. 519

Registrar-General (1978). *Decennial Supplement for England and Wales, 1970-72: Occupational Mortality*. Office of Population Censuses and Surveys, HMSO, London, ch. 5, p. 115; ch. 4, p. 48

Ron, E. and Modan, B. (1980). Benign and malignant thyroid neoplasms after childhood irradiation for tinea capitis. *Journal of the National Cancer Institute*, 65: 7-11

Rothman, K. and Keller, A. (1972). The effect of joint exposure to alcohol and tobacco on risk of cancer of the mouth and pharynx. *Journal of Chronic Diseases*, 25: 711-16

―――― Cann, C.I., Flanders, D. and Fried, M.P. (1980). Epidemiology of laryngeal cancer. *Epidemiologic Reviews*, 2: 195-209

Sanghvi, L.D. (1981). Cancer epidemiology: The Indian scene. *Journal of Cancer Research and Clinical Oncology*, 99: 1-14

Shanmugaratnam, K. (1982). Nasopharynx. In: Schottenfeld, D. and Fraumeni, J.F. (eds.), *Cancer Epidemiology and Prevention*, Saunders, Philadelphia, ch. 30, p. 536

Simons, M.J., Chan, S.H., Wee, G.B., Shanmugaratnam, K., Goh, E.H., Ho, J.H.C. *et al.* (1978). Nasopharangeal carcinoma and histocompatibility antigens. In: de-The, G. and Ito, Y. (eds.) *Nasopharyngeal Carcinoma: Etiology and Control*, International Agency for Research on Cancer, Lyon, ch. 20, p. 271

Smith, C.J. (1973). Global epidemiology and etiology of oral cancer. *International Dental Journal*, 23: 82-93

South Australian Central Cancer Registry (1982). *Cancer in South Australia: Incidence, Mortality and Survival, 1977-1980*. S.A. Health Commission, Cancer Series No. 3, Government Printer, Adelaide

Stokinger, H.E. (1977). Routes of entry and modes of action. In: Key, M.M., Henschel, A.F. and Butler, J. (eds.), *Occupational Diseases: A Guide to Their Recognition*, DHEW, Washington, DC, ch. 2, p. 11

Sundby, P. (1967). *Alcoholism and Mortality*, Rutgers Center on Alcohol Studies, New Brunswick, p. 82

Tuyns, A.J. and Audigier, J.C. (1976). Double wave cohort increase for oesophageal and laryngeal cancer in France in relation to reduced alcohol intake during the second world war. *Digestion*, 14: 197-208

―――― Pequinot, G. and Jensen, O.M. (1977). Oesophageal cancer in Ille-et-Vilaine in relation to alcohol and tobacco consumption: Multiplicative risks. *Bulletin of Cancer*, 64: 45-60

―――― Pequinot, G. and Abbatucci, J.S. (1979). Oesophageal cancer and alcohol consumption: Importance of type of beverage. *International Journal of Cancer*, 23: 443-7

van Rensburg, S.J. (1981). Epidemiological and dietary evidence for a specific nutritional predisposition to esophageal cancer. *Journal of the National Cancer Institute*, 67: 243-51

Waterhouse, J., Muir, C., Correa, P. and Powell, J. (1976). *Cancer Incidence in Five Continents*, Vol. III, International Agency for Research on Cancer, Lyon

Winn, D.M., Blot, W.J., Shy, C.M., Pickle, L.W., Toledo, A. and Fraumeni, J.F. (1981). Snuff dipping and oral cancer among women in the Southern United States. *New England Journal of Medicine*, 304: 745-9

Wynder, E.L., Bross, I.D.J. and Feldman, R.M. (1957). A study of the etiological factors in cancer of the mouth. *Cancer*, 10: 1300-23

―――― Covey, L.S., Mabuchi, K. and Mushinski, M. (1976). Environmental factors in cancer of the larynx: A second look. *Cancer*, 38: 1591-601

―――― and Stellman, S.D. (1977). Comparative epidemiology of tobacco related cancer. *Cancer Research*, 37: 4608-22

Yu, M.C., Ho, J.H.C., Ross, R.K. and Henderson, B.E. (1981). Nasopharyngeal carcinoma in Chinese — salted fish or inhaled smoke? *Preventive Medicine*, 10: 15-24

Ziegler, R.G., Morris, L.E., Blott, W.J., Pottern, L.M., Hoover, R. and Fraumeni, J.F. (1981). Esophageal cancer among black men in Washington, D.C., II. Role of Nutrition. *Journal of the National Cancer Institute*, 67: 1199-206

5 CANCER OF THE LUNG

A. Smith and P.A. Troop

Introduction

Lung cancer has attracted a remarkable amount of epidemiological attention and the vast literature of the subject includes a number of substantial reviews. Doll and Peto (1981) devote considerable attention to lung cancer in their recent review of the avoidable causes of cancer. The literature is unusually contentious and the principal findings have endured a disproportionate amount of criticism — much of it ill-considered. Although there have been few more successful attempts to identify a preventable cause of ill-health by epidemiological inquiry, there has been a notable reluctance to embark on appropriate public action. In spite of the relative absence of public resolve there has been encouraging evidence in some countries that individual members of the public have taken appropriate personal steps. Nevertheless, there must be real anxiety that the incidence and mortality from this disease will continue to increase on a world scale.

Trends and Variations in Incidence

Unqualified reference to lung cancer usually implies primary carcinoma of the bronchus and although other important cancers — both secondary and primary — occur in the lung, we shall here restrict our attention to primary carcinoma. As with many diseases, comparative secular or geographical studies of incidence are made difficult and inconclusive by the problems of securing complete or representative reporting of the diagnosed condition. In the case of lung cancer, the relatively invariable course of the disease and the uniformly high case fatality rate mean that data on mortality provide a useful substitute for incidence data. Even so, there is undoubtedly substantial under-reporting of lung cancer mortality in many parts of the world.

Lung cancer was relatively rarely recorded either in clinical practice or on death certificates before the beginning of the present century. Part of the substantial increase in recorded mortality in Britain since 1911 is reasonably attributable to improvements in diagnostic technique and to an increased awareness of the importance of the condition, but it is not really possible to doubt that cancer of the lung has undergone a substantial change in true incidence that is only partly explained by changes in the age structure of the population and reductions in the incidence of competing causes of death. It seems entirely reasonable to refer to an epidemic of this disease having arisen some 60 to 70 years ago and continuing to flourish globally.

Examination of trends in age- and sex-specific rates in the mortality from this disease reveals a number of particularly interesting patterns. In Britain, as in most countries for which data are available, the rise in recorded mortality attributed to lung cancer began some 30 years later for women than for men (Doll, 1982) and total mortality remains less for women than for men at all ages. In Britain, the gap is closing, however, because while rates for women continue to increase at most ages the rates for younger men ceased to rise some 30 years ago (Smith, 1963) and for the last few years have shown a distinct fall at ages below 50 years. There is now evidence that mortality rates in women under 50 years of age may be beginning to show similar changes.

Cohort analysis of these rates in England and Wales (Case, 1956) shows that for both sexes, successive generations experienced both higher rates and a steeper rise of mortality with age until about the middle of the present century. Since then, successive male generations have ceased to exhibit these earlier trends and there is now clear evidence that younger generations of males are showing both lower death rates at all ages and a less steep rise of mortality with age. There is now suggestive evidence of incipient changes of a similar kind in women (Table 5.1).

Internationally, considerable variation in mortality is reported. It is generally the case that the disease is more common in industrialised countries and there can be little doubt that much of the variation in reported mortality is attributable to variations in diagnosis and recording. The difficulties of obtaining reliable data on either incidence or mortality make international comparisons difficult to interpret. For most countries the best evidence is from mortality data but there can be little doubt that there is substantial under-reporting of lung cancer mortality in many countries. This results from the substantial variations in quality and completeness of mortality registration and certification and in the availability of health services.

Table 5.1: Cohort Mortality for Lung Cancer, England and Wales (rates per million population)

			Age in years			
	40-44	45-49	50-54	55-59	60-64	65-69
Birth cohort	Males					
1891			626	1,375	2,575	3,941
1901	203	555	1,232	2,326	3,673	5,281
1911	250	594	1,226	2,208	3,522	5,061
1921	225	532	1,074	1,907		
1931	178	422				
	Females					
1891			102	176	288	384
1901	39	77	139	243	424	662
1911	52	106	218	402	677	972
1921	68	157	331	546		
1931	68	172				

Source: OPCS, 1981a.

Aetiology

Lung cancer is a disease in which the distinction between aetiology and pathogenesis is particularly important and instructive. We are not yet in a position to identify specific compounds which initiate or promote the development of malignant change in the bronchial epithelium and the role of squamous metaplasia remains unclear. In spite of this there is little room for doubt that the principle cause of lung cancer has been identified even if we remain remarkably unable to protect the population from exposure to it.

Tobacco

Most discussion of the aetiology of lung cancer has centred on the role of tobacco and particularly of cigarettes. Evidence suggesting that smoking might be a causal influence began to be reported on a substantial scale in the 1950s (Wynder and Graham, 1950; Doll and Hill, 1952) but earlier clinical impressions had prompted the investigation of this hypothesis. These early epidemiological reports were mainly based on retrospective inquiries (e.g. Doll and Hill, 1952) in which lung cancer patients and suitably selected controls were interviewed concerning their smoking habits and cases and controls were compared in respect of the intensity of their reported exposure, the kind of tobacco product involved, the duration of exposure, the age at which smoking began and in some cases the reported extent of inhalation. These early retrospective studies all reported similar findings and showed that cases when compared with controls included:

  (a) more smokers;
  (b) more cigarette smokers;
  (c) more heavy smokers;
  (d) more who had started smoking at an early age;
  (e) fewer who had stopped smoking.

In most of the individual studies the size of the differences and the volume of data available rendered these findings unlikely to be due to chance and the consistency across the studies further strengthened the rejection of the chance hypothesis. In most studies there was reasonable attention to the methodological problems of obtaining valid data on both diagnosis and smoking habits. Most of these early studies were open to a number of possible criticisms, however, and these have continued to be stressed by those who are disinclined to accept the aetiological role of tobacco smoking. Although later studies have largely met them, the criticisms are nevertheless worth listing and considering.

Perhaps the most consistent criticism is that retrospectively obtained data on personal habits may not be reliable. Smoking is a habit which may be variably indulged in and there may be considerable difficulty in either recalling or recording the detailed complexity of a possibly long-term history. At the time of these early studies smoking was widely prevalent – particularly in males – and the possibility of establishing a clear difference between cases and controls was seriously affected by the possible vagaries of recollection and recall. Some of the early studies had paid careful attention to the need to avoid undue emphasis on smoking during the interviews at which data were collected (e.g. Doll and Hill, 1952), although as the central findings became public knowledge this became more difficult. The possibility remained that patients who knew they had a serious chest illness might modify their statements about their smoking history – possibly in the hope of persuading themselves that their illness was 'only' a smoker's cough –

or they might have been particularly prone to recall influences that might be relevant to chest disease. In one early study (Doll and Hill, 1952) the opportunity was taken to examine data from a subset of patients in whom the diagnosis had been revised subsequent to the collection of data on smoking behaviour. Patients wrongly considered to have had lung cancer at the time of interview were shown to resemble controls more than cases in their smoking habits.

Nevertheless, the importance of the issue and the substantial scale of the economic, social and personal investment in the smoking habit led to the elaboration of ingenious alternative interpretations of the observed association. Some critics who were prepared to accept the data as valid, and that the different smoking experiences of cases and controls were real, were nevertheless prepared to entertain a variety of non-causal explanations. The main tenor of this kind of criticism was the possibility that the association of lung cancer with smoking was the consequence of an association of both smoking and cancer with a third factor. For example, the possibility was raised that those who were constitutionally disposed to contract cancer might also be con-stitutionally prone to the tobacco habit. Studies of personality type were invoked as evidence that smokers and lung cancer patients might share a common genotype. Another line of criticism was to suggest that smoking might simply determine the site at which a tumour would develop but not whether the individual would develop cancer. Although most of these alternative interpretations of the data are incompatible with evidence now available they persist as comforting options for those who are not disposed to accept the causal hypothesis.

Later studies have largely met the earlier methodological criticisms. At least eight large prospectively-based inquiries, in which causes of mortality have been compared in groups differentiated by smoking histories recorded while their members were still well, have uniformly confirmed the association identified in the earlier retrospective studies and have largely vindicated the care that went into these earlier designs.

One of the most important and widely cited of these studies has followed a large cohort of British doctors for more than 20 years (Doll and Peto, 1976). These doctors completed detailed questionnaires on their smoking habits and their subsequent mortality has been moni-tored. The results have been reported in a series of papers which have not only clearly established that the risk of death from lung cancer is consistently associated with amount and duration of cigarette smoking and that the risk progressively declines in those who give up the habit, but have also identified associations of smoking with other mortality risks – notably ischaemic heart disease. Similarly based studies on other defined groups in a number of different countries have produced similar findings (e.g. Rogot and Murray, 1980). There can no longer be any legitimate doubt that smokers of cigarettes have a raised risk of lung cancer which is clearly related to the duration and intensity of exposure to the habit.

It is an important feature of the substantial evidence now on record that the degree of risk of developing lung cancer has always shown a clear association with the duration and intensity of exposure to cigarette smoke to which the group under study has been subject (US Surgeon General, 1979). Naturally, no group has been studied as closely as it is usually possible to study dose-response phenomena in animal experimentation but there can be few dose-response phenomena of any importance that have been as critically studied in man.

At the simplest level, risk of dying of lung cancer shows a straightforward and consistent relationship with the stated daily number of cigarettes smoked (Doll and Peto, 1976; Hammond, 1972; Kahn, 1966). Although such a piece of evidence is subject to the limitation that smoking almost certainly varies both over the short and longer terms and may be consciously or unconsciously over- or underestimated by respondents, the relationship holds throughout a wide range of studies employing various data collection devices in a wide range of groups of people. The slope of the association of risk with daily consumption shows some variation but much of the variation of slope is probably consistent with known variations in inhalation habits and in tar content of cigarettes.

Duration of exposure to the smoking habit has been recorded by direct interrogation on this point and by recording the age at which the habit was initiated. In most studies the risk is quite sharply related both to total duration of the habit and to age at initiation (Kahn, 1966; Hammond, 1972). Some studies have sought to estimate total lifetime tobacco consumption (e.g. Edwards, 1957), taking into account daily number of cigarettes and duration of the habit as well as the amount of tobacco in tipped and plain cigarettes (e.g. Wald, 1976). What is quite clear is that such refinements in the estimation of dose do nothing at all to invalidate the early use of data on habitual daily number of cigarettes and duration of the habit.

Inhalation of smoke has been the most controversial issue (Doll and Peto, 1976; Hammond, 1972). It seems improbable that many cigarette smokers refrain from inhaling since it is the rapid absorption of nicotine from alveolar capillaries that makes nicotine such a satisfying and addictive drug. Nevertheless, statements about inhalation are not always consistent. Most data do show a strong association of lung cancer risk with self-reported inhalation behaviour and this is maintained when data are available on the degree of inhalation as well as on the simple issue of inhaling or not. The evidence is complicated by an association between inhalation and amount smoked — heavy smokers more often inhale and inhale deeply — and by sex differences in reported inhalation. Much has been made of one study in which findings on inhalation were anomalous (Doll and Peto, 1976).

Cigarette smoking has almost universally been found to be more sharply associated with lung cancer risk than have other forms of tobacco consumption. Pipe and cigar smoking seem less associated with the risk of cancer of the bladder and pancreas as well as of lung cancer. Of the many physical and chemical differences between cigarette smoke and other types of tobacco smoke, Doll and Peto (1981) select the relative alkalinity of the latter. They suggest that alkalinity favours the absorption of nicotine into the bloodstream thus making deep inhalation less necessary while it also increases the irritating effect of the smoke and so makes it less likely to be deeply inhaled. There is now good evidence that cigarettes vary in their tar content and that there has been a general trend to the use of lower-tar cigarettes. This trend is consistent with secular trends in lung cancer mortality, although the issue is very complicated.

The risk of dying of lung cancer in later life (over 60 years of age) is related to the exposure to cigarette smoke in the previous decade. This is suggested strongly by the evidence that those who have given up smoking during the previous ten years and those who have changed to brands yielding less tar seem to enjoy a reduced risk compared with those whose smoking continued unchanged (Rogot and Murray, 1980; Hammond *et al.*, 1977). However, it is also the case that the risk of dying of lung cancer in later life is influenced by earlier smoking habits — especially in those who continue to smoke. Thus the effects of smoking may be observed many years afterwards although the reduced risk associated with reductions in smoking in the decade before death are clearly demonstrable.

From the point of view of attempts to interpret or predict trends in the level and age distribution of lung cancer mortality these observations are important since they make such interpretation or prediction extremely difficult. They also complicate the elaboration of any detailed hypotheses about the mechanisms of tumour induction linking smoking and lung cancer. Doll and Peto (1981) devote considerable space to this problem without completely clarifying the issues but certainly without offering much comfort to those concerned with predicting worldwide consequences of current developments in the marketing and use of tobacco products.

Lung Cancer in Women

In most countries, women took up the cigarette habit on a large scale at least 20 years later than men and in most countries fewer women smoke than men and those who do smoke less. The hypothesis that cigarette smoking is the principal cause of lung cancer would require that corresponding differences should be observed in mortality from the disease in women. There is no doubt that the history of lung cancer in women is fully in accordance with the causal hypothesis, the only important departure from strict correspondence of female experience with that of males in an earlier period is that female mortality rates have generally not yet reached the high levels recorded for men. Since women seem to experience a somewhat lower risk of lung cancer at any given level of reported exposure to cigarette smoking, the suggestion has been made that they might be less susceptible to the disease or to its principal cause. Recently Doll (1982) has provided a persuasive explanation for the different experience in terms of a lower reported frequency of inhaling, the later age at which women start to smoke, and the lower tar content of more recent cigarettes. This latter point is controversial and based on the observation of Wald and his colleagues (1981) that tar yields of stored cigarettes from earlier periods are higher than for most recent examples. This point is persuasive rather than convincing since it is difficult to be sure of the effect of time on tar yields of stored tobacco products.

What seems quite clear is that we must expect a continuing rise in mortality from lung cancer among those generations of women who have been substantially exposed to cigarette smoking over the past 30 years whether present or future cigarettes are safer or not.

Other Relevant Data

Other data that have since become available are almost entirely supportive of the simple causal hypothesis. For example, the low rate of cancer in people whose religious custom proscribes tobacco is difficult to reconcile with the hypothesis that genotype may determine an association between lung cancer and proneness to tobacco addiction. A variety of studies in which dose levels have been differentiated have consistently demonstrated a positive association of dose with cancer risk.

An interesting sequence of findings followed a report by Kreyberg (1956) that the relative proportion of adenocarcinomas to other types of lung cancer had changed in published reports over a period of some 30 years. These reports dated from before the emergence of the aetiological hypothesis relating to cigarette smoking. Further studies on cigarette smoking in relation to histological tumour type showed that there was little if any association of smoking with adenocarcinoma – a much rarer type than the others. This provides a satisfying explanation of the changing distribution of tumour types since it is now quite plausible that adenocarcinoma should have remained at a fairly constant frequency while other types have shown an increase.

More recent studies have sought to identify the aetiologically significant elements in cigarette smoke. There is fairly consistent evidence that for a given cigarette consumption the cancer risk is associated with tar levels as indicated by choice of cigarette brand (Hammond *et al.*, 1977; Wynder *et al.*, 1970). The value of low tar cigarettes is compromised somewhat by the evidence that the number of cigarettes smoked is a more important determinant of risk (Hammond *et al.*, 1977) and that a switch to lower tar brands may often be associated with an increased cigarette consumption.

Cessation of Smoking

Because there is a widely prevalent belief that little purpose is served by giving up what has been a long-established habit (because 'the damage is done') it is important to take note of the considerable evidence that giving up the habit reduces the risk compared with that of continuing to smoke (Doll and Peto, 1976; Rogot and Murray, 1980). Demonstration of this relationship has been difficult because a significant proportion of those who give up have done so because they were ill – often with chest disease. The apparent risk increases in the first year after giving up – presumably because of inclusion of sick individuals (US Surgeon General, 1979). The relative decline in risk after the first year of cessation is clear in all studies but is not, surprisingly, related to total consumption before cessation. The relationship is complicated by the fact that even in non-smokers the risk of lung cancer increases with advancing age – although much less steeply and at a much lower level than in those who continue to smoke (Enstrom, 1980).

This presumably reflects a small increase in age-specific cancer risk which is largely independent of exposure to the causal agent. Ex-smokers experience a mortality which is initially similar to that in smokers but which changes with the passage of time and moves closer to the risk curve for non-smokers (US Surgeon General, 1979). After 10 to 15 years the risk for ex-smokers is little more than for non-smokers, although the end-point attainable varies somewhat with the duration and intensity of exposure during the smoking period.

Evidence on the aetiological significance of 'passive' smoking remains unconvincing. Studies of the lung cancer rates in non-smoking spouses of smokers have so far produced contradictory findings (Garfinkel, 1981; Hirayama, 1981).

Genetics

It is likely that any subgroup of the population selected for having undergone a major, potentially lethal, biological experience will be genotypically more homogeneous than the population to which they belong. It is therefore surprising how little support has been adduced for the hypothesis that patients with lung cancer share an especial inherited disposition to tobacco addiction.

One major study whose results have sometimes been misinterpreted, if not misquoted, has been based on the Swedish Twin Registry (Ceder-löf *et al.*, 1977). Within this registry has been identified a group of twin pairs discordant as to smoking habits. These consist both of pairs in which only one member smokes and pairs in which, although both smoke, smoking consumption is substantially different. In all cases pairs have been categorised as dizygotic and monozygotic. The hypothesis under test is that in discordant twin pairs the smoker should die first. So far as lung cancer is concerned this hypothesis is not refuted by the very small body of available data. In dizygotes, six cases occurred in smokers and one in non-smokers. There was only one case among monozygotes and that was in a smoker. There is certainly no evidence that death from lung cancer is more concordant in monozygotic twin pairs. What is also of interest is the evidence that discordance for smoking is as common in monozygotic as in dizygotic pairs.

Other Causes

Air Pollution

Evidence that general air pollution might be a contributory cause has been intensely debated. Lung cancer mortality has been reported in some studies to be higher in urban than in rural areas and some reports have noted that this difference is greater among smokers (US Surgeon

General, 1979). The issue is complicated by the tendency of smoking to be more common and heavier in urban than rural communities and for the habit to be begun at an earlier age, but such data as have been examined suggest that any independent effect of air pollution must be small. For example, comparison of data from the United Kingdom (UK) and Finland (Doll and Peto, 1981) where air pollution levels are very different show very similar associations of cancer incidence with cigarette consumption. It remains possible that cigarette smoking and air pollution may act synergistically.

Occupation

Early clinical observations identified a number of occupations that carried an apparently raised risk of lung cancer for those engaged in them. In the sixteenth century, a disease which was probably lung cancer had been identified as a particular hazard to miners of mineral ores with a high level of radioactivity and this risk remains well recognised (Wagoner *et al.*, 1965).

Lung cancer mortality shows a general association with social class (OPCS, 1978), which is mainly accounted for by well-documented class variations in smoking prevalence (e.g. Capell, 1978). In so far as these may reflect differences in the need for other sources of gratification for people whose employment offers little intrinsic reward, these differences could be viewed as having an occupational origin.

However, the best documented evidence of direct occupational causation of lung cancer is in relation to the processing of asbestos (Liddell, 1981) and of fossil fuels (Doll *et al.*, 1972). The relationship between asbestos and smoking is of interest since the evidence suggests that exposure to asbestos may enhance the effect of smoking as well as cause bronchial carcinoma in the absence of smoking (Saracci, 1977). Asbestos is clearly implicated as a main cause of pleural mesothelioma. More study is required of asbestos in the aetiology of bronchial carcinoma since the evidence is not altogether consistent and is difficult to interpret. In the past there has been a demonstrable risk of lung cancer for nickel workers. It is important to ensure that the known and substantial risk associated with cigarette smoking is not allowed to mask other hazards both now and in the future. Nevertheless, smoking remains overwhelmingly more important as a cause of lung cancer than any direct occupational hazard so far identified.

Diet

Evidence that vitamin A and beta-carotene intake may exert a protective effect (Peto *et al.*, 1981) is of considerable interest at the level of cancer pathogenesis but does not seem to offer a worthwhile preventive strategy at the present time (Doll and Peto, 1981). Cancer death rates are probably higher in people with very low blood retinol levels but such low levels must be rare in developed countries. Excess vitamin A intake does not seem to have any protective effect.

Epidemic Spread

Although a decline in smoking prevalence is now well established in many industrialised countries, this is not universal and there is now substantial evidence that cigarette smoking is increasing in the developing world (WHO, 1979; Taha and Ball, 1980). There is also evidence that the tar content of tobacco retailed in developing countries is much higher than is now usual in developed countries (Wickström, 1979). This is perhaps part of a wider problem which arises when profitable industrial and commercial operations that have become less acceptable in the developed world seek outlets in countries whose state of political and economic development renders them vulnerable to exploitation.

Such data as are reliably available suggest that smoking-related diseases are increasing in frequency in developing countries. The apparent decline in lung cancer that has begun among men in some developed countries must be seen against the continuing risk in women in these countries and the potentially enormous epidemic which is likely to be incurred in the world as a whole.

Prevention of Lung Cancer

For all practical purposes the prevention of lung cancer involves avoidance of cigarette smoking, although control of occupational hazards in relation to asbestos and coal products will continue to be important. Probably more than 80 per cent of lung cancer would not occur in the absence of cigarette smoking (Doll and Peto, 1981). In this sense smoking is the main cause of the disease and must be identified as the main target of any preventive action.

It has always been an attractive possibility that the responsible element in tobacco smoke might be identified and eliminated so that people might continue to smoke without harm to their health. This possibility has been rendered more elusive by evidence that those elements that are harmful to health may be necessary ingredients of the pleasure or the addictive need to smoke, and that the various elements each have different harmful effects on health (Wald, 1976). Reductions in one element may lead to compensatory increases in tobacco consumption which in turn may increase the hazards. The most straightforward advice that can be given to an individual is not to smoke. Two considerations render this less than helpful as advice to the public in general. One is the addictive nature of smoking which makes it difficult to give up the habit when it is once acquired. The other is the sustained social and economic pressure exerted on individuals to take up and maintain the habit.

In most industrialised countries, and increasingly in the developing world, the production and retail of tobacco products is a major industry sustaining a substantial workforce, returning considerable profit to investors and providing an important source of tax revenue to the state. A serious attempt to reduce the prevalence of smoking is likely to encounter resistance in the interests of employment, profit and taxation since alternatives are in each case politically difficult to provide. Effective control of cigarette advertising has been very difficult to achieve even in the relatively few countries that have attempted it.

Nevertheless there has been a marked decline in smoking prevalence among men in Britain which has been only partly offset by an increase among women. The latest evidence reports a decline for women too. Reductions in smoking seem to be partly offset by heavier consumption in smokers so that the total consumption of tobacco is maintained at profitable levels. The shape of the dose-response curve indicates that for a given national consumption of cigarettes a smaller prevalence at higher levels of individual consumption would be less harmful to the national health. It is therefore not clear that a high-pricing policy would improve health and there is little evidence that it is the relatively high price in the UK that discourages smoking. In any case the price in real terms has fallen in the UK as in many other countries.

The social climate has been favourable to the spread of cigarette smoking which is widely associated with life style images that can be presented as attractive. Advertising of tobacco products stresses the association of cigarettes with success in life and sport as well as with sexual satisfaction and independence. In the UK the tobacco advertisers have responded to the ban on television cigarette advertising by sponsorship of popular sporting and other similar events that gain substantial television coverage.

In spite of the pressures from the tobacco interests there is evidence that the habit is generally in decline in some developed countries. In the UK there have been marked reductions in smoking prevalence in recent years — particularly marked in the professional classes and in men but also to a smaller extent among working-class people and recently among women (OPCS, 1981b). There remain some curious anomalies. While doctors of both sexes smoke much less than most other groups and very much less than they did 20 years ago (Royal College of Physicians, 1977), nurses continue to smoke relatively heavily and have so far shown little sign of change (OPCS, 1977). Their role as exemplars is difficult to ascertain but is likely to be significant. Medical students smoke a little less than other students (Knopf and Wakefield, 1974) but seem surprisingly unaware that doctors smoke very much less than others (Elkind, 1982). However, as they proceed through the medical course medical students do come to consider it appropriate for doctors to advise against smoking, especially for pregnant women and patients with lung disease (Elkind, 1982).

In the UK the Health Education Council (HEC) has established an educational programme with three objectives:

1. to promote an image of smoking as an abnormal and unpleasant activity;
2. to discourage non-smokers from taking up smoking;
3. to help smokers to give up.

Recently ASH (Action on Smoking and Health, an independent body sponsored by the Royal College of Physicians) has devised and publicised a programme for district health authorities to implement as a campaign against smoking at district level. Its objectives are similar to those of the HEC.

It remains difficult to persuade national governments to take positive action — perhaps because they see anti-smoking activity as electorally disadvantageous in spite of the fact that only a minority of adults now smoke in many industrialised countries. A major problem for political parties in countries where tobacco products yield a high tax revenue is the devising of electorally acceptable alternative revenue sources.

Early Detection and Screening

Lung cancer has a very high case fatality rate and a very poor response to most therapeutic approaches. The difficulty of primary resection and the early stage at which metastatic spread often occurs have meant that successful treatment is relatively uncommon when diagnosis results from the investigation of reported symptoms. The situation is not helped by the frequently long history of symptoms referable to smoking-induced, non-malignant disease of the lungs which may obscure the early symptoms of the malignant lesion. Many patients with lung cancer have had a long history of obstructive lung disease with acute infective exacerbations and the early symptoms and signs of a tumour are easily interpreted as part of the chronic condition. It is also not uncommon for the presenting symptoms of lung cancer to derive from metastatic disease.

Screening for lung cancer has also been disappointing (Woolner *et al.*, 1981). Early studies based on periodic chest X-ray suggested that unequivocal radiological evidence of lung cancer might not appear early enough for intervention to be effective and more recent studies do not so far suggest that better screening methods are yet available (Grant, 1982). Sputum cytology may be diagnostic but also seems to yield positive results too late for useful intervention.

Advances in Treatment

The surgical treatment of lung cancer remains a hazardous process in itself — especially when the disease is advanced — and up to 50 per cent of cases are generally judged to be unsuitable for resection. Radiotherapy does not usually provide a satisfactory radical treatment although it may be a valuable palliative for patients who are too old or whose tumours are unsuitable for resection. It is too early to assess the potential of chemotherapy but there is evidence (MRC, 1979) that it is sometimes successful in inducing remission for some types of tumour and can be effective in the palliative control of metastatic disease.

Terminal care presents very variable problems depending on whether the fatal processes arise from the primary lesion or from metastases. Death from an unresected primary may be particularly distressing and this indicates the general desirability of resection when it is technically possible. Unfortunately, the generally unfavourable prognosis in this disease engenders a fatalism among doctors which may result in care being far less effective than it might be.

Summary

Bronchial carcinoma became common in industrialised countries during the present century although there is evidence that the epidemic may have begun to decline in those countries. Unfortunately, there is little ground for optimism that the epidemic will be avoided elsewhere.

Evidence is overwhelming that cigarette smoking is the principal cause of the disease and that although the habit may be beginning to be controlled in industrialised countries it has already spread to the developing world.

The disease is difficult to treat and relatively unamenable to improved prognosis by means of earlier detection. Prevention involves abstention from cigarette smoking with some small useful contribution from reduction of occupational exposure to asbestos and coal processes.

Past and present smoking makes it certain that substantial suffering and death from this disease will continue for at least several decades and it is important that societies that have profited from the promotion of the tobacco habit should accept a responsibility for providing palliative and terminal care.

References

Capell, P.J. (1978). Trends in cigarette smoking in the United Kingdom. *Health Trends*, 10: 49-54

Case, R.A.M. (1956). Cohort analysis of cancer mortality in England and Wales, 1911-1954 by site and sex. *British Journal of Preventive and Social Medicine*, 10: 172-99

Cederlöf, R., Friberg, L. and Lundman, T. (1977). The interactions of smoking, environment and heredity and their implications for disease aetiology. *Acta Medica Scandinavica*, Suppl. 612, ch. 7.3, pp. 94-104

Doll, R. (1982). Trends in mortality from lung cancer in women. In: Knut Magnus (ed.), *Trends in Cancer Incidence: Causes and Practical Implications*, Hemisphere Publishing Corporation, Washington, New York, London, Pt. 4, pp. 223-30

——— and Hill, A.B. (1952). A study of the aetiology of carcinoma of the lung. *British Medical Journal*, 2: 1271-86

——— Vessey, M.P., Beasley, R.W.R., Buckley, A.R., Fear, E.C., Fisher, R.E.W. *et al.* (1972). Mortality of gasworkers – final report of a prospective study. *British Journal of Industrial Medicine*, 29: 394-406

——— and Peto, R. (1976). Mortality in relation to smoking: 20 years' observations on male British doctors. *British Medical Journal*, 2: 1525-36

——— and Peto, R. (1981). *The Causes of Cancer: Quantitative Estimates of Avoidable Risks of Cancer in the United States Today*, Oxford University Press, ch. 5, pp. 1220-56

Edwards, J.H. (1957). Contribution of cigarette smoking to respiratory disease. *British Journal of Preventive and Social Medicine*, 11: 10-21

Elkind, A.K. (1983). Smoking: how medical students see the doctor's role. *Public Health*, 97: 38-45

Enstrom, J.E. and Godley, F.H. (1980). Cancer mortality among a representative sample of non-smokers in the United States during 1966-68. *Journal of the*

National Cancer Institute, 65: 1175-83

Garfinkel, L. (1981). Time trends in lung cancer mortality among non-smokers and a note on passive smoking. *Journal of the National Cancer Institute*, 66: 1061-6

Grant, I.W.B. (1982). Screening for lung cancer, *British Medical Journal*, 284: 1209-10

Hammond, E.C. (1972). Smoking habits and air pollution in relation to lung cancer. In: Lee, H.K. (ed.), *Environmental Factors in Respiratory Disease*, New York Academic Press, ch. 12, pp. 177-98

—— Garfinkel, L., Seidman, H., and Lew, E.A. (1977). Some recent findings concerning cigarette smoking. In: Hiatt, H.H., Watson, J.D. and Winsten, J.A. (eds.), *Origins of Human Cancer*, Cold Spring Harbor Laboratory, Cold Spring Harbor, New York, pp. 101-12

Hirayama, T. (1981). Non-smoking wives of heavy smokers have a higher risk of lung cancer: a study from Japan. *British Medical Journal*, 282: 183-5

Kahn, H.A. (1966). The Dorn study of smoking and mortality among US veterans: report on eight and one half years observation. In: Haenszel, W. (ed.), *Epidemiological Approaches to the Study of Cancer and Other Chronic Diseases*, National Cancer Institute Monograph No. 19, pp. 1-125

Knopf, A. and Wakefield, J. (1974). Effect of medical education on smoking behaviour. *British Journal of Preventive and Social Medicine*, 28: 246-51

Kreyberg, L. (1956). Occurrence and aetiology of lung cancer in Norway in the light of pathological anatomy. *British Journal of Preventive and Social Medicine*, 10: 145-58

Liddell, D. (1981). Asbestos and public health. *Thorax*, 36: 241-4

Medical Research Council Lung Cancer Working Party (1979). Radiotherapy alone or with chemotherapy in the treatment of small-cell carcinoma of the lung. *British Journal of Cancer*, 40: 1-10

Office of Population Censuses and Surveys (1977). *Smoking and Professional People*, HMSO, London

—— (1978). *Occupational Mortality: Decennial Supplement*, HMSO, London, pp. 48-9, 51

—— (1981a). *Cancer Statistics: Incidence, Survival and Mortality in England and Wales*. Studies on medical and population subjects No. 43. HMSO, London, p. xii

—— (1981b). *Cigarette Smoking: 1972-1980*, OPCS Monitor GHS 81/2, p. 5

Peto, R., Doll, R., Buckley, J.D. and Sporn, M.B. (1981). Can dietary beta-carotene materially reduce human cancer rates? *Nature*, 290: 201-8

Rogot, E. and Murray, J.L. (1980). Smoking and causes of death among US veterans: 16 years of observation. *Public Health Reports*, 95: 213-22

Royal College of Physicians (1977). *Smoking or Health*. Pitman Medical, London

Saracci, R. (1977). Asbestos and lung cancer: an analysis of the epidemiological evidence on the asbestos–smoking interaction. *International Journal of Cancer*, 20: 323-31

Smith, A. (1963). Trends in mortality from respiratory disease. Supplement to *Annual Report of the Registrar for Scotland for 1961*, HMSO, Edinburgh, pp. 5-8

Taha, A. and Ball, K. (1980). Smoking and Africa: the coming epidemic. *British Medical Journal*, 280: 991-3

United States Public Health Service (1979). *Smoking and Health*. A report of the Surgeon General. Washington DC, US Government Printing Office, ch. 5, pp. 5-1 to 5-74

Wagoner, J.K., Archer, V.E., Lundin, F.E., Holaday, M.A. and Lloyd, J.W. (1965). Radiation as the cause of lung cancer among uranium miners. *New England Journal of Medicine*, 273: 181-8

Wald, N.J. (1976). Mortality from lung cancer and coronary heart disease in relation to changes in smoking habits. *Lancet*, 1: 136-8

—— Doll, R. and Copeland, G. (1981). Trends in the tar, nicotine and carbon monoxide yields of UK cigarettes manufactured since 1934. *British Medical Journal*, 282: 763-5

Wickström, B.O. (1979). *Cigarette Smoking and the Third World*. University of Gothenberg, Sweden

Woolner, L.B., Fontana, R.S. and Sanderson, D.R. (1981). Evaluation of lung cancer screening through December 1979. *Mayo Clinic Proceedings*, 53: 544-55

World Health Organization (1979). Tobacco smoking in the third world. *WHO Chronicle*, 33: 94-7

Wynder, E.L. and Graham, E.A. (1950). Tobacco smoking as a possible etiological factor in bronchogenic carcinoma. *Journal of the American Medical Association*, 143: 329-36

—— Mabuchi, K. and Beattie, E.J. (1970). The epidemiology of lung cancer: recent trends. *Journal of the American Medical Association*, 213: 2221-8

6 CANCER OF THE SKIN

F. Urbach

Introduction

Examination of the sun's role in the production of human skin cancer does not lend itself to direct experimentation. However, extensive astute observations have strongly suggested the aetiological significance of light energy in the induction of these tumours. Blum (1959), Urbach *et al.* (1972; 1975) and Emmett (1974) have reviewed the evidence supporting the role of sunlight in human skin cancer development. Briefly, the main arguments are:

1. It is clearly established that superficial skin cancers occur most frequently on the head, neck, arms and hands, parts of the body habitually exposed to sunlight.
2. Pigmented races, who sunburn much less readily than people with white skin, have very much less skin cancer, and when it does occur, it most frequently affects areas not exposed to sunlight.
3. Skin cancer is more common in white-skinned people living in areas where insolation is greater.
4. Genetic diseases resulting in greater sensitivity of skin to the effect of solar ultra-violet (UV) radiation are associated with marked increases in and premature skin cancer development (albinism; xeroderma pigmentosum).
5. Skin cancer can be produced readily on the skin of mice and rats with repeated doses of UV radiation and the upper wavelength limit of the most effective cancer producing radiation is about 320 nm, that is, the same spectral range that produces erythema solare in human skin, ultra-violet B (UVB) radiation.

Though these arguments do not constitute absolute proof, there is excellent epidemiological evidence supporting the role of sunlight in three types of skin cancers: basal cell carcinomas, squamous cell carcinomas, (non-melanoma skin cancer — NMSC), and although less clearly, malignant melanomas (MM).

Together the first two types of skin cancer add up to the most frequently detected cancer in man and have an increased incidence over the past decade. They are also the most easily and most successfully treated human cancers. The quantitative extent to which agents other than UV exposure cause non-melanoma skin cancer in the white population has not been established. It is, however, believed to be small. Some non-melanoma skin cancer is caused by exposure to arsenic, pitch and X-rays, often in the course of work and sometimes following treatment of skin disorders. This latter group of tumours is found among patients of all degrees of skin pigmentation who happen to be exposed to these agents, and in some less developed countries it mostly seems to arise in neglected wounds.

There are important differences between many aspects of natural history of non-melanoma and melanoma skin cancer. For NMSC, three kinds of evidence — latitude dependence, body location and relation to outdoor sunlight dependence — all combine to point closely to exposure to solar UV radiation as the prime cause.

The situation is different for MM. The latitude dependence, only recently pointed to as the prime indicator of relationship to solar UV radiation, is becoming less striking and indeed in some areas invalid as better epidemiological studies become available (Teppo *et al.*, 1978). The body location does not fit areas of maximal solar exposure, and differs greatly from NMSC. In contrast to NMSC, malignant melanoma appears to have a predilection for middle-class, primarily indoor workers and their wives.

There is a general consensus among those who have studied the natural history of malignant melanoma that if there is a relationship to solar UV radiation exposure the mechanisms involved must be very different from those operating in NMSC, and that the cumulative effect of chronic repeated UV radiation exposure cannot be held responsible for malignant melanoma induction. The present lack of an animal model for malignant melanoma and the uncertainties regarding dose-response characteristics prevent the conversion of projections of change in UV radiation intensity to estimates of extra deaths.

Geographical Distribution and Incidence of Non-melanoma Skin Cancer

Incidence data for skin cancer, other than melanoma, must be treated with considerable reserve. Many cancer registries do not register non-melanoma skin cancer and those that do are uniformly incomplete since most of these tumours are treated in doctors' offices and either not reported at all or are reported without histological verification.

United States of America

The main sources for incidence data of skin cancer in the USA come from the National Cancer Survey performed in eight cities in 1947, a survey in Iowa performed in 1950 and in New York State (excluding New York City) in 1960 (Haenszel, 1963). The most extensive data are those of the Texas Tumor Registry obtained by MacDonald and Bubendorf (1964) covering the years 1944 to 1964, and the most recent are those of the Third National Cancer Survey (Scotto *et al.*, 1974, 1981). All these data show a marked increase in the incidence of skin cancer in the past three decades and a pronounced north–south gradient. The most recent USA data (Scotto *et al.*, 1981) show a 15-20 per cent increase in NMSC in the six-year period between 1972 and 1978, unaccompanied by any increase in measured UV radiation. However, this 3 per cent per year increase was limited to basal cell carcinoma; squamous cell carcinoma showed no significant increase (Fears and Scotto, 1982).

South America

The only reasonably accurate data are available from Brazil. Lopes de Faria *et al.* (1982) estimate for white Brazilians a NMSC incidence of 27.5 per 100,000 for males, and 24/100,000 for females. Skin cancer was the most common neoplasm in males, and second in rank for females. NMSC was more common in the north (nearest the equator) than in the south of Brazil.

Europe

The data available for incidence and prevalence of skin cancer in Europe are fragmentary and extremely difficult to interpret since surveys, such as they are, were performed by variously rigorous methods, and over at least three decades, during which the incidence of skin cancer has greatly increased. However, it is clear that just as in the USA and Australia, a marked north–south gradient exists (Doll *et al.*, 1966).

Africa

Information relating to skin cancer in Africa shows that the native Africans have extremely low rates of non-melanoma as well as melanoma skin cancer (Öettle, 1963; Davies *et al.*, 1968).

The incidence rates in the Johannesburg Bantus and in Uganda are of the same order (1-2 per 100,000 population) as for Soweto (South Africa) blacks. The exceptions are albino natives, who are extremely prone to the development of skin cancer. Öettle (1963) estimated a crude annual incidence rate of 579 per 100,000 population for male and 408 per 100,000 for female albino Bantus for squamous cell carcinomas of the skin. Only one basal cell carcinoma was found in this study.

India

Incidence data for skin cancer in India are not available. However, it is clear that the majority of skin cancers seen in hospitals occur in whites. Among native Indians special types of squamous cell carcinomas of the skin are found, which are presumably due to extreme heat, combustion and chronic friction (Mulay, 1963).

Japan and Taiwan

Skin cancer is uncommon in Japan and Taiwan. Squamous cell carcinomas are two to three times more common than basal cell cancers, and may arise at the site of premalignant skin changes such as burns, chronic trauma, or secondary to arsenic ingestion (Yeh, 1963; Miyaji, 1963).

Australia

Probably the best skin cancer surveys of recent years have been carried out in Australia, particularly in Queensland (Silverstone and Searle, 1970). The effect of latitude within Australia can be approximated. If the male incidence in Hobart is unity, in Brisbane it is four and in Townsville it is eight. These places correspond to south latitudes of about 43°, 28° and 19°, respectively. If one plots the global distribution of annual UV solar radiation as put forward by Schulze and Gräfe (1969) against incidence of skin cancer on a global basis, a case can be made that a doubling of incidence occurs for every 10° decrease in latitude. The Australian data would approximate to this, particularly in Queensland where the difference in incidence between Brisbane and Townsville is about two to one and the difference in latitude about 9°.

New Zealand

Not as much work has been done on skin cancers as in Australia; however, estimates of skin cancer incidence were reported by Eastcott (1963). These were for basal cell carcinoma 113 per 100,000 population, for squamous cell carcinoma 38 per 100,000, and for malignant melanoma 5.5 per 100,000. A comprehensive NMSC survey was performed between 1978 and 1980 by Freeman (1981), who found an annual skin cancer incidence even greater than that of Australia (basal cell carcinoma 316 per 100,000 population and for squamous cell carcinoma 165 per 100,000).

Malignant Melanoma

The two major findings that support the contention that NMSC is primarily caused by chronic exposure to solar UV radiation are the anatomical distribution of the cancers and their striking latitude gradient. However, the anatomical distribution of MM does not clearly parallel the presumed sites of maximum solar exposure. In the case of one type of malignant melanoma, Lentigo Malignant Melanoma (LMM), the characteristics of age distribution and histological evidence of solar connective tissue damage all seem, for practical purposes, to be identical to the features of squamous cell carcinoma of the skin. It must thus be assumed that solar UV radiation exposure is the primary cause of LMM (Larsen and Grude, 1979).

Cutchis (1978) was one of the first to point out that the geographic distribution of MM (Doll *et al.*, 1970) shows important anomalies if the assumption is made that exposure to solar UV radiation is the most significant factor in the causation of MM.

If solar UV radiation is the primary cause of MM then, as in NMSC, there should exist recognisable latitude gradients for the incidence and mortality of MM, with rates increasing toward the tropics. The existence of such latitude gradients has been reported from Norway (Magnus, 1973; 1975), Sweden (Magnus, 1977; Teppo *et al.*, 1975; Eklund and Malec, 1978), Finland (Teppo *et al.*, 1980), and the USA (Fears *et al.*, 1976; Cutler and Young, 1975).

There are, however, inconsistencies in a number of these studies which have recently been noticed. Of great importance have been the observations that major cities show a disproportionately high incidence of MM, which could not be explained on latitude alone, and that most Nordic countries show incidence rates for MM greater than can be expected based on their latitude (Crombie, 1979; Jensen and Bolander, 1980; Houghton *et al.*, 1980; Lee and Issenberg, 1972; Eklund and Malec, 1978; Viola and Houghton, 1978).

Most recently, Crombie (1979) examined data from a large series of tumour registries for Europe and concluded that the incidence of MM increased with increasing latitude in central Europe from Italy to Germany, the reverse of that found in England and Wales, the Nordic countries and the USA. He concluded that this latitude reversal may be due to darker pigmentation of southern Europeans' skin, but pointed out that the effect of change in susceptibility would have to be very large to overcome a latitude effect.

Lee (1977) was the first to point out a peculiar association in incidence of MM with certain, unexpected, occupational groups. He observed that the occupational groups that suffered the highest mortality from melanomas of the skin were clerical and professional workers and their wives. This initial finding has been confirmed by Viola and Houghton (1978) for Connecticut, by Holman *et al.* (1980) for Western Australia, and summarised by Lee and Strickland (1980).

The size and consistency of the relationship of MM risks to some factors associated with better education, high social status, or more money, and the presence of the relationship in both employed men and their wives suggests that the effect is real, and that the relationship is a biological one between MM incidence and some feature of life associated with improved education or economic status. A very recent report suggests that exposure to fluorescent lighting at work in offices may be the common denominator (Beral *et al.*, 1982).

The incidence of MM has been rising rapidly in white populations for many years. For example, in Norway a continuous rise in incidence of about 7 per cent per year has been observed since 1955 (Magnus, 1981). A major component of the causation of this rising incidence is a systematic increase in risk of successively later born cohorts (Holman *et al.*, 1980; Lee *et al.*, 1979; Elwood and Lee, 1975; Magnus, 1975; Eklund and Malec, 1978; Lee and Carter, 1970). The increase and cohort variations seem to be much greater for MM of trunk and lower limbs than for MM of the face and neck area (Magnus, 1981).

Age, Sex, Social Group

Non-melanoma Skin Cancer

The most recent age-specific incidence rates for NMSC have been published for eight areas of the United States by Scotto *et al.* (1981). It has long been known that whites have a much higher incidence of NMSC than pigmented races (Öettle, 1963). The higher incidence observed in sun-exposed areas of skin of whites and albinos is attributable to the chronic effects of UV radiation. Basal cell carcinoma in particular is very rare in pigmented races (Atkinson *et al.*, 1963; Mora and Burris, 1980; Matsuoka *et al.*, 1981; Higginson and Öettle, 1960).

In contrast to the anatomical distribution of squamous cell carcinoma in whites (70 per cent on head and neck), Isaacson *et al.* (1978) found only one-third of squamous cell carcinomas in urban blacks in South Africa to be on the head and neck. Furthermore, the male-female ratio was 60:40, as compared to 85:15 in whites. Basal cell carcinoma was almost absent.

In controlled studies, skin cancer patients as a group had greater frequencies of light eyes, complexion and hair colour than controls. They also sunburned more frequently and tanned less easily than controls, though the degree of tan achieved was only marginally less. Male cancer patients experienced greater cumulative outdoor exposure than male controls. The proportion of Irish and English (including Scots and Welsh) ancestry was greater in cancer patients, while that of Slavic and 'other' categories of national origin was smaller (Urbach *et al.*, 1972; O'Beirn *et al.*, 1968; Gellin *et al.*, 1965).

Patients with basal cell and squamous cell carcinoma differed with respect to age and sex distribution. In the case of basal cell carcinoma, the two sexes were almost equally represented; almost 15 per cent of the patients were less than 50 years of age, and nearly 65 per cent were less than 70 years old. In the squamous cell carcinoma group, on the other hand, males outnumbered females by more than 6 to 1, and all patients were at least 50 years of age, with more than 70 per cent of them being over 70 years.

Malignant Melanoma

In recent reports of several large series of cases of MM, certain observations occur uniformly. These are: a consistent, worldwide increase in MM, primarily in lesions involving the backs of men and the lower legs of women (Magnus, 1977; Holman *et al.*, 1980); a progressive decrease of age of onset (Lee *et al.*, 1979; Malec and Eklund, 1978), again worldwide and great differences in incidence and localisation of MM between white and non-white populations.

It also appears that in spite of significant increases of MM approximately doubling each decade, the site distribution does not change with latitude or geography at any one time (Lee, 1972; Lee and Merrill, 1971). Furthermore, differences in trends of incidence of age for various sites are marked. Thus, MM on the head and neck has a low incidence until about age 45, after which there is a progressive, steep increase in both males and females to advanced age. In contrast, MM affecting the trunk begins to rise in incidence earlier, at about age 30, is much more frequent in males than females, and declines in frequency after age 50 to 60 years. MM of the upper limbs is more frequent in females than in males, rises sharply about age 30 to level off at about age 50. The incidence of MM of the lower limbs rises rapidly in females from puberty to age 30, reaches a plateau at a high level and rises slightly higher in old age. In males, MM of the lower limbs rises very gradually with age, to reach an incidence about equal to that of females at age 70 (Magnus, 1981; Beardmore, 1972; Houghton *et al.*, 1980).

Among non-Caucasians, malignant melanoma is much less frequent than among white-skinned people. Scotto *et al.* (1975) reported an incidence in the USA of 4.47 per 100,000 population in whites, and 0.8 per 100,000 in blacks. Thus, the incidence in US blacks was about 18 per cent of that in whites, a relatively much higher proportion than that found for NMSC. In sharp contrast to the distribution in whites, non-Caucasians (and blacks in particular) have a very high incidence of malignant melanoma on the foot (whites, 10-15 per cent; blacks 60-75 per cent; Asians, 30-35 per cent). It has been suggested that this disproportionate incidence on the foot is due to a relative absence of nevus-cell nevi on the skin of non-Caucasians excepting palms and soles (Coleman *et al.*, 1980; Van Scott *et al.*, 1957; Kenney, 1982). Thus, if nevus-cell nevi sometimes are precursors or can be stimulated to develop MM, this maldistribution could in part account for this phenomenon.

There is now clear evidence that a real genetic element is among the factors responsible for the causation of malignant melanoma. Estimates that 6 to 11 per cent of malignant melanomas are of genetic origin have been made by various authors (Anderson *et al.*, 1967; Wallace and Exton, 1972; Clark *et al.*, 1978). Familial patients manifest a younger age distribution, an earlier average age at first diagnosis, increased frequency of multiple primary melanomas and a significantly higher survival rate (Clark *et al.*, 1978).

There is excellent, although circumstantial, evidence that NMSC is primarily due to repeated exposure of the skin to solar ultra-violet radiation. The situation is somewhat different where MM is concerned. The question is of great importance, since MM is a serious, often fatal cancer. Because of its seriousness, recording of cases of MM is usually very good, so that epidemiological studies that are quite reliable have been carried out in many countries in the past three decades. Very briefly, the following are the salient findings:

1.   There has been a consistent, worldwide increase in MM, incidence rates increasing 3 to 7 per cent annually, leading to a doubling

in 10 to 15 years.

2. There are striking differences in anatomical distribution by sex — MM is much more frequent on the backs of men and the lower legs of women.

3. In contrast to NMSC, only about 10 per cent of MM (a subtype that closely resembles squamous cell cancer in its biological behaviour) shows important evidence of chronic solar skin damage (McGovern, 1977).

4. While there are latitude gradients for MM within some countries, the normal gradient of increasing incidence from higher to lower latitudes is reversed in Central Europe.

5. From available data, it appears that the latent period for MM development is short, perhaps even 3 to 5 years.

6. In contrast to NMSC, which affects mainly those chronically exposed to sunlight, i.e., outdoor workers, MM is much more frequent in white-collar, educated, more affluent city dwellers (Lee, 1977).

7. As yet, no animal model for experimental production of MM exists using UV radiation.

It is obvious that, if UV radiation is causally related to the development of MM, the mechanisms are very different. The various theories that have been proposed for the aetiology of MM related to UV radiation are:

1. Intermittent, high dose exposure, presumably due to social changes (Fears *et al.*, 1976).

2. Production by UV radiation of a 'circulating factor' which causes distant effects on precursor lesions (Lee, 1977).

3. 'Initiation' of melanocytes, either by chemicals or UV radiation with either acting as a 'promoter'.

4. 'Promotion' of pre-existing, abnormal precursor cells or lesions by UV radiation with precursor lesions perhaps genetically determined (Houghton and Viola, 1981).

Implications for Prevention

Since the majority of NMSC is due to chronic exposure to solar UV radiation (Vitaliano and Urbach, 1980), the obvious most successful method for prevention of development of NMSC is avoidance of sunlight exposure. Since 40 to 80 per cent of erythema effective (and probably carcinogenic) UV radiation reaches the ground between 10 a.m. and 2 p.m., avoidance of outdoor exposure for two hours about noon would significantly decrease NMSC incidence (Scotto and Fears, 1977; Scotto *et al.*, 1975).

An alternative would be the liberal use of sunscreening agents which act as UV radiation filters if used properly. That clothing also protects against solar UV radiation was shown by Berne and Fisher (1980); with the exception of women's thin stockings, most clothing tested was as efficient as most chemical sunscreens. Finally, Kaidbey *et al.* (1979) showed that black epidermis also was an impressive sunscreening material. Thus the rarity of NMSC in pigmented races is also evidence that physical filters (sunscreens) should, if used constantly and properly, result in a significant reduction of the incidence of NMSC.

Summary and Conclusions

Repeated ultra-violet B (UVB) exposure, prolonged over many years, can result in chronic degenerative changes in the skin, characterised by skin 'ageing' and the development of premalignant and malignant skin lesions. The skin cancer of man can be broadly divided into two types: non-melanoma skin cancer (NMSC) and malignant melanoma (MM).

There is reason to believe that most NMSC, but not all, is causally related to chronic, repeated UVB exposure. In contrast, MM is a relatively uncommon tumour, primarily occurring in man. The sex ratio varies from 1:1 to 1:1.2 in favour of females. The anatomical distribution of MM does not follow the most UV radiation-exposed sites. While NMSC is extremely uncommon in pigmented races, MM occurs about one-fifth as frequently in such people as in those with white skin and is mostly found on the foot and lower leg. Ten to 15 per cent of MM are of the lentigo maligna type and most likely due to chronic UVB exposure. Another 6 to 11 per cent of MM appears to be of genetic origin, as evidenced by familial and multiple lesions and peculiar precursors found early in life (B-K mole). The remaining 75-80 per cent approximately of MM in white persons has interesting attributes: the incidence rises sharply from adolescence to early adult life (particularly on the legs of women), reaches a plateau through middle age, and rises again in old age. The male/female incidence shows a preponderance of young females and the sites of greatest incidence differ, being trunk in males and lower legs in females. Of interest is the observation that, although the various populations studied live in such disparate areas as Finland and Australia, and thus are exposed to hugely different amounts of solar UV radiation, the relative proportion of MM affecting various body sites has remained quite stable until recently.

Latitude gradients of incidence and mortality of MM exist within certain countries, but not in others. In contrast to NMSC, the populations most affected are not the outdoor workers, but rather the white-collar, more educated, more affluent people, and the demonstrable concentration of MM in large cities cancels out a latitude gradient in such places as Finland and Western Australia, where this has been investigated.

The lack of evidence for chronic solar damage of skin in which MM appears, the young age of a majority of patients, the variation in latitude gradients, the peculiar anatomical distribution not matching most exposed skin areas and the preponderance in city dwellers suggest very strongly a significant difference in pathogenesis of NMSC and MM, at least as far as solar UV radiation is concerned.

References

Anderson, D.E., Smith, L., Jr. and McBride, C.M. (1967). Hereditary aspects of malignant melanoma. *Journal of the American Medical Association*, 200: 741-6

Atkinson, L., Farago, C., Forbes, B.R.V. and ten Seldam, R.E.J. (1963). In: Urbach, F. (ed.), *The Biology of Cutaneous Cancer*, National Cancer Institute, Monograph No. 10, US Government Printing Office, Washington, DC, pp. 153-66

Beardmore, G.L. (1972). The epidemiology of malignant melanoma in Australia. In: *Melanoma and Skin Cancer*, New South Wales Government Printer, Sydney, pp. 39-64

Beral, V., Evans, S., Shaw, H. and Milton, G. (1982). Malignant melanoma and exposure to fluorescent lighting at work. *Lancet*, 2: 290-3

Berne, B. and Fischer, J. (1980). Protective effects of various types of clothes against ultraviolet radiation. *Acta Dermato-Venereologica*, 60: 459-60

Blum, H.F. (1959). *Carcinogenesis by Ultraviolet Light*. Princeton University Press, Princeton, New Jersey, ch. 17, pp. 285-305

Clark, W.H., Jr., Reiner, R.R., Greene, M., Ainsworth, A.M. and Mastrangelo, M.J. (1978). Origin of familial malignant melanoma from heritable melanocytic lesions. *Archives of Dermatology*, 114: 732-8

Coleman, W.P., Lorig, P.R., Teed, R.J. and Krementz, E.J. (1980). Acral lentiginous melanoma. *Archives of Dermatology*, 116: 773-6

Crombie, J.K. (1979). Racial differences in melanoma incidence. *British Journal of Cancer*, 40: 774-81

Cutchis, P. (1978). *On the Linkage of Solar Ultraviolet Radiation to Skin Cancer*. Institute for Defense Analysis, United States Department of Transportation, Washington, DC, pp. 105-6

Cutler, S.J. and Young, J.L. (1975). *Third National Cancer Survey: Incidence Data*. National Cancer Institute Monograph Number 41, Department of Health, Education and Welfare Publication Number (NIH) 75-787, US Government Printing Office, Washington, DC

Davies, J.N.P., Tauk, R., Meyer, R. and Thursten, P. (1968). Cancer of the integumentary tissues in Ugandan Africans. *Journal of the National Cancer Institute*, 41: 31-51

Doll, R., Payne, P. and Waterhouse, J. (1966). *Cancer Incidence in Five Continents*. Vol. I. International Union Against Cancer, Springer Verlag, Berlin, pp. 210-98

—— Muir, C. and Waterhouse, J. (1970). *Cancer Incidence in Five Continents*. Vol. II. International Union Against Cancer, Springer Verlag, Berlin

Eastcott, D.F. (1963). Epidemiology of skin cancer in New Zealand. In: Urbach, F. (ed.), *The Biology of Cutaneous Cancer*, National Cancer Institute Monograph Number 10, US Government Printing Office, Washington, DC, pp. 141-51

Eklund, G. and Malec, B. (1978). Sunlight and incidence of cutaneous malignant melanoma. *Scandinavian Journal of Plastic and Reconstructive Surgery*, 12: 231-41

Elwood, J.M. and Lee, J.A.H. (1975). Recent data on the epidemiology of malignant melanoma. *Seminars in Oncology*, 2: 149-54

Emmett, E.A. (1974). Ultraviolet radiation as a cause of skin tumors. *CRC Critical Reviews of Toxicology*, 2: 211-55

Fears, T.R., Scotto, J. and Schneiderman, M.A. (1976). Skin cancer, melanoma and sunlight. *American Journal of Public Health*, 66: 461-4

—— and Scotto, J. (1982). Personal communication

Freeman, N.R. (1981). Personal communication

Gellin, G.A., Kopf, A.W. and Andrade, R. (1965). Basal cell epitheliomas: A controlled study of associated factors. *Archives of Dermatology*, 91: 38-45

Haenszel, W. (1963). Variations in skin cancer incidence within the U.S. In: Urbach, F. (ed.), *The Biology of Cutaneous Cancer*, National Cancer Institute Monograph Number 10, US Government Printing Office, Washington, DC, pp. 225-43

Higginson, J. and Öettle, A.G. (1960). Cancer incidence in the Bantu and 'Cape colored' races of South Africa. *Journal of the National Cancer Institute*, 24: 589-671

Holman, C.D.J., Mulroney, C.D. and Armstrong, P.K., (1980). Epidemiology of preinvasive malignant melanoma in Australia. *International Journal of Cancer*, 25: 317-23

Houghton, A., Flannery, J. and Viola, M.V. (1980). Malignant melanoma in Connecticut and Denmark. *International Journal of Cancer*, 25: 95-104

—— and Viola, M.V. (1981). Solar radiation and malignant melanoma of the skin. *Journal of the American Academy of Dermatology*, 5: 477-83

Isaacson, C., Selzer, G., Kaye, V., Greenberg, M., Woodruff, J., Davies, J. *et al.* (1978). Cancer in urban blacks of South Africa. *South African Cancer Bulletin*, 22: 49-62

Jensen, O.M. and Bolander, A.M. (1980). Trends in malignant melanoma of the skin. *World Health Statistics Quarterly*, 33: 2-26

Kaidbey, K.H., Agin, P.P., Sayre, R.M. and Kligman, A.M. (1979). Photoprotection by melanin – a comparison of black and Caucasian skin. *Journal of the American Academy of Dermatology*, 1: 249-60

Kenny, J. (1982). Personal communication

Larsen, T. and Grude, T.J. (1979). A retrospective histological study of 669 cases of primary malignant melanoma in clinical stage I. VI. The relations of dermal solar elastosis to sex, age, and survival of the patient, and to localization, histological type and level of invasion of the tumor. *Acta Pathologica et Micro-biologica Scandinavica, Section A* 87: 361-6

Lee, J.A.H. (1972). Sunlight and the etiology of melanoma. In: *Melanoma and Skin Cancer*, New South Wales Government Printer, Sydney, pp. 83-94

——— (1977). Current evidence about the causes of malignant melanoma. In: Ariel, I.M. (ed.), *Progress in Clinical Cancer*, 6: 151-61, Grune and Stratton, New York, Vol. 6, pp. 151-61

——— and Carter, A.P. (1970). Secular trends in mortality from malignant melanoma. *Journal of the National Cancer Institute*, 45: 91-7

——— and Merrill, J.M. (1971). Sunlight and melanoma. *Lancet*, 1: 550-1

——— and Issenberg, H.J. (1972). A comparison between England and Wales and Sweden in the incidence and mortality of malignant skin tumours. *British Journal of Cancer*, 26: 59-66

——— Petersen, G.R., Stevens, R.G. and Vesanen, K. (1979). The influence of age, year of birth and date on mortality from malignant melanoma in the populations of England and Wales, Canada and the white populations of the U.S. *American Journal of Epidemiology*, 110: 734-9

——— and Strickland, D. (1980). Malignant melanoma: Social status and outdoor work. *British Journal of Cancer*, 41: 757-63

Lopes de Faria, J., Milani, J.P., Albino Filho, J. and Moreira Filho, D.J.C. (1982). Geographic pathology and epidemiology of cancer in Brazil. In: Grundmann, E. (ed.), *Cancer Campaign, Volume 6, Cancer Epidemiology*, Gustav Fischer Verlag, Stuttgart

MacDonald, E.J. and Bubendorf, E. (1964). Some epidemiologic aspects of skin cancer. In: *Tumors of the Skin*, Yearbook Medical Publisher, Chicago, pp. 23ff.

Magnus, K. (1973). Incidence of malignant melanoma of the skin in Norway 1955-1970. *Cancer*, 32: 1275-86

——— (1975). Epidemiology of malignant melanoma of the skin in Norway with special reference to the effect of solar radiation. In: *Biological Characterization of Human Tumors*, Excerpta Medica International Congress Series #375, Excerpta Medica, Amsterdam, pp. 249-59

——— (1977). Incidence of malignant melanoma of the skin in the five Nordic countries. *International Journal of Cancer*, 20: 477-85

——— (1981). Habits of sun exposure and risk of malignant melanoma. *Cancer*, 48: 2329-35

Malec, E. and Eklund, G. (1978). The changing incidence of malignant melanoma of the skin in Sweden 1959-1968. *Scandinavian Journal of Plastic and Reconstructive Surgery*, 12: 19-27

Matsuoka, L.Y., Schauer, P.K. and Sordillo, P.P. (1981). Basal cell carcinoma in black patients. *Journal of the American Academy of Dermatology*, 4: 670-2

McGovern, V.J. (1977). Epidemiologic aspects of melanoma: A review. *Pathology*, 9: 223-41

Miyaji, T. (1963). Skin cancer in Japan: A nationwide five year survey 1956-60. In: Urbach, F. (ed.), *The Biology of Cutaneous Cancer*, National Cancer Institute, Monograph No. 10, US Government Printing Office, Washington, DC, pp. 55-70

Mora, R.G. and Burris, R. (1980). Cancer of the skin in blacks. *Cancer*, 47: 1436-8

Mulay, D.M. (1963). Skin cancer in India. In: Urbach, F. (ed.), *The Biology of Cutaneous Cancer*, National Cancer Institute, Monograph No. 10, US Government Printing Office, Washington, DC, pp. 215-24

O'Beirn, S.F., Judge, P., Urbach, F., MacCon, C.F. and Martin, F. (1968). Skin cancer in County Galway, Ireland. In: *Sixth National Cancer Conference Proceedings*, Lippincott, Philadelphia, pp. 489-500

Oettle, A.C. (1963). Skin cancer in Africa. In: Urbach, F. (ed.), *The Biology of Cutaneous Cancer*, National Cancer Institute, Monograph Number 10, US Government Printing Office, Washington, DC, pp. 197-214

Schulze, R. and Gräfe, K. (1969). Consideration of sky ultraviolet radiation in the measurement of solar UVR. In: Urbach, F. (ed.), *The Biologic Effects of Ultraviolet Radiation*, Pergamon Press, Oxford, pp. 369-73

Scotto, J., Kopf, A.W. and Urbach, F. (1974). Nonmelanoma skin cancer in four areas of the U.S. *Cancer*, 34: 1333-8

———— Fears, T.R. and Gori, G.B. (1975). *Measurements of Ultraviolet Radiation in the U.S. and Comparison to Skin Cancer Data*. United States Department of Health, Education and Welfare Publication Number (NIH) 76-1092, Washington, DC, pp. 3.7-3.8

———— and Fears, T.R. (1977). Intensity patterns of solar ultraviolet radiation. *Environmental Research*, 14: 113-27

———— Fears, T.R. and Fraumeni, J.F., Jr. (1981). *Incidence of Nonmelanoma Skin Cancer in the United States*. Department of Health, Education and Welfare Publication No. (NIH) 82-2433, US Department of Health and Human Services, National Institute of Health, National Cancer Institute, Washington, DC, pp. 11-13

Silverstone, H. and Searle, J.H.A. (1970). The epidemiology of skin cancer in Queensland. *British Journal of Cancer*, 24: 235-53

Teppo, L., Hakema, M., Hakulinen, T., Lehtonen, J. and Saxen, E. (1975). Cancer in Finland. *Acta Pathologica et Microbiologica Scandinavica*, Section A, Suppl. 252, pp. 1-79

———— Pakkanen, M. and Hakulinen, T. (1978). Sunlight as a risk factor of malignant melanoma of the skin. *Cancer*, 41: 2018-27

———— Pukkala, E., Hakama, M., Hakulinen, T., Herva, A. and Saxen, E. (1980). Way of life and cancer incidence in Finland: A municipality based ecological analysis. *Scandinavian Journal of Social Medicine*, Suppl. 19, pp. 50-4

Urbach, F., Rose, D.B. and Bonnem, M. (1972). Genetic and environmental interactions in skin carcinogenesis. In: *Environment and Cancer*, Williams and Wilkins, Baltimore, pp. 355-71

———— Davies, R.E. and Berger, D. (1975). Estimation of the effect of ozone reduction in the stratosphere on the incidence of skin cancer in man. In: Grobecker, A. (ed.), *Impacts of Climatic Change on the Biosphere*, Climatic Impact Assessment Program Monograph Number 5, Part One, National Technical Information Service, Springfield, Virginia, pp. 7-42 to 7-60

Van Scott, E.J., Reinertson, R.P. and McCall, C.B. (1957). The growing prevalence, histologic type and significance of palmar and plantar nevi. *Cancer*, 1: 363-7

Viola, M.V. and Houghton, A. (1978). Melanoma in Connecticut. *Connecticut Medicine*, 42: 268-9

Vitaliano, P.P. and Urbach, F. (1980). The relative importance of risk factors in non-melanoma carcinoma. *Archives of Dermatology*, 116: 454-6

Wallace, D.C. and Exton, L.A. (1972). Genetic predisposition to development of malignant melanoma. In: McCarthy, W.H. (ed.), *Melanoma and Skin Cancer*, New South Wales Government Printer, Sydney, pp. 65-82

Yeh, S. (1963). Relative incidence of skin cancer in Chinese in Taiwan: with special reference to arsenical cancer. In: Urbach, F. (ed.), *The Biology of Cutaneous Cancer*, National Cancer Institute, Monograph No. 10, US Government Printing Office, Washington, DC, pp. 81-108

7 CANCER OF THE STOMACH

A. Oshima and I. Fujimoto

Introduction

Stomach cancer is still a major medical problem in Japan, where it occurs with the greatest frequency in the world, although its incidence and mortality have recently been declining in almost all countries. In order to understand and control this disease, a great number of clinical, pathological and epidemiological studies have been carried out, and many excellent reviews on the epidemiology of stomach cancer have been published (Wynder *et al.*, 1963; Bjelke, 1974; Haenszel and Correa, 1975; Piper, 1978; Pfeiffer, 1979).

Incidence and Mortality

Inter-country Variation

There is a marked inter-country variation in stomach cancer mortality, as shown in Figure 7.1 (Segi *et al.*, 1981). Japan, Chile, Cost Rica and Eastern Europe are high-risk areas, and the mortality rates in these areas are considerably higher than those in low-risk areas, such as the United States of America (USA) and Australia. Similar inter-country variation is also seen in stomach cancer incidence, although data are limited to those areas having population-based cancer registries (Waterhouse *et al.*, 1976).

Time Trends

Figure 7.2 shows the trends of age-standardised cancer incidence rates of selected sites in Osaka, Japan. Recently the incidence rate of stomach cancer has been declining in Osaka where this rate for both sexes is the highest in the world. This declining tendency of stomach cancer incidence has been observed over the past 40 years in the USA (Devesa and Silverman, 1978) and in Denmark (Clemmesen, 1977).

Segi *et al.* (1981) calculated age-standardised cancer mortality rates during the period from 1954/5 to 1974 in 23 countries of the world. They observed that stomach cancer mortality had decreased by 20 to 60 per cent during this period in all countries except Portugal.

Figure 7.1: Age-standardised Death Rates of Stomach Cancer by Country, 1975

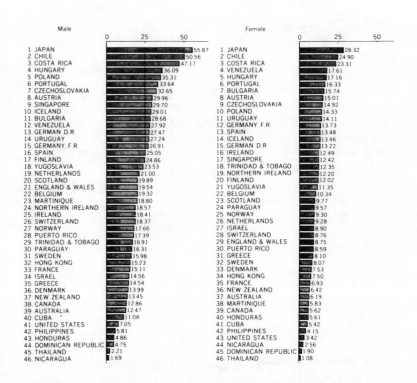

Male		Female	
1. JAPAN	55.87	1. JAPAN	28.32
2. CHILE	50.56	2. CHILE	24.90
3. COSTA RICA	47.17	3. COSTA RICA	23.31
4. HUNGARY	36.09	4. VENEZUELA	17.61
5. POLAND	35.31	5. HUNGARY	17.16
6. PORTUGAL	33.64	6. PORTUGAL	16.33
7. CZECHOSLOVAKIA	32.65	7. BULGARIA	15.74
8. AUSTRIA	29.96	8. AUSTRIA	15.01
9. SINGAPORE	29.70	9. CZECHOSLOVAKIA	14.92
10. ICELAND	29.01	10. POLAND	14.33
11. BULGARIA	28.68	11. URUGUAY	14.11
12. VENEZUELA	27.92	12. GERMANY, F.R.	13.73
13. GERMAN D.R.	27.47	13. SPAIN	13.48
14. URUGUAY	27.24	14. ICELAND	13.46
15. GERMANY, F.R.	26.91	15. GERMAN D.R.	13.22
16. SPAIN	25.05	16. IRELAND	12.49
17. FINLAND	24.86	17. SINGAPORE	12.42
18. YUGOSLAVIA	23.53	18. TRINIDAD & TOBAGO	12.35
19. NETHERLANDS	21.00	19. NORTHERN IRELAND	12.20
20. SCOTLAND	19.89	20. FINLAND	12.02
21. ENGLAND & WALES	19.54	21. YUGOSLAVIA	11.35
22. BELGIUM	19.32	22. BELGIUM	10.34
23. MARTINIQUE	18.80	23. SCOTLAND	9.77
24. NORTHERN IRELAND	18.57	24. PARAGUAY	9.57
25. IRELAND	18.41	25. NORWAY	9.30
26. SWITZERLAND	18.37	26. NETHERLANDS	9.28
27. NORWAY	17.66	27. ISRAEL	8.90
28. PUERTO RICO	17.39	28. SWITZERLAND	8.76
29. TRINIDAD & TOBAGO	16.91	29. ENGLAND & WALES	8.75
30. PARAGUAY	16.31	30. PUERTO RICO	8.59
31. SWEDEN	15.98	31. GREECE	8.10
32. HONG KONG	15.23	32. SWEDEN	8.07
33. FRANCE	15.11	33. DENMARK	7.53
34. ISRAEL	14.56	34. HONG KONG	7.50
35. GREECE	14.54	35. FRANCE	6.93
36. DENMARK	13.99	36. NEW ZEALAND	6.42
37. NEW ZEALAND	13.45	37. AUSTRALIA	6.19
38. CANADA	12.86	38. MARTINIQUE	5.83
39. AUSTRALIA	12.47	39. CANADA	5.62
40. CUBA	11.08	40. HONDURAS	5.61
41. UNITED STATES	7.05	41. CUBA	5.42
42. PHILIPPINES	5.81	42. PHILIPPINES	4.15
43. HONDURAS	4.86	43. UNITED STATES	3.42
44. DOMINICAN REPUBLIC	4.75	44. NICARAGUA	2.56
45. THAILAND	2.21	45. DOMINICAN REPUBLIC	1.90
46. NICARAGUA	1.69	46. THAILAND	1.08

Note: Rates per 100,000 population. Standard population: UICC's world population.

Source: Segi, M. *et al.* (1981) (By kind permission of the publisher: Japanese Scientific Societies Press).

Age and Sex

In general, the overall male: female mortality ratio of stomach cancer is roughly 2.0 to 1.5 (Figure 7.1) and is rather stable in most countries. The sex- and age-specific incidence rates of stomach cancer in Osaka, Japan, are shown in Figure 7.3 where it will be seen that the incidence rate increases with age in both sexes. However, in a log-log scale the

Figure 7.2: Time Trends of Age-standardised Cancer Incidence Rates of Selected Sites in Osaka, Japan, 1963-1977

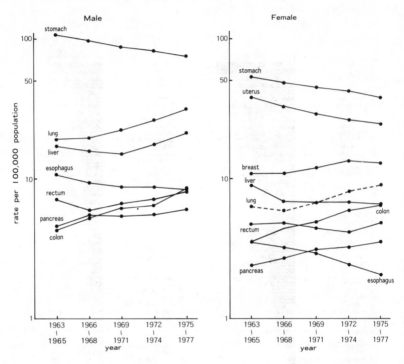

Source: Osaka Cancer Registry

incidence rate curve becomes approximately linear as in the case of most epithelial carcinomas (Peto, 1977). The male:female ratio is less than 1.0 under 40 years of age and exceeds 2.0 in the age range 50-84 years.

Migrant Studies

The inter-country variation and time trends of stomach cancer mortality and incidence suggest that environmental factors play a more important role in the aetiology of stomach cancer than genetic factors. Studies of Japanese migrants in the USA (Buell and Dunn, 1965; Haenszel and Kurihara, 1968) have shown that the stomach cancer mortality rate among Japanese migrants 'Issei' (i.e. first generation born in Japan) was almost as high as that among Japanese in Japan, and that the rate among Japanese migrants 'Nisei' (i.e. second generation born in the

USA) reduced towards the lower rate among Caucasians in the USA. These findings suggest that dietary experience in early life is critical in determining the level of risk. Similar findings were observed among migrants in Australia from high-risk countries (Staszewski *et al.*, 1971; McMichael *et al.*, 1980) and among migrants to a low-risk area from a high-risk area within Columbia (Correa *et al.*, 1970).

Figure 7.3: Sex- and Age-specific Incidence Rates of Stomach Cancer in Osaka, Japan, 1973-1977

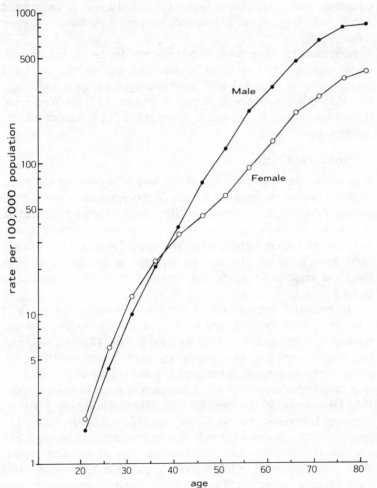

Source: Osaka Cancer Registry.

Aetiological Considerations

Descriptive Epidemiology

Geographical variation, time trends and migrant studies of stomach cancer all suggest that dietary factors are important in its development. It is plausible to consider that dietary factors are aetiologically associated with stomach cancer because gastric mucosa is directly exposed to ingested foods. Haenszel and Correa (1975) outlined the following three general categories of diet effect: (1) presence of a carcinogen or carcinogens in foods; (2) introduction of carcinogens during food preparation; (3) absence of protective factors in some foods.

Hirayama (1977) reported that the recent decrease in the stomach cancer mortality rate in Japan is associated with an increase in the consumption of milk and milk products, eggs, oil, meat and fruits, and that this cancer has decreased in parallel with the Westernisation of the dietary intake and with the wider distribution of electric refrigerators.

Analytic Epidemiology

A great number of case-control studies have been conducted in many countries in order to elucidate dietary factors associated with stomach cancer. Table 7.1 is a summary of the results of some such studies. In general, it can be said that stomach cancer is associated with a food pattern high in carbohydrates and salted foods, and low in fresh fruits and vegetables. This latter association of low intake of fresh fruits and vegetables suggests that vitamin C may act as a protective factor.

The estimated relative risk of the 'risk-heightening foods' (Table 7.1) are at most two-fold, and no specific risk factors like cigarette smoking in lung cancer have been detected to date. There are methodological difficulties in researching dietary histories retrospectively, and problems remain concerning the reliability and validity of the results.

A large-scale prospective study has been in progress in Japan since 1965 (Hirayama, 1975), when about 265,000 people aged 40 years and over were interviewed and they have been followed up since then. The interview form contained not only data on smoking and drinking habits but also on dietary history (e.g. the frequency of ingestion of rice, meat, fish, milk, green-yellow vegetables, pickles and miso-soup). This study suggests that milk and green-yellow vegetables may be protective factors against stomach cancer.

Table 7.1: Dietary Factors and Stomach Cancer — Summary of Results of Recent Case-control Studies

Author (year of publication)	Place of study	Risk-heightening foods	Risk-lowering foods
Wynder *et al.* (1963)	Iceland, Japan, Slovenia, USA	None identified	None identified
Hirayama and Yusa (1963)	Japan	Salted foods	Milk
Acheson and Doll (1964)	England	None identified	None identified
Higginson (1966)	USA	Fried foods	None identified
Graham *et al.* (1967, 1972)	USA	Potatoes	Raw vegetables
Haenszel *et al.* (1972)	Hawaii (Japanese migrants)	Pickled vegetables, salted/dried foods	Western vegetables (lettuce, celery)
Haenszel *et al.* (1976a)	Japan	None identified	Western vegetables
Bjelke (1974)	USA (Norwegian migrants), Norway	Cooked cereals, soup, salted fish	Vegetables, fruits (Vit. C)
Modan (1974)	Israel	Carbohydrates	None identified
Kurita (1974)	Japan	Rice, salted foods, hot foods	None identified

Some Important Findings from Recent Histological and Experimental Studies

Laurén (1965) proposed a classification of stomach cancer into two main histological types: the intestinal and diffuse. Muñoz *et al.* (1968) reported that the intestinal type is dominant in high-risk areas of stomach cancer. Moreover, it was shown from hospital-based data that the proportion of the intestinal type in all stomach cancer has been decreasing in Norway (Muñoz *et al.*, 1968) and in the USA (Muñoz and Asvall, 1971). Similar findings were also observed in Japan both from hospital-based (Nagayo and Yokoyama, 1978; Kato *et al.*, 1981) and from population-based data (Hanai *et al.*, 1982). Correa *et al.* (1973) estimated the age-specific incidence rate of stomach cancer by histological type among Japanese in Hawaii and in Japan. They showed that the incidence rate curve of the diffuse type has a more gradual slope than that of the intestinal type, i.e. that the rate for the diffuse type increases more slowly with age. These findings suggest that the two types of stomach cancer are different aetiologically as well as histologically.

Precursor Lesions

It was shown by histo-pathological examination of stomach cancer at a very early stage in Japan that intestinal metaplasia co-exists frequently with stomach cancer, especially with the intestinal type (Nakamura *et al.*, 1968; Nagayo, 1975). Examination of autopsy material showed that the frequency of chronic gastritis is higher in Japanese who have a high risk of stomach cancer than in Caucasians in the USA who have a low risk (Imai *et al.*, 1971). Similar findings were also observed in a high- and low-risk area within one country (Correa *et al.*, 1970).

These findings suggest that atrophic gastritis and/or intestinal meta-plasia may be a precursor to stomach cancer. This was also suggested by Siurala *et al.* (1974) who followed atrophic gastritis patients for over 20 years. They observed that the incidence rate of stomach cancer among atrophic gastritis patients was much higher than that among subjects with normal mucosa and with superficial gastritis (Ihamäki *et al.*, 1978).

If intestinal metaplasia is in fact a precursor, then the epidemiology of this condition can be used to study stomach cancer epidemiology. Haenszel *et al.* (1976b) conducted a case-control study of atrophic gastritis and/or intestinal metaplasia and observed a negative association of a Western-type diet which included fresh green vegetables (e.g. lettuce) with these conditions.

Besides atrophic gastritis and/or intestinal metaplasia, pernicious anaemia, gastric surgical stumps and certain type of gastric polyp are regarded as precursor lesions of stomach cancer (Morson *et al.*, 1980). However, they seem to play only a minor role in the aetiology of stomach cancer as a whole. The positive association between benign gastric ulcer and cancer, which was often suspected histo-pathologically, has recently been denied clinically and epidemiologically (Hirohata, 1968; Oshima *et al.*, 1978).

Animal Models and Mutagenicity Tests

Sugimura and Fujimura (1967) devised a very successful model for the development of gastric cancer. They found that stomach cancer could be induced easily in rats, hamsters and dogs by administering N-methyl-N'-nitro-N-nitrosoguanidine and related chemicals. By using this animal model, many studies have been conducted to elucidate the carcinogenic process and to examine factors influencing carcinogenesis (Sugimura and Kawachi, 1979).

On the other hand, the Ames test has enabled easy measurement of the mutagenicity level of foods, which parallels the carcinogenicity level (Ames *et al.*, 1973). Using this test, Sugimura *et al.* (1977) detected very potent mutagens-carcinogens in broiled foods including pyrolysed substances of some aminoacids.

By adding to the epidemiology the techniques and findings of the recent laboratory studies, the aetiology of stomach cancer will be further elucidated in the near future. Based on epidemiological studies in Columbia (Cuello *et al.*, 1976) and laboratory studies, Tannenbaum *et al.* (1977) have recently proposed a hypothesis for the development of stomach cancer, in which chronic gastritis leads to colonisation of the stomach by both oral and intestinal micro-organisms due to high pH. These organisms reduce nitrate to nitrite. By the reaction of the nitrite with appropriate nitrogen compounds, N-nitroso compounds are formed, which are potential carcinogens for the stomach. This hypothesis, if correct, could provide a clue for the prevention of stomach cancer by modification of the environment.

Early Detection and Screening

Advances in Diagnostic Techniques

In Japan three remarkable advances have been made in diagnostic techniques for stomach cancer: the development of double contrast radiology (Murakami, 1971a), X-ray television (Matsuda, 1967) and endoscopy (Murakami, 1971b). By wide application of these advanced diagnostic techniques, many cases of early gastric cancer have been detected in Japan. According to the population-based Osaka Cancer Registry, 62.8 per cent of all stomach cancer cases diagnosed in 1978 underwent surgery, and the percentage of early gastric cancer in all surgical cases was as high as 16.9. Early gastric cancer is defined as that in which the infiltration of cancer cells is limited to the mucosal or submucosal layer. The five-year survival rate of early gastric cancer cases, when resected surgically, is over 90 per cent (Murakami, 1971c).

Early gastric cancer is not a peculiar type of cancer which can be diagnosed only in Japan, it can be diagnosed everywhere in the world by means of the above-mentioned techniques. Recently the number of early gastric cancer cases detected has increased in countries other than Japan, for example in Britain (Evans *et al.*, 1978; Fielding *et al.*, 1980), Sweden (Öhman *et al.*, 1980) and in the USA (Green *et al.*, 1981), in parallel with the application of double contrast radio-logical techniques, fibreoptic endoscopy and endoscopic biopsy.

Mass Screening Programmes for Stomach Cancer in Japan

In Japan, mass screening programmes with the use of photofluoro-graphy are being widely used to detect stomach cancer in the early stages. Most of the screening tests are carried out by staff in specially equipped mobile units. According to the Japanese Society of Gastric Mass Survey, about 3.6 million people were screened in 1978, and 3,676 stomach cancer cases were detected. About one-third of the cancer cases detected by the screening were early gastric cancer cases (Table 7.2).

Table 7.2: Results of Mass Screening Programmes for Stomach Cancer in Japan, 1978

	No.	%
Total screened	3,640,123	100.0
Further examinations recommended	516,817	14.2
Further examinations performed	391,849	10.8
Stomach cancer cases detected		
Early cancer cases	1,103	0.03
Advanced cancer cases	2,573	0.07
Total	3,676	0.10

Source: Japanese Society of Gastric Mass Survey.

Various indicators of the effectiveness of the mass screening pro-grammes are shown in Table 7.3. Stomach cancer cases detected by screening have a relative five-year survival rate of over 60 per cent, much higher than that of cancer cases diagnosed under usual medical care which is about 20 per cent as described later (Table 7.4). In this comparison, however, lead time bias and length bias should be taken into consideration (Cole and Morrison, 1980).

In Japan, the mortality rate from stomach cancer has been gradually decreasing since around 1960. This secular trend, however, cannot be a direct reflection of either the recent advances in diagnostic techniques or of the efforts in mass screening only. According to the Osaka Cancer Registry, the mortality rate has been declining in parallel with the incidence rate (Oshima *et al.*, 1979). Therefore, the decline in the

Table 7.3: Indicators of Effectiveness of Mass Screening Programmes for Stomach Cancer

---

Survival rates of stomach cancer

Cases detected by screening *vs.* cases diagnosed under usual medical care

Mortality rates from stomach cancer in the target population

Secular trend: before *vs.* after the introduction of the screening

Geographical comparisons

Screened *vs.* unscreened sectors of the population

Randomised controlled trial

---

mortality rate should be considered to be mainly due to such factors as changes in dietary habits.

There are some data showing that stomach cancer deaths have been decreasing more rapidly in areas with intensive screening programmes than in other areas (Ichikawa, 1978). There is, however, still some uncertainty because the areas may be different in many social and environmental characteristics.

Oshima *et al.* (1979) followed up for approximately six years about 18,000 persons aged 40-59 years who had been screened and they observed a decrease of about 25 per cent in stomach cancer deaths among them, as compared with the expected deaths calculated on the basis of sex- and age-specific rates among the general population. It must be said, however, that there was some bias in the selection of those screened.

The indicators in Table 7.3 can, as described above, give only circumstantial evidence of the effectiveness of the screening, without a randomised controlled trial. The time has passed, however, when it is possible to conduct a randomised controlled trial of screening for stomach cancer in Japan.

Tsukuma *et al.* (1983) studied the natural history of early gastric cancer without a randomised controlled trial. They followed up those patients who had been diagnosed endoscopically as early gastric cancer cases and who had had histological evidence of cancer by biopsy, but on whom surgical resection had been delayed for over six months or had not been conducted because of complications or refusal of surgical resection by the patients. The survivorship function for the duration of early gastric cancer and the survival rate curve of early gastric cancer patients on whom surgical resection had not been conducted were observed. It was estimated that half of early gastric cancer cases, if left alone, will progress to advanced cancer in 37 months and will die of stomach cancer in 77 months from the time of the endoscopic diagnosis. These findings confirm the impression of the natural history upon which early detection and screening are based.

In Japan much effort is now being made to extend the screening programmes to ensure wide coverage of persons at risk. In low-risk countries, however, careful prior consideration (including a cost-benefit analysis) should be given to the introduction of a screening programme.

Prognosis

The five-year relative survival rates for three categories of stomach cancer patients in Osaka are seen in Table 7.4. The survival rates are closely related to the proportion of early gastric cancer cases. Table 7.5 shows the comparison of five-year survival rates for stomach cancer patients from four population-based cancer registries. The better prognosis in Osaka probably reflects the wide distribution of diagnostic techniques for early detection.

Summary and Conclusions

Although stomach cancer has recently been decreasing in almost all countries in the world, it is still one of the most important medical problems in many countries. We have as yet no specific primary preventive measures against stomach cancer. It is, however, clear that risk factors exist in foods. Recent advances in laboratory studies have provided many important clues in elucidating dietary risk factors and the pathogenesis of human stomach cancer.

On the other hand, remarkable advances have been made in diagnostic techniques. By applying these advanced techniques, many cases of early gastric cancer have been detected not only in Japan but also in many other countries of the world. We have now evidence that the secondary preventive measures, by early detection and screening, will lead to an even more rapid reduction in the stomach cancer mortality rate.

Table 7.4: Five-year Relative Survival Rate of Stomach Cancer Patients in Osaka, Japan

Category of cases	No. of cases	5-year relative survival rate (%)	Proportion of early gastric cancer (%)
All incident cases (1970-1972)	12,267	18.7	10.6[a]
Cases detected by screening, Center for Adult Diseases, Osaka (1961-1979)	841	66.2	38.0
Cases diagnosed at the out-patient department of Center for Adult Diseases, Osaka (1970-1972)	905	49.3	33.4[b]

Notes: a. Estimate from the survey in 1978.
 b. Estimate from the data of cases diagnosed in 1976.
Source: Osaka Cancer Registry.

Table 7.5: Comparison of Five-year Relative Survival Rates for Stomach Cancer among Four Registries

Cancer registry (year)	5-year relative survival rate (%)	
	Male	Female
Osaka, Japan (1970-1974)[a]	20.9	16.7
United States (1970-1973)[b]	12.0	14.0
England and Wales (1971-1973)[c]	7.4	7.3
Norway (1972-1975)[d]	14.0	14.0

Source: a. Osaka Cancer Registry.
 b. Myer, M.H. and Hankey, B.F.: *Cancer Patients Survival Experience*. US DHHS, Washington, 1980.
 c. OPCS: *Cancer Statistics, Survival, 1971-73 Registrations*. HMSO, London, 1980.
 d. Cancer Registry of Norway: *Survival of Cancer Patients, Cases Diagnosed in Norway 1968-1975*. The Norwegian Cancer Registry, Oslo, 1980.

References

Acheson, E.D. and Doll, R. (1964). Dietary factors in carcinoma of the stomach: a study of 100 cases and 200 controls. *Gut*, 5: 126-31

Ames, B.N., Durston, E., Yamasaki, E. and Lee, F.D. (1973). Carcinogens are mutagens: a simple test system for combining liver homogenates for activation and bacteria for detection. *Proceedings of the National Academy of Science*, 70: 2281-5

Bjelke, E. (1974). Epidemiologic studies of cancer of the stomach, colon, and rectum: with special emphasis on the role of diet. *Scandinavian Journal of Gastroenterology*, 9 (Suppl. 31): 1-253

Buell, P. and Dunn, J.E. (1965). Cancer mortality among Japanese Issei and Nisei of California. *Cancer*, 18: 656-64

Clemmesen, J. (1977). Gastric carcinoma decreasing in incidence? *Acta Pathologica et Microbiologica Scandinavica*, Suppl. 261: 65-75

Cole, P. and Morrison, A. (1980). Basic issues in population screening for cancer. *Journal of the National Cancer Institute*, 64: 1263-72

Correa, P., Cuello, C. and Duque, E. (1970). Carcinoma and intestinal metaplasia of the stomach in Columbian migrants. *Journal of the National Cancer Institute*, 44: 297-306

——— Sasano, N., Stemmerman, G.N. and Haenszel, W. (1973). Pathology of gastric carcinoma in Japanese population: comparisons between Miyagi prefecture, Japan and Hawaii. *Journal of the National Cancer Institute*, 51: 1449-59

Cuello, C., Correa, P., Haenszel, W., Gordillo, G., Brown, C., Archer, M. *et al.* (1976). Gastric cancer in Columbia, I. Cancer risk and suspect environmental agents. *Journal of the National Cancer Institute*, 57: 1015-21

Devesa, S.S. and Silverman, D.T. (1978). Cancer incidence and mortality trends in the United States: 1935-74. *Journal of the National Cancer Institute*, 60: 545-71

Evans, D.M.D., Craven, J.C., Murphy, F. and Cleary, B.K. (1978). Comparison of early gastric cancer in Britain and Japan. *Gut*, 19: 1-9

Fielding, J.W.L., Ellis, D.J., Jones, B.G., Power, D.J., Waterhouse, J.A.H. and Brookes, V.S. (1980). Natural history of 'early' gastric cancer: results of a 10-year regional survey. *British Medical Journal*, 281: 965-7

Graham, S., Lilienfeld, A.M. and Tidings, J.E. (1967). Dietary and purgation factors in the epidemiology of gastric cancer. *Cancer*, 20: 2224-34

——— Schotz, W. and Martino, P. (1972). Alimentary factors in the epidemiology of gastric cancer. *Cancer*, 30: 927-38

Green, P.H.R., O'Toole, K.M., Weinberg, L.M. and Goldfarb, J.P. (1981). Early gastric cancer. *Gastroenterology*, 81: 247-56

Haenszel, W. and Kurihara, M. (1968). Mortality from cancer and other diseases among Japanese in the United States. *Journal of the National Cancer Institute*, 40: 43-68

——— Kurihara, M., Segi, M. and Lee, R.K.C. (1972). Stomach cancer among Japanese in Hawaii. *Journal of the National Cancer Institute*, 49: 969-88

——— and Correa, P. (1975). Developments in the epidemiology of stomach cancer over the past decade. *Cancer Research*, 35: 3452-9

——— Kurihara, M., Locke, F.B., Shimizu, K. and Segi, M. (1976a). Stomach cancer in Japan. *Journal of the National Cancer Institute*, 56: 265-78

——— Correa, P., Cuello, C., Guzman, N., Burbano, L.C., Lores, H. *et al.* (1976b). Gastric cancer in Columbia, II. Case-control epidemiologic study of precursor lesions. *Journal of the National Cancer Institute*, 57: 1021-6

Hanai, A., Fujimoto, I. and Taniguchi, H. (1982). Trends of stomach cancer incidence and histologic types in Osaka. In: Magnus, K. (ed.), *Trends in Cancer Incidence*, Hemisphere Publishing Corporation, Washington, Part 3, p. 143

Higginson, J. (1966). Etiologic factors in gastro-intestinal cancer in man. *Journal of the National Cancer Institute*, 37: 527-45

Hirayama, T. (1975). Prospective studies on cancer epidemiology based on census population in Japan. In: Bucalossi, P., Veronesi, U. and Caseinelli, N. (eds.), *Proceedings of XI International Cancer Congress Florence 1974 Volume 3*, Excerpta Medica, Amsterdam, p. 27

—— (1977). Changing patterns of cancer in Japan with special reference to the decrease of stomach cancer mortality. In: Hiatt, H.H., Watson, J.D. and Winsten, J.A. (eds.), *Origins of Human Cancer*, Cold Spring Harbor Laboratory, New York, Section 2, p. 55

—— and Yusa, Y. (1963). The epidemiology of cancer of the stomach in Japan with special reference to the role of diet. *Kosei no Shihyo*, 10: 10-15 (in Japanese)

Hirohata, T. (1968). Mortality from gastric cancer and other causes after medical or surgical treatment for gastric ulcer. *Journal of the National Cancer Institute*, 41: 895-908

Ichikawa, H. (1978). Mass screening for stomach cancer in Japan. In: Miller, A.B. (ed.), *Screening in Cancer, UICC Technical Report Series*, Volume 40, International Union Against Cancer, Geneva, p. 279

Ihamäki, T., Saukkonen, M. and Siurala, M. (1978). Long term observation of subjects with normal mucosa and with superficial gastritis: results of 23-27 years' follow-up examinations. *Scandinavian Journal of Gastroenterology*, 13: 771-5

Imai, T., Kubo, T. and Watanabe, H. (1971). Chronic gastritis in Japanese with reference to high incidence of gastric carcinoma. *Journal of the National Cancer Institute*, 47: 179-95

Kato, Y., Kitagawa, T., Nakamura, K. and Sugano, H. (1981). Changes in the histologic types of gastric carcinoma in Japan. *Cancer*, 48: 2084-7

Kurita, H. (1974). Clinico-epidemiological study of stomach cancer considering sex and age differences. *Japanese Journal of Cancer Clinics*, 20: 580-93 (in Japanese)

Laurén, P. (1965). The two histological main types of gastric carcinoma: diffuse and so-called intestinal type carcinoma. *Acta Pathologica et Microbiologica Scandinavica*, 64: 31-49

Matsuda, H., Takai, G., Inui, Y. and Ninomiya, K. (1967). Studies on application of remote control X-ray television for examination of the stomach and duodenum. *American Journal of Roentgenology, Radium Therapy and Nuclear Medicine*, 100: 711-16

McMichael, A.J., McCall, M.G., Hartshorne, J.M. and Woodings, T.L. (1980). Pattern of gastro-intestinal cancer in European migrants to Australia. The role of dietary change. *International Journal of Cancer*, 25: 431-7

Modan, B. (1974). The role of starches in the etiology of gastric cancer. *Cancer*, 34: 2087-92

Morson, B.C., Sobin, L.H., Grundman, E., Johansen, A., Nagayo, T. and Serck-Hanssen, A. (1980). Precancerous condition and epithelial dysplasia in the stomach. *Journal of Clinical Pathology*, 33: 711-21

Muñoz, N., Correa, P., Cuello, C. and Duque, E. (1968). Histological types of gastric carcinoma in high- and low-risk areas. *International Journal of Cancer*, 3: 809-18

—— and Asvall, J. (1971). Time trends of intestinal and diffuse types of gastric cancer in the United States. *International Journal of Cancer*, 8: 158-64

Murakami, T. (ed.) (1971a). *Early Gastric Cancer. GANN Monograph on Cancer Research No. 11*, University of Tokyo Press, Tokyo, ch. 3, p. 93
────── (ed.) (1971b). Ibid., ch. 4, p. 145
────── (ed.) (1971c). Ibid., ch. 1, p. 45.
Nagayo, T. (1975). Microscopical cancer of the stomach – a study on histogenesis of gastric carcinoma. *International Journal of Cancer*, 16: 52-60
────── and Yokoyama, H. (1978). Recent changes in the morphology of gastric cancer in Japan. *International Journal of Cancer*, 21: 407-12
Nakamura, K., Sugano, H. and Takagi, K. (1968). Carcinoma of the stomach in incipient phase. Its histogenesis and histological appearances. *Gann*, 59: 251-8
Öhman, U., Emäs, S. and Rubio, C. (1980). Relation between early and advanced gastric cancer. *American Journal of Surgery*, 140: 351-5
Oshima, A., Kawasaki, T., Sakagami, F., Hanai, A., Fujimoto, I., Hashimoto, T. *et al.* (1978). High-risk group of stomach cancer and screening. *Igan to Shudankenshin*, No. 40: 27-34 (in Japanese)
────── Hanai, A. and Fujimoto, I. (1979). Evaluation of a mass screening program for stomach cancer. *National Cancer Institute Monograph*, 53: 181-6
Peto, R. (1977). Epidemiology, multi-stage models, and short-term mutagenecity tests. In: Hiatt, H.H., Watson, J.D. and Winsten, J.A. (eds.), *Origins of Human Cancer*, Cold Spring Harbor Laboratory, New York, Section 15, p. 1403
Pfeiffer, C.J. (ed.) (1979). *Gastric Cancer. Etiology and Pathogenesis*, Gerhard Witzstrock Publishing House, New York, Part I, p. 13
Piper, D.W. (ed.) (1978). *Stomach Cancer. UICC Technical Report Series*, Volume 34, International Union Against Cancer, Geneva, ch. 2, p. 5
Segi, M., Aoki, K. and Kurihara, M. (1981). World cancer mortality. In: Segi, M., Tominaga, S., Aoki, K. and Fujimoto, I. (eds.), *Cancer Mortality and Morbidity Statistics, Japan and the World. GANN Monograph on Cancer Research No. 26.*, Japan Scientific Societies Press, Tokyo, ch. 3, p. 121
Siurala, M., Lehtola, J. and Ihamäki, T. (1974). Atrophic gastritis and its sequelae. Results of 19-23 years' follow-up examinations. *Scandinavian Journal of Gastroenterology*, 9: 441-6
Staszewski, J., McCall, M.G. and Stenhouse, N.S. (1971). Cancer mortality in 1962-66 among Polish migrants to Australia. *British Journal of Cancer*, 25: 599-610
Sugimura, T. and Fujimura, S. (1967). Tumor production in glandular stomach of rat by N-methyl-N'-nitroso-N-nitrosoguanidine. *Nature*, 216: 943-4
────── Nagao, M., Kawachi, T., Honda, M., Yahagi, T., Seino, Y. *et al.* (1977). Mutagen-carcinogens in food, with special reference to highly· mutagenic pyrolytic products in broiled foods. In: Hiatt, H.H., Watson, J.D. and Winsten, J.A. (eds.), *Origins of Human Cancer*, Cold Spring Harbor Laboratory, New York, Section 17, p. 1561
────── and Kawachi, T. (1979). Experimental induction of gastric cancer. In: Pfeiffer, C.J. (ed.), *Gastric Cancer Etiology and Pathogenesis*, Gerhard Witzstrock Publishing House, New York, Part III, p. 231
Tannenbaum, S.R., Archer, M.C., Wishnok, J.S., Correa, P., Cuello, C. and Haenszel, W. (1977). Nitrate and the etiology of gastric cancer. In: Hiatt, H.H., Watson, J.D. and Winsten, J.A. (eds.), *Origins of Human Cancer*, Cold Spring Harbor Laboratory, New York, Section 17, p. 1609
Tsukuma, H., Mishima, T. and Oshima, A. (1983). Prospective study of 'early' gastric cancer. *International Journal of Cancer*, 31: 421-6
Waterhouse, J., Muir, C., Correa, P. and Powell, J. (eds.) (1976). *Cancer Incidence in Five Continents*, Volume III, IARC Scientific Publications No. 15, IARC, Lyon, ch. 9, p. 453
Wynder, E.L., Kmet, J., Dungal, N. and Segi, M. (1963). An epidemiological investigation of gastric cancer. *Cancer*, 16: 1461-96

8 CANCER OF THE PANCREAS

K. Mabuchi

Introduction

Cancer of the pancreas is a highly fatal disease, and only 50 per cent of patients with the disease survive two or more years after the diagnosis is made (Levin *et al.*, 1981). Although it is still relatively uncommon, an increasing trend in mortality and incidence as reported from various countries is alarming (Levin *et al.*, 1981; Aoki and Ogawa, 1978). Therefore, cancer of the pancreas presents a significant medical and public health problem, but very few efficient preventive or control measures are currently available.

Pathology

A vast majority (from 70 to 90 per cent) of carcinomas of the pancreas are adenocarcinomas arising in the exocrine component of the pancreas. These mainly originate from the ductal epithelial cells while a small proportion is believed to be of acinar cell origin (Macdonald *et al.*, 1982). Islet cell tumours and other less frequent types of tumour usually have a more favourable prognosis than adenocarcinomas, but this review focuses on adenocarcinoma. Although histological distinction is not always clear in the epidemiological literature, cancer of the pancreas may be considered equivalent to adenocarcinoma for this discussion because of the preponderance of the latter tumours. However, it must be remembered that clinical and epidemiological features do differ among different histological types of pancreatic neoplasm.

At the time of diagnosis, pancreatic cancer is most frequently found in the head of the pancreas (50-70 per cent), and less frequently in the body (10-40 per cent) and the tail (4-10 per cent) (Macdonald *et al.*, 1982; Wynder *et al.*, 1973). This distribution is at least in part due to the fact that lesions in the head more frequently present symptoms (e.g. obstructive jaundice) while other lesions tend to be less symptomatic at early stages. Thus, carcinomas of the head of the pancreas are smaller than those of the body or tail when detected (Macdonald *et al.*, 1982).

Accuracy of Diagnosis and Reporting

Carcinoma of the exocrine pancreas is asymptomatic at early stages, presumably because of the deep location of the organ. The presenting features include jaundice, pain, weight loss, anorexia, nausea, vomiting and weakness, most of which are non-pathognomonic. Because of the vague symptomatologies, the recognition of pancreatic cancer is often delayed until the lesion has advanced or disseminated. When pancreatic cancer is suspected, histological confirmation may not be feasible. Obstructive jaundice occurs relatively early in patients with carcinoma of the head of the pancreas, but even in such cases the differential diagnosis of other tumours in the preampullary region (i.e. the ampulla of Vater, bile duct and preampullary duodenum) is often difficult.

Several studies estimated that from 40 to 50 per cent of pancreatic cancer cases as diagnosed at autopsy have incorrect clinical diagnosis (Bauer and Robbins, 1972; Leach, 1950; Mack, 1982). These percentages probably overstate true false-negativity since cases presenting difficult diagnostic problems are likely to be subjected to autopsy. An estimate of false-positivity is even more difficult to obtain since a substantial proportion of pancreatic cancer patients never undergo autopsy or histological confirmation. Of special interest to the epidemiologist examining mortality statistics is the accuracy of information on death certificates. A study of death certificates in Canada during 1950-56 showed that 23 per cent of the 375 patients dying from pancreatic cancer as reported on death certificates did not have pancreatic cancer when their medical records were reviewed (Barclay and Phillips, 1962). Also, 2 per cent of the 383 patients' deaths not mentioning pancreatic cancer had resulted from this condition. Despite some methodological limitations inherent in these types of studies, the data support the general scepticism about the accuracy of diagnosis and reporting of pancreatic cancer.

Incidence and Mortality

In the United States of America (USA) approximately 21,000 persons are reported to die from pancreatic cancer each year (Silverberg, 1980). As expected from the very high case fatality, mortality statistics for pancreatic cancer closely approximate the morbidity statistics. Thus about 24,000 new (incidence) cases of pancreatic cancer are estimated to occur each year in the USA (Silverberg, 1980). In terms of the magnitude of mortality, pancreatic cancer usually ranks fifth or sixth in the USA and many other countries, being exceeded by malignancies of the lung, breast, large bowel and prostate (Levin *et al.*, 1981).

International Variation

The international distribution of pancreatic cancer is derived from recent incidence data reported from cancer registries around the world (Table 8.1). The incidence is generally higher in Western European countries and the USA than in the Eastern European or Asiatic countries. A similar pattern is found for the mortality (Aoki and Ogawa, 1978). In view of the serious diagnostic difficulties, some of the inter-country differences or even inter-ethnic differences within the same country are likely to be explained by diagnostic and reporting differences. Nevertheless, some of the specific findings are intriguing and perhaps worthy of further investigations. These include the high incidence in the Maoris in New Zealand and native Hawaiians, both of whom are of Polynesian descent (Fraumeni, 1975), the black versus white rates in the USA and the higher incidence in Israeli Jews migrated from Europe and the USA than in other Jews in Israel.

Perhaps more intriguing is the similarity of pancreatic cancer mortality and incidence reported from different populations. Analysis of cancer mortality in 24 countries showed pancreatic cancer to have one of the lowest degree of variability as measured by the ratio of standard deviation to mean (Kurihara, 1976). Similarly, incidence of pancreatic cancer shows an eight-fold differential internationally whereas that of other cancers shows from 25-fold to 300-fold differentials (Doll, 1980).

Time Trends

An increasing trend of pancreatic cancer mortality has been observed in many countries during the last few decades. The trends are gradual and steady. The rate of increase is greater for countries where the mortality was previously low than those with higher previous mortality, thus demonstrating a general converging pattern. However, since around 1969 the rising trend has begun to level off in some countries (Mack, 1982). In the USA little or no change has occurred in either the incidence or mortality since 1969 (Pollack and Horm, 1980). A likely

Table 8.1: International Distribution of Incidence of Pancreatic Cancer (rates per 100,000 adjusted for world population)

	Incidence	
Area and population	Male	Female
Hawaii: Hawaiian	15.8	5.3
California, Bay area: Black	15.2	9.0
Detroit: Black	14.9	7.2
California, Alameda: Black	13.9	9.4
New Zealand: Maori	13.0	4.5
Israel: Jews born in Europe/USA	10.1	6.7
California, Bay area: White	9.9	6.2
Finland	9.8	5.4
New Mexico: Non-Spanish white	9.7	6.1
New Mexico: Spanish	9.6	5.4
California, Bay area: Chinese	9.6	5.4
California, Alameda: White	9.5	6.3
Israel: Jews born in Israel	9.5	6.2
Hawaii: White	9.5	7.4
Canada	6.2-9.5	3.5-5.9
New York State	9.3	5.4
Detroit: White	8.9	5.8
United Kingdom	6.9-8.7	3.7-5.0
Connecticut	8.6	5.8
El Paso: Spanish	8.5	9.2
Sweden	8.3	5.7
Poland	3.6-8.1	2.6-5.1
Denmark	8.0	5.4
Iceland	7.9	7.6
Norway	7.9	4.7
West Germany	6.0-7.8	3.1-4.2
Japan	3.8-7.3	2.3-4.5
New Zealand: Non-Maori	7.3	3.8
Hungary	1.5-7.2	1.7-5.1
Hawaii: Japanese	7.0	4.7
El Paso: Non-Spanish white	6.9	3.8
Israel: Jews born in Africa/Asia	6.1	5.0
East Germany	6.1	3.6
Hawaii: Chinese	6.0	4.6
Yugoslavia: Slovenia	4.7	2.9
Puerto Rico	4.2	3.1
Hawaii: Filipino	4.1	3.7
Colombia: Cali	3.7	3.4
New Mexico: American Indian	2.4	6.2
India: Bombay	1.8	0.9
Nigeria: Ibadan	1.7	1.7

Source: Waterhouse *et al.*, 1976.

explanation for these phenomena seems to be a recent improvement in diagnosis, but the effect of other factors such as smoking and occupational exposures must also be considered (Moolgavkar and Stevens, 1981).

Age, Sex and Socioeconomic Factors

As with many adult types of cancer, the incidence of pancreatic cancer increases with age in approximately log-linear fashion (Mack, 1982). This is compatible with the notion that cancer results from continued exposure to carcinogenic stimuli over an extended period of time (Doll, 1968). In a few population groups, such as the US blacks, the age-specific incidence sharply declines in the oldest age groups, most likely due to errors in the estimate of denominators.

Cancer of the pancreas occurs more frequently in males than females in most population groups, except for American Indians and possibly the Hispanic in El Paso, Texas (Table 8.1) in which the female preponderance of this cancer is noteworthy. No consistent association exists between pancreatic cancer and socioeconomic status as measured by income, education, occupation or urbanisation (Levin *et al.*, 1981; Mack, 1982).

Risk Factors and Aetiology

Tobacco

The association between cigarette smoking and pancreatic cancer has been extensively examined in various epidemiological studies, both prospective and case-control, conducted in USA, Canada, England, Sweden and Japan (US Public Health Service, 1979). Virtually all studies demonstrated a significantly increased risk of pancreatic cancer among cigarette smokers, although the magnitude of relative risk is modest, ranging from 1.5 to 3.0. A few studies have also shown increased risk with an increasing number of cigarettes smoked, thus establishing a dose-response relationship, a requisite for causal association (Wynder *et al.*, 1973; MacMahon *et al.*, 1981). Evidence on cigar and pipe smoking is less clear, mainly because of the smaller number of smokers of such tobacco products.

The proportion of pancreatic cancer attributable to cigarette smoking has not been well estimated, although the relative risk of the above magnitude suggests that it is small. Also unclear is the extent to which smoking explains time- and space-variation of pancreatic cancer. One study showed no correlation between pancreatic cancer mortality and *per capita* tobacco consumption (Stocks, 1970), whereas a statistical model applied to mortality and cigarette consumption data in England and Wales suggested that cigarette smoking explains the temporal trend as well as the male-female differential in pancreatic cancer mortality (Moolgavkar and Stevens, 1981).

Table 8.2: Occupations Reported to be Associated with Pancreatic Cancer

Relative risk ≥ 2.0	Relative risk 1.4-1.9
Aircraft mechanics	Cannery workers
Aluminium workers	Chemists
Atomic energy workers	Civil servants
Beta-naphthylamine/benzidine workers	Clothing workers
Cement workers	Coal, gas or coke workers
Chemists	Cranemen and derrickmen
Construction workers	Delivery men
Dentists	Dentists
Dry cleaners, service station workers and garage workers	Electrical fitters
Engineers	Electrical machine manufacturers
Hairdressers	Farmers
Machine operators	Fishermen
Managers and administrators	Fruit warehousemen
Metal craftsmen and workers	Furniture store workers
Motion picture projectionists	Insurance agents
Nurserymen	Jewellers
Oil refinery workers	Managers and administrators
Printing workers	Merchant seamen
Professionals and technicians	Metal workers
Radiologists	Mine workers
Service workers	Paper mill workers
Stationery workers	Produce buyers and shippers
Stonecutters	Sawmill workers
Telegraph operators	Sheet metal workers

Source: Mack, 1982 (modified data).

Occupations

A list of occupations reported to be associated with pancreatic cancer is rather long (Table 8.2). One of the difficulties in interpreting findings from occupational studies derives from the fact that large numbers of occupations and industries are examined in such studies so that some of the significant findings can be expected by statistical chance alone. Furthermore, some of the excess cancer risks may only reflect the life style or other characteristics of workers rather than specific carcinogenic hazards in the work place. Of interest from the viewpoint of identifying specific carcinogens are the excess pancreatic cancer risks found in metal industry workers (Decoufle *et al.*, 1977; Dörken, 1964), chemists (Li *et al.*, 1969), coke-oven and coke by-product workers (Redmond *et al.*, 1976; Registrar-General, 1954), and sawmill workers (Milham, 1976). However, among coke-oven workers, the excess mortality was confined to those working in 'non-oven' areas where exposure to the suspect carcinogen was minimal (Redmond *et al.*, 1976).

Specific exposure to beta-naphthylamine and benzidine, known carcinogens, is associated with increased mortality from pancreatic cancer, but the finding is based on too few deaths to be conclusive (Mancuso and El-Atter, 1967). A case-control study of 109 pancreatic cancer patients and the same number of demographically comparable controls demonstrated a significantly increased odds ratio for cancer for individuals employed in the dry cleaning business and service station and garage workers (Lin and Kessler, 1981). Common exposure among these workers is to petroleum products. The odds ratio also increased with increasing duration of employment, providing evidence for causal association.

Alcohol

Despite the general suspicion of the role of alcohol in pancreatic cancer, epidemiological evidence does not support this. The association between alcohol consumption and pancreatic cancer as reported in early studies (Burch and Ansari, 1968; Ishii *et al.*, 1968) is regarded as inconclusive because the possible confounding effect of smoking was not addressed. More recent case-control studies, one involving 142 pancreatic cancer patients and 275 age-, sex- and race-matched controls (Wynder *et al.*, 1973), and the other including 369 cases and 644 controls (MacMahon *et al.*, 1981), revealed no association between alcohol drinking and pancreatic cancer. Furthermore, cohort studies of 1,382 alcoholics in Massachusetts (Monson and Lyon, 1975) and of 205,000 males convicted for drunkenness in Finland (Hakulinen *et al.*, 1974) showed no significant excess risk of pancreatic cancer.

Coffee

Internationally, there is a statistical correlation between pancreatic cancer mortality and *per capita* coffee consumption (Stocks, 1970). No such correlation is found with tea or cigarette consumption. One of the case-control studies described above demonstrated a significant, moderately elevated odds ratio (from 2 to 3) for pancreatic cancer associated with coffee drinking. The significantly increased odds ratio persisted after the effect of smoking was controlled for and a dose-response relationship was observed (MacMahon *et al.*, 1981). While no carcinogens have been identified in coffee, caffeine and other xanthines are mutagenic (Kuhlmann *et al.*, 1968).

In another case-control study of pancreatic cancer, a significant association was found with caffeine-free coffee, but not with regular coffee (Lin and Kessler, 1981). The finding led the authors to suspect the presence of carcinogenic agents in coffee, such as trichloroethylene which was once widely used in the decaffeination process. Trichloroethylene and certain other chlorinated hydrocarbons are laboratory carcinogens. At the present time, these epidemiological findings should be interpreted cautiously since some of the patients, particularly those with pancreatic cancer, may change their coffee consumption because of their gastrointestinal symptoms. This possibility has not been investigated in previous studies.

Diet

Statistical correlations also exist between pancreatic cancer mortality and *per capita* consumption of certain dietary components, including fats and oil, sugar, animal protein, eggs and milk (Lea, 1967; Wynder *et al.*, 1973). A case-control study in Japan suggested a high dietary intake of fat and a low intake of vegetables to be associated with pancreatic cancer (Ishii *et al.*, 1968), and a prospective study in the same country showed increased mortality from pancreatic cancer among individuals with high meat consumption (Hirayama, 1967).

Associated Diseases

Clinical studies have suggested certain diseases to be associated with pancreatic cancer. Some diseases are present when pancreatic cancer is found while others may have preceded cancer. Temporal associations are not always clear in the clinical literature so that the nature of the association is difficult to determine.

Diabetes mellitus or hyperglycaemia is a relatively frequent finding in pancreatic cancer patients (Bell, 1957). Since pancreatic cancer may itself interfere with glucose tolerance, the temporal relation between the two diseases of the pancreas needs to be assessed. A prospective study of 21,447 diabetics registered at a Boston clinic showed a significantly increased mortality from pancreatic cancer in both males and females (Kessler, 1970). However, after eliminating patients in whom cancer occurred within a year of the first clinic visit, the excess mortality was significant only for females. Similarly, the association between prior diabetes and pancreatic cancer was limited to females in the case-control study (Wynder *et al.*, 1973). Therefore, diabetes may have aetiological significance at least in women. It is of interest that certain populations with unusually high pancreatic cancer incidence, such as the Maoris and native Hawaiians, have a high prevalence of diabetes (Fraumeni, 1975), and that the geographical correlation of the two diseases is also limited to females (Blot *et al.*, 1978).

A possible role of endocrine factors in pancreatic cancer has been suggested by several studies. In one case-control study, significantly more pancreatic cancer patients than controls reported a history of uterine myoma, spontaneous abortion and oophorectomy (Lin and Kessler, 1981). An autopsy study suggested an increased frequency of hyperplasia of the ovarian corticostroma and endometrium and neoplasms of the breast, ovary and uterus in pancreatic cancer patients (Soloway and Sommers, 1966). Whether or not these findings point to some common endocrine aetiology is yet to be investigated.

Pancreatitis and pancreatic calcification are apparently prevalent in autopsy and clinical series of pancreatic cancer patients (Mikal and Campbell, 1950; Gambill, 1971; Bartholomew *et al.*, 1958; Paulino-Netto *et al.*, 1960; Johnson and Zintel, 1963). However, no significant association with a history of either condition was found in case-control studies (Wynder *et al.*, 1973; Lin and Kessler, 1981). Also, the clinical association of gall-bladder disease with pancreatic cancer (Bell, 1957) was not supported by controlled studies (Wynder *et al.*, 1973; Lin and Kessler, 1981).

Radiation

A small excess mortality from pancreatic cancer has been found in patients receiving therapeutic radiation for ankylosing spondylitis (Court-Brown and Doll, 1965), among radiologists (Court-Brown and Doll, 1958) and US atomic energy workers (Mancuso *et al.*, 1977). Such a small excess mortality may actually be due to some other factors such as concomitant chemical exposure or biased ascertainment of cancer (Hutchison *et al.*, 1979).

Familial Background

The familial aggregation of adenocarcinoma of the pancreas is very rare, but has been documented in several families with or without hereditary pancreatitis (MacDermott and Kramer, 1973; Friedman and Fialkow, 1976; Kattwinkel *et al.*, 1973).

Aetiological Hypotheses

On the basis of the epidemiological evidence discussed, one may conclude that cigarette smoking is most likely to play a role in the aetiology of pancreatic cancer. Occupational exposures may also have aetiological significance in human pancreatic carcinogenesis, although more studies are needed to define specific agents. The aetiological significance of other potential risk factors needs to be further investigated, including coffee, dietary components and diabetes mellitus.

Several mechanistic hypotheses have been offered concerning human pancreatic cancer. It has been proposed that bile containing carcinogens originating from cigarettes, occupational environments or even diet may be refluxed into the pancreas where their carcinogenic effect is exerted (Wynder *et al.*, 1973). This hypothesis is tenable because bile reflux has been demonstrated in certain individuals (Hansson, 1967), but it remains to be shown that bile reflux is indeed more prevalent in pancreatic cancer patients than normal subjects. The hypothesis also explains why cancer is more frequent in the head of the pancreas than in the body or tail. On the other hand, such chemical carcinogens as nitrosamines and other nitroso compounds show a distinct site-specificity in laboratory animals (Reddy, 1975; Pour *et al.*, 1981). Nitrosamines are present, though in small amounts, in cigarettes and these may reach the pancreas via the bloodstream. Furthermore, it has been suggested that cigarette smoking may stimulate the secretion of gastrointestinal hormones such as gastrin and cholecystokinin (Murthy *et al.*, 1977), and that these hormones in turn induce hyperplasia (McMichael, 1981). Gastrin and cholecystokinin are potent stimulators of pancreatic hyperplasia in animals (Johnson, 1981). Coffee drinking may also stimulate the secretion of the gastrointestinal hormones (Cohen, 1980).

Secondary Prevention

As noted at the beginning, the prognosis of pancreatic cancer patients is extremely grave. Despite the recent improvement in their survival experience, the median survival time is currently four months and the two-year survival is only 5 per cent (Levin *et al.*, 1981). The introduction and wide acceptance of several new diagnostic procedures such as ultrasonography, endoscopic retrograde cholangiopancreatography, cytology, computed tomography and angiography have improved the accuracy of diagnosis in symptomatic patients (Moosa and Levin, 1981; Liang *et al.*, 1981). However, these procedures are clearly not applicable to the detection of early cancer in a large number of asymptomatic individuals. Currently available screening tests (e.g. carcinoembryonic antigen, alpha-fetoprotein, pancreatic oncofetal antigen, peptide hormones and pancreatic ribonuclease) have limited usefulness because of their low sensitivity and specificity (Moosa and Levin, 1981). Further research in this area is urgently needed.

Comment

It is widely appreciated that the carcinogenic process of initial exposure leading to cancer formation represents many stages or steps in cellular evolution, involving a multiplicity of synergistic and antagonistic interactions among various factors (Farber, 1981). This view is compatible with the fact that cancer formation takes so many years and that only a small fraction of persons exposed to carcinogens (e.g. cigarettes) develop cancer. In view of the very small relative risk of pancreatic cancer associated with smoking, it would appear that factors modifying the initial or early carcinogenic events are particularly important in pancreatic carcinogenesis. While continued efforts are needed to identify additional carcinogens, another area of research should be directed at defining early carcinogenic or premalignant changes as well as factors associated with each stage of carcinogenesis. The latter approach clearly demands that epidemiologists work closely with clinical oncologists, pathologists, biochemists and researchers of other disciplines.

References

Aoki, K. and Ogawa, H. (1978). Cancer of the pancreas, international mortality trends. *World Health Statistical Reports*, 31: 2-27

Barclay, T.H.C. and Phillips, A.J. (1962). The accuracy of cancer diagnosis on death certificates. *Cancer*, 15: 5-9

Bartholomew, L.G., Gross, J.B. and Comfort, M.W. (1958). Carcinoma of the pancreas associated with chronic relapsing pancreatitis. *Gastroenterology*, 35: 473-7

Bauer, F.W. and Robbins, S.L. (1972). An autopsy study of cancer patients. *Journal of the American Medical Association*, 221, 1471-4

Bell, E.T. (1957). Carcinoma of the pancreas. I. A clinical and pathologic study of 609 necropsied cases. II. The relation of carcinoma of the pancreas to diabetes mellitus. *American Journal of Pathology*, 33: 499-523

Blot, W.J., Fraumeni, J.F., Jr. and Stone, B.J. (1978). Geographic correlates of pancreas cancer in the United States. *Cancer*, 42: 373-80

Burch, E.G. and Ansari, A. (1968). Chronic alcoholism and carcinoma of the pancreas. *Archives of Internal Medicine*, 122: 273-5

Cohen, S. (1980). Pathogenesis of coffee-induced gastrointestinal symptoms. *New England Journal of Medicine*, 303: 122-4

Court-Brown, W.M. and Doll, R. (1958). Expectation of life and mortality from cancer among British radiologists. *British Medical Journal*, 2: 181-7

——— and Doll, R. (1965). Mortality from cancer and other causes after radiotherapy for anklylosing spondylitis. *British Medical Journal*, 2: 1327-32

Decoufle, P., Stanislawczyk, K., Houten, L., Bross, I.D.J. and Viadana, E. (1977). *A Retrospective Survey of Cancer in Relation to Occupation*, US Government Printing Office, Washington, DC

Doll, R. (1968). The age distribution of cancer in man. In: Eagel, A. and Larsson, T., (eds.), *Cancer and Aging*, Nordiska Bokhandelas Förlag, Stockholm, Sweden, p. 15

——— (1980). The epidemiology of cancer. *Cancer*, 45: 2475-85

Dörken, H. (1964). Einige daten bei 280 patienten mit pankreaskrebs. *Gastroenterologica*, 102: 47-77

Farber, E. (1981). Chemical carcinogenesis. *New England Journal of Medicine*, 305: 1379-89

Fraumeni, J.F., Jr. (1975). Cancers of the pancreas and biliary tract: Epidemiological considerations. *Cancer Research*, 35: 3437-46

Friedman, J.M. and Fialkow, P.J. (1976). Familial carcinoma of the pancreas. *Clinical Genetics*, 9: 463-9

Gambill, E.E. (1971). Pancreatitis associated wtih pancreatic carcinoma: A study of 26 cases. *Mayo Clinic Proceedings*, 46: 174-7

Haklulinen, T., Lehtimähki, L., Lehtonen, M. and Teppo, L. (1974). Cancer morbidity among two male cohorts with increased alcohol consumption in Finland. *Journal of the National Cancer Institute*, 52: 1711-14

Hansson, K. (1967). Experimental and clinical studies in aetiologic role of bile reflux in acute pancreatitis. *Acta Chirurgica Scandinavica*, Suppl. 375: 1-120

Hirayama, T. (1967). Smoking in relation to the death rates of 265,118 men and women in Japan. National Cancer Center Research Institute, Tokyo, p. 14

Hutchison, G.B., MacMahon, B., Jablon, S. and Land, C.E. (1979). Review of report by Mancuso, Stewart and Kneale of radiation exposure of Hanford workers. *Health Physics*, 37: 207-20

Ishii, K., Nakamura, K, Ozaki, H., Yamada, N. and Takeuchi, T. (1968). Epidemiological problems of pancreatic cancer. *Nippon Rinsho*, 26: 1839-42

Johnson, J.R. and Zintel, H.A. (1963). Pancreatic calcification and cancer of the pancreas. *Surgery, Gynecology and Obstetrics*, 117: 585-8

Johnson, L.R. (1981). Effects of gastrointestinal hormones on pancreatic growth. *Cancer*, 47: 1640-5

Kattwinkel, J., Lopey, A., Disant'Agnese, P.A., Edwards, W.A. and Huffey, M.P. (1973). Hereditary pancreatitis: three new kindreds and a critical review of the literature. *Pediatrics*, 51: 55-9

Kessler, I.I. (1970). Cancer mortality among diabetics. *Journal of the National*

Cancer Institute, 44: 673-86

Kuhlmann, W., Fromme, H.G., Heege, E.M. and Ostertag, N. (1968). The mutagenic action of caffeine in higher organisms. *Cancer Research*, 28: 2375-89

Kurihara, M. (1976). Geographical pathology of cancer. *Igaku-No-Ayumi*, 96: 330-8

Lea, A.J. (1967). Neoplasms and environmental factors. *Annals of the Royal College of Surgeons of England*, 41: 432-7

Leach, W.B. (1950). Carcinoma of the pancreas. A clinical and pathological analysis of 39 autopsied cases. *British Journal of Pathology*, 26: 333-47

Levin, D.L., Connelley, R.R. and Devesa, S.S. (1981). Demographic characteristics of cancer of the pancreas. Mortality, incidence and survival. *Cancer*, 47: 1456-68

Li, F.P., Fraumeni, J.F., Jr., Mantel, N. and Miller, R.W. (1969). Cancer mortality among chemists. *Journal of the National Cancer Institute*, 43: 1159-64

Liang, V., Taylor, W.F. and DiMagno, E.P. (1981). Efforts at early diagnosis of pancreatic cancer. The Mayo Clinic experience. *Cancer*, 47: 1698-703

Lin, R.S. and Kessler, I.I. (1981). A multifactorial model for pancreatic cancer in man. Epidemiologic evidence. *Journal of the American Medical Association*, 245: 147-52

MacDermott, R.P. and Kramer, P. (1973). Adenocarcinoma of the pancreas in four siblings. *Gastroenterology*, 65: 137-9

Macdonald, J.S., Gunderson, L.L. and Cohn, I., Jr. (1982). Cancer of the pancreas. In: DeVita, V.T., Jr., Hellman, S. and Rosenberg, S.A. (eds.), *Cancer. Principles and Practice of Oncology*, Lippincott Company, Philadelphia, ch. 18, p. 563

Mack, T. (1982). Pancreas. In: Schottenfeld, D. and Fraumeni, J.F., Jr. (eds.), *Cancer Epidemiology and Prevention*, Saunders, Philadelphia, ch. 36, p. 638

MacMahon, B., Yen, S., Trichopoulos, D., Warren, K. and Nardi, G. (1981). Coffee and cancer of the pancreas. *New England Journal of Medicine*, 304: 630-3

Mancuso, T.F. and El-Attar, A.A. (1967). Cohort study of workers exposed to beta-naphthylamine and benzidine. *Journal of Occupational Medicine*, 9: 277-85

—— Stewart, A. and Kneale, G. (1977). Radiation exposures of Hanford workers dying from cancer and other diseases. *Health Physics*, 33: 369-84

McMichael, A.J. (1981). Coffee, soya, and pancreatic cancer. *Lancet*, 2: 689-90

Mikal, S. and Campbell, J.A. (1950). Carcinoma of the pancreas: Diagnostic and operative criteria based on one hundred consecutive autopsies. *Surgery*, 28: 963-9

Milham, S. (1976). Neoplasia in the wood and pulp industry. *Annals of the New York Academy of Sciences*, 271: 294-300

Monson, R.R. and Lyon, J.L. (1975). Proportional mortality among alcoholics. *Cancer*, 36: 1077-9

Moolgavkar, S.H. and Stevens, R.G. (1981). Smoking and cancers of bladder and pancreas: Risks and temporal trends. *Journal of the National Cancer Institute*, 67: 15-23

Moosa, A.R. and Levin, B. (1981). The diagnosis of 'early' pancreatic cancer. *Cancer*, 47: 1688-97

Murthy, S.N.S., Dinoso, V.P., Clearfield, H.R. and Chey, W.Y. (1977). Simultaneous measurement of basal pancreatic, gastric acid secretion, plasma gastrin, and secretion during smoking. *Gastroenterology*, 73: 758-61

Paulino-Netto, A., Dreiling, D.A. and Baronofsky, I.D. (1960). The relationship between pancreatic calcification and cancer of the pancreas. *Annals of Surgery*,

151: 530-7

Pollack, E.S. and Horm, J.W. (1980). Trends in cancer incidence and mortality in the United States, 1969-76. *Journal of the National Cancer Institute*, 64: 1091-103

Pour, P.M., Runge, R.G., Birt, D., Gingell, R., Lawson, T., Nagel, D. *et al.* (1981). Current knowledge of pancreatic carcinogenesis in the hamster and its relevance to the human disease. *Cancer*, 47: 1573-87

Reddy, J.K. and Rao, M.S. (1975). Pancreatic adenocarcinoma in guinea pigs induced by N-methyl-N-nitrosurea. *Cancer Research*, 35: 2269-77

Redmond, C.K., Strobino, B.R. and Cypess, R.H. (1976). Cancer experience among coke by-product workers. *Annals of the New York Academy of Sciences*, 271: 102-15

Registrar-General (1954). *Decennial Supplement, England and Wales, 1951. Part I, Occupational Mortality*, HMSO, London

Silverberg, E. (1980). Cancer statistics, 1980. *Ca—A Cancer Journal for Clinicians*, 30: 39-44

Soloway, H.B. and Sommers, S.C. (1966). Endocrinopathy associated with pancreatic carcinomas: Review of host factors including hyperplasia and gonadotropic activity. *Annals of Surgery*, 164: 300-4

Stocks, P. (1970). Cancer mortality in relation to national consumption of cigarettes, solid fuel, tea and coffee. *British Journal of Cancer*, 24: 215-25

US Public Health Service (1979). *Smoking and Health. A Report of the Surgeon General*, US Government Printing Office, Washington, DC, pp. 5-50

Waterhouse, T., Muir, C., Correa, P. and Powell, J. (1976). *Cancer Incidence in Five Continents*, Volume III, International Agency for Research on Cancer, Lyon

Wynder, E.L., Mabuchi, K., Maruchi, N. and Fortner, J.G. (1973). Epidemiology of cancer of the pancreas. *Journal of the National Cancer Institute*, 50: 645-67

9 CANCER OF THE COLON AND RECTUM

A.B. Miller

Introduction

Cancer of the colon and rectum together constitute the second most important cancer in each sex in most Western countries. However, because in males lung is the most frequently diagnosed cancer and in females breast, when both sexes are considered together, colo-rectal cancer becomes the most frequently diagnosed cancer, though lung usually exceeds the total of the two sites in numbers of deaths. This is because the large majority of cases of lung cancer are fatal, whereas approximately 60 per cent of patients with colo-rectal cancer die of their disease.

This review will largely concentrate on the aetiology of cancer of the colon and rectum, and particularly the importance of dietary factors. Familial and hereditary factors will not be considered, nor the risk associated with inflammatory bowel disease (Crohn's disease and ulcerative colitis) which have been reviewed elsewhere (Lynch *et al.*, 1981; Schottenfeld and Winawer, 1982).

Incidence and Mortality

Migrants from Italy, Norway, Poland and the Soviet Union have rates of colon and rectal cancer resembling more that of the host country than the country of origin (Haenszel, 1961). Changes occurring rapidly on migration have been noted frequently, for example in southern Europeans migrating to Australia (McMichael *et al.*, 1980).

The mortality from colo-rectal cancer is higher in urban than rural regions. In the United States of America (USA) those born in urban regions who migrate to rural areas acquire the lower mortality of the rural areas, with the reverse for those who migrate from rural to urban areas (Haenszel and Dawson, 1965). Among long-term residents, mortality is higher in the north of the USA than in the south. Mortality from colo-rectal cancer is elevated in counties in the USA where there are large populations of Irish, German or Czechoslovakian descent (Blot *et al.*, 1976).

Internationally the highest rates of colon cancer are found in North America and New Zealand, the lowest in Asia and the Caribbean, intermediate in Scandinavia and England (deJong *et al.*, 1972). In high- and intermediate-risk areas there is decreasing incidence from the ascending to the descending colon, with an increase at the sigmoid colon, and rectal cancer rates being generally higher than the sigmoid. In low-incidence areas there may be a deficit of sigmoid cancers. At older ages, the sex ratio for colon cancer shows a male preponderance, due to an excess in the descending and sigmoid colon. Rectal cancer is commoner in males.

Over the period 1952-3 to 1966-7, Scotland showed the highest reported death rate, though the rates were falling, as were those for England and Wales (Berg and Howell, 1974). USA white rates appeared stable, but those for West Germany, Italy and Japan were rising. A strong correlation in international incidence rates for colon and rectal cancer was found and it was suggested that while much of rectal cancer is caused by the same factors that cause colon cancer, there is a second set of rectal cancers of different aetiology.

Since then, mortality rates for large bowel cancer have remained relatively stable in the USA (Doll and Peto, 1981) and Canada (Miller, 1982). However, since World War II the death rates from large bowel cancer have risen rapidly in Japan, with a greater rate of increase for cancers of the colon than rectum in both sexes (Lee, 1976). Each birth cohort showed an increase in rates of colon cancer suggesting the effect of a secular change affecting all birth cohorts simultaneously, rather than an effect on successive birth cohorts. This adds support to the migrant studies which suggest that changing environmental factors have a relatively rapid effect on rates of colon cancer.

The incidence of large bowel cancer in Cali, Colombia, was higher in the upper socioeconomic classes (Haenszel *et al.*, 1975). The gradients were most marked for cancer of the ascending through rectosigmoid colon and were minimal for cancer of the caecum and rectum. Lynch *et al.* (1975) found a greater frequency of colon cancer in patients living in census tracts with higher average income in the Omaha-Douglas County, Nebraska population. Blot *et al.* (1976) also found that colon and rectal cancer mortality were associated with higher income and education levels in the USA. Similar findings were reported from the Finnish Cancer Registry (Teppo *et al.*, 1980).

Similar frequencies for different diseases imply common aetiological factors. Berg (1975) pointed out that international incidence rates for the endocrine-dependent cancers (i.e. breast, corpus uteri and ovarian cancers in females and testis and prostate cancers in males) were closely correlated with the rates for large bowel cancers. Miller (1982) found a high correlation between males and females in the same registry for incidence of colon cancer; significant positive correlations within the same sex for colon and rectal cancer, for both sites combined with pancreatic cancer and negative correlations between colon and stomach cancer. In women, liver cancer is negatively correlated with colon and rectal cancer, and colon and to a lesser extent rectal cancer are positively correlated with breast, endometrial and ovarian cancers.

Studies of Special Religious Goups

Studies in Seventh-Day Adventists support a protective effect of a lacto-ovo-vegetarian diet against colon cancer (Phillips, 1975; Phillips *et al.*, 1980). Mormons also have a lower incidence of cancer of the colon than the United States average (Lyon *et al.*, 1980; Enstrom, 1980). However, a preliminary dietary survey found little difference in meat, fat and fibre consumption between the population of Utah and that of the USA as a whole (Lyon and Sorenson, 1978).

Malhotra (1977) suggested that the virtual absence of colon cancer in Punjabis from the north of India is due to a diet rich in roughage, cellulose and vegetable fibre and short-chain fermented milk products, almost completely absent from south Indian diets. Vegetable fibres are abundant in the stools of north Indians but absent from those of south Indians.

Correlations with Dietary Variables

Studies of the incidence and mortality of large bowel cancer internationally in relation to dietary variables strongly support an association of colon cancer, and to a lesser extent rectal cancer, with total dietary fat intake (Armstrong and Doll, 1975). Knox (1977) suggested that associations between total fat intake and cancer of the large intestine, and between beer intake and cancer of the rectum, were causal. Kolonel *et al.* (1981), however, found no association of fat intake and differences in ethnic-specific incidence rates for colon cancer in Hawaii, in contrast to a positive finding for breast cancer.

Correlations with other dietary factors have also been evaluated. Thus, Irving and Drasar (1973) failed to find a correlation of cancer of the colon with different fibre-containing foods internationally, though they demonstrated a high correlation with fat and animal protein intake. Berg and Howell (1974) reported the highest correlation internationally for colon cancer mortality rates for meat consumption, and within individual types of meat, for beef. In contrast, trends in beef and fat consumption in the USA do not correlate with trends in incidence and mortality of colo-rectal cancer (Enstrom, 1975).

Jansson *et al.* (1978) found the mean mortality rate for colo-rectal cancer increased with increasing selenium levels in the drinking water, in contrast to a negative correlation between dietary selenium and cancer in general. MacLennan *et al.* (1978) evaluated the diet in samples of men from Copenhagen, Denmark and Kuopio, Finland, with fourfold differences in colon cancer incidence. The high-incidence group consumed more white wheat breads, meat (especially pork) and beer, but less potatoes and milk than the low-incidence group. The estimated consumption of fat was similar, but the consumption of fibre was higher in the low-incidence group. Stool weights were also higher in the low-incidence group, but intestinal transit time was similar.

Bingham *et al.* (1979) related the average intake of foods, nutrients and dietary fibre in different regions of Great Britain to regional patterns of death from colo-rectal cancer. They found no significant associations with the consumption of fat, animal protein or beer nor with total dietary fibre. However, intake of the pentose fraction of dietary fibre and of vegetables other than potatoes were negatively correlated with death rates for colon cancer.

Lui *et al.* (1979) evaluated food disappearance data for 1954-65 and mortality from colon cancer in 1967-73 from 20 industrialised countries. The term 'food disappearance' related to estimates of the amounts of food produced, imported and sold in a country. As this includes food that is wasted and not eaten, it is not identical to food intake, but for most foods is reasonably well correlated with consumption levels. Data for total fat, saturated fat, mono-unsaturated fat and cholesterol were positively, and fibre intake negatively, correlated with colon cancer mortality. The partial correlation of dietary cholesterol and colon cancer remained highly significant when fat or fibre were controlled. However, the partial correlations of fat or of fibre with colon cancer mortality were no longer significant when cholesterol was controlled.

Dietary correlation studies produce evidence for groups, rather than individuals. Although variation among dietary factors internationally is great, it may be much smaller for groups within countries. The variation of incidence and mortality within countries may also be low. Further-more, dietary information is generally derived from food disappearance data, and not necessarily from food consumption data, and may be correlated with current information on incidence or mortality. It may be more appropriate to take dietary information some 20 or 30 years ago and correlate this with current incidence or mortality rates. Hence lack of correlation, either nationally or internationally, does not suffice to disprove an hypothesis. Conversely, one should not rely too heavily on observed correlations in case they are confounded by some factor that could not be studied or has not yet been identified.

Colon Cancer and Cholesterol

Support for the possible importance of dietary cholesterol (Lui *et al.*, 1979) comes from the correlation between mortality from colon cancer and coronary heart disease (Rose *et al.*, 1974; Lipworth and Rice, 1979). Japanese migrants to Hawaii have high rates of colon cancer and a high frequency of myocardial infarction, severe athero-sclerosis, diverticulosis and polyposis of the colon compared to Japanese in Japan (Stemmermann *et al.*, 1979). These changes may be related to the consumption of characteristically Western foods by Hawaiian Japanese.

There have been a number of studies of cardiovascular disease during which information on the association of colon cancer and cholesterol blood levels has been obtained. Pearce and Dayton (1971) reported a greater incidence of cancer in men on a diet high in polyunsaturated vegetable oils and low in saturated fat and cholesterol than in the control group in an eight-year controlled trial of 846 men. Ederer *et al.* (1971), however, after combining data from five controlled trials of cholesterol-lowering diets (including that of Pearce and Dayton, 1971) found no evidence of increased cancer incidence or mortality. Rose *et al.* (1974) reported an association between colon cancer and blood cholesterol in men, using pooled data from six cohort studies. There were 90 cases of colon cancer, their initial levels of blood cholesterol being lower than expected. Rose and Shipley (1980) subsequently reported that the inverse association between plasma cholesterol and non-coronary heart disease deaths was confined to the first two years of follow-up. Hence the association of low cholesterol and bowel cancer mortality could have resulted from the metabolic consequences of cancer present but unsuspected at the time of examination. Two other studies, however, have cast doubt on this explanation. Thus, in a community sample of 3,102 individuals from Evans County, Georgia, followed for 12-14 years (Kark *et al.*, 1980), 129 incident cases of cancer (including six of colon cancer) were ascertained. Cases diagnosed 12 months or more following the initial examination had significantly lower mean serum cholesterol levels at entry than the control population. Williams *et al.* (1981) performed a similar analysis for 5,209 subjects followed for 24 years in the Framingham study. Of 691 incident cancers observed 88 were in the colon. Only two were diagnosed in the first two years after entry and only three in the next two years. The initial serum cholesterol level was inversely associated with incidence of colon cancer only in men. Colon cancer rates in men with serum cholesterol levels less than 190mg/dl were about three times those seen in men with higher levels.

In studies in Yugoslavia (Kozareric *et al.*, 1981), Puerto Rico (Garcia-Palmieri *et al.*, 1981) and in Sweden (Peterson *et al.*, 1981) an inverse relationship between cancer death and serum cholesterol was also seen, but deaths from colon cancer were not separately reported.

In a study of 8,006 Hawaiian Japanese men, aged 45-68 years, followed for 14 years, 80 cases of colon cancer were observed (Stemmermann *et al.*, 1981). Serum cholesterol levels below 180 mg/dl predicted high rates of colon cancer, men who died from colon cancer having the lowest levels. A lack of a similar association with other cancers (including rectal cancer) and the finding of the inverse association in men diagnosed 5 to 9.9 years after examination suggested to the authors that the low serum cholesterol was not due to pre-existing disease, though an inverse association was not seen in men diagnosed with colon cancer 10 or more years after the cholesterol levels were measured. In contrast, serum cholesterol was not associated with risk of death from cancer, including colon cancer, in three studies of Chicago men (Dyer *et al.*, 1981).

Serum cholesterol levels were lower in 133 cases of colon cancer than their matched controls (Miller *et al.*, 1981). However, significant differences in cholesterol levels were found only for cases with advanced tumours and controls and only women had significantly lower serum cholesterol levels with advancing disease. The lack of an association in early disease supports the concept that low serum cholesterol levels observed in colon cancer patients may be the result of a metabolic change due to advanced tumours.

The relationship between serum cholesterol and colo-rectal cancer is thus obscure. It is possible that high fat (and/or cholesterol) levels in the diet in individuals with a metabolism that maintains a low serum cholesterol result in reduced biosynthesis of cholesterol and a high excretion of cholesterol breakdown products in the intestine (Lin and Connor, 1980).

Faecal Flora and Intestinal Contents

There has been much interest in the possibility that differences in the bacterial flora in the large intestine in groups at high risk of colon cancer compared to those at low risk are clues to the mechanism of large bowel carcinogenesis. Thus, Hill *et al.* (1971) found that faeces from people in Britain and the USA had higher counts of bacteroides and lower counts of aerobic bacteria than people in Uganda, south India or Japan. They also found higher concentrations of steroids in faeces from people in Western countries than in African and Eastern countries.

However, studies by Finegold *et al.* (1975) did not show the same bacteriological differences, while others have concentrated on bile acid metabolism, which seems to be influenced by dietary fat intake. Thus, Reddy and Wynder (1973) found that Americans who ate a Western-type diet excreted high levels of bile acids and more microbially degraded bile acids than American vegetarians and Seventh-Day Adventists, Japanese and Chinese. Reddy *et al.* (1978) found that the average daily intake of dietary fat and protein was the same in a high-risk population in New York and a low-risk population in rural Kuopio, Finland, but a greater proportion of fat came from dairy products in Kuopio where there was a high dietary intake of cereal products rich in fibre. The daily stool output and faecal fibre excretion were greater in Kuopio and the concentration of faecal secondary bile acids and bacterial beta-glucuronidase activity was lower, though the total daily excretion was the same in the two populations. The similarity in the total bile acid secretion may be due to a similar total dietary fat intake. The difference in concentration in bile acids and their breakdown products was probably because of the difference in fibre intake.

Hill *et al.* (1978) have postulated an adenoma-carcinoma sequence influenced by external, probably dietary, factors on a genetic background of varying individual susceptibility. Other groups (Bruce *et al.*, 1981) have been attempting to evaluate faecal mutagens and endogenously produced nitrosamines, but so far with no conclusive agreement on their relevance or on the pathogenesis of the disease.

Because of the possible association of colon cancer and bile acids, there has been interest in cholecystectomy and cancer of the colon. In two studies (Linos *et al.*, 1981; Vernick and Kuller, 1981; 1982) an association of right-sided colon cancer and cholecystectomy was found, in one (Linos *et al.*, 1981) in females only. Markman (1982), while confirming this, also noted an association of colon cancer with appendicectomy in females. Thus, the nature of the relationship of cholecystectomy with colon cancer remains unclear.

Reproduction and Parity

McMichael and Potter (1980) suggested an association between parity and a woman's subsequent risk of developing colon cancer. Nuns have a higher mortality from colon cancer than women in the general population (Fraumeni *et al.*, 1969). This of course could be a dietary or a socioeconomic effect. In Norway and Minnesota, Bjelke (1974) found a smaller proportion of women with colon, but not rectal, cancer than controls had three or more births. In Dales *et al.*'s (1979) study, 60 per cent of the women with colo-rectal cancer had been parous compared to 81 per cent of the controls. Miller *et al.* (1980) found an association between parity and incidence of gastrointestinal cancers as a group, but not for large intestine or rectal cancer individually. Weiss *et al.* (1981) found that women with colon cancer had given birth to fewer children than had controls, but no association between parity and rectal cancer. McMichael and Potter (1980), showed that birth cohorts in women characterised by high parity had slightly lower rates of colon cancer than earlier cohorts, whereas men from the same cohorts had increased rates compared to earlier ones. They proposed that the physiological events accompanying pregnancy and changes in hormone profile protect against the development of colon cancer through a decrease in bile acid secretion.

Occupation

Few studies, except those of cohorts of men occupationally exposed to asbestos (Miller, 1978a), have indicated a specific association with colon and rectal cancer. Berg and Howell (1975) pointed to a 30 per cent rise in mortality from bowel cancer in men but not women and suggested an occupational explanation. They pointed to an excess for white-collar workers and for workers in certain manufacturing industries, but the levels of increased risk were low; it is possible, therefore, that dietary differences associated with socioeconomic status could largely explain the findings.

Case-control Studies of Diet and Large Bowel Cancer

Wynder and Shigematsu (1967) conducted a study involving 791 patients with large bowel cancer and age- and hospital-matched controls and concluded that, apart from the established high risk for patients with ulcerative colitis and familial polyposis, no environmental factors could be identified that differed significantly between cases and controls. However, the dietary inquiry only enabled them to determine an average intake of certain specified foods.

A study of 179 Japanese patients with bowel cancer and 357 hospital controls in Hawaii revealed excess risk for persons who regularly ate Western-style meals (Haenszel *et al.*, 1973). The bowel cancer patients ate meats, legumes and starches more frequently with beef and string beans major contributors to the first two effects. Nevertheless, a study using similar methodology in Japan of 588 patients with colo-rectal cancer and 1,176 hospitalised controls did not replicate these findings (Haenszel *et al.*, 1980). An association was found, however, of reduced risk with consumption of cabbage.

Modan *et al.* (1975) conducted a case-control study in Israel of 198 cases of cancer of the colon, 77 cases of rectal cancer, and matched neighbourhood and surgical controls. They found a lower frequency of consumption of fibre-containing food items in cases of colon cancer compared to each control group, but no differences for the cases of cancer of the rectum. They found no differences in the consumption frequency of fat-containing food items.

Studies in Norway and Minnesota showed slightly lower intakes of cereal products, milk and coffee by colo-rectal cancer cases compared to controls (Bjelke, 1978). Several vegetables were used less frequently by the cases who had lower indices of intakes of vitamin A and crude fibre, both being correlated with vegetable intake. The cases did not differ from controls in total meat or beef intake. However, the younger cases had a higher intake of processed meats than their controls.

Phillips (1975) reported a case-control study of 41 cases of colon cancer in Seventh-Day Adventists each matched to three Seventh-Day Adventist controls. The consumption of beef, lamb, fish and the heavy use of dairy products apart from milk and other high-fat foods were significantly related to risk of colon cancer. Milk, vegetarian protein products and green leafy vegetables showed a non-significant negative association with colon cancer.

Dales *et al.* (1979) carried out a study of black colo-rectal cancer patients and matched controls from hospitals and multiphasic health check-up clinics. The 72 colon cancer cases reported less frequent use of foods with at least 0.5 per cent fibre content than the 202 controls, with a consistent dose-response relationship. The 77 colon and recto-sigmoid junction cancer cases had eaten foods with at least 5 per cent saturated fat more often than their 215 controls. Significantly more colon cancer patients than controls reported a high saturated fat:low fibrous-food eating pattern, as opposed to a low saturated fat:high fibrous-food pattern.

Martinez *et al.* (1979) reported a case-control study of 461 patients with adenocarcinoma of the large bowel and 461 community controls in Puerto Rico. Cases had a significantly higher frequency of consumption of meats, cereals, total fats, total residue and fibre. The higher total residue and fibre consumption of cases compared to controls in this study raises the possibility that a systematic bias may have affected the reporting of all the food frequencies presented.

Graham *et al.* (1978) analysed the interviews of 256 white patients with cancer of the colon, 330 with cancer of the rectum and 783 controls with non-neoplastic non-digestive system diseases for the colon cancer cases and 628 for the cases of cancer of the rectum. A decrease in risk of colon cancer was found to be associated with frequent ingestion of vegetables, especially cabbage, Brussels sprouts and broccoli. For cancer of the rectum decreased risk was only for frequent ingestion of raw vegetables and cabbage.

Jain *et al.* (1980) studied 348 cases of cancer of the colon and 194 cases of cancer of the rectum individually matched to 542 neighbourhood controls and frequency-matched to 535 hospital controls. A detailed quantitative dietary history directed to a two-month period six months prior to the interview was used. Increased risk of both colon and rectal cancer was found for elevated intakes of calories, total fat, total protein, saturated fat, oleic acid and cholesterol, with evidence of dose-response relationships, but no association with consumption of crude fibre, vitamin C and linoleic acid. The nutrients for which an increased risk was demonstrated were highly correlated, though a logistic regression analysis indicated highest risk for saturated fat. The population-attributable risk for saturated fat intake for colon and rectal cancer combined was 41 per cent for males and 44 per cent for females, using the neighbourhood control data as an approximation to the population exposure. The high-risk group of males consumed more than 100g total fat per day, and the high risk females, more than 70g. These intake levels comprised 36 per cent or more of the total caloric intake of both sexes.

Alcohol, Especially Beer

Rectal cancer has been associated with beer consumption in some (Breslow and Enstrom, 1974; Enstrom, 1977; Dean *et al.*, 1979) but not all studies (Jensen, 1979; Schmidt and Popham, 1981). McMichael *et al.* (1979) suggested that there is a better correlation of trends in rectal cancer mortality with changes in beer consumption than with saturated fat. However, the trends for consumption of beer in Australia, USA, New Zealand and Canada do not correlate well with rectal cancer mortality either; it is the trends from the United Kingdom that are largely supportive of the hypothesis (Jain *et al.*, 1980).

In their case-control study of colo-rectal cancer, Wynder and Shige-matsu (1967) showed a significantly higher proportion of beer drinkers compared to one control group, but no differences with a second control group. Among 166 male intestinal cancer patients in England and Wales, Stocks (1957) demonstrated a significant association with beer drinking. Bjelke (1973) reported a dose-response relationship for the risk of colo-rectal cancer and the frequency of beer and liquor consumption in a prospective study of 12,000 middle-aged Norwegian men. A steeper gradient was exhibited with beer consumption. Conversely, case-control studies of intestinal cancer in Finland, Kansas and Norway (Pernu, 1960; Higginson, 1966; Bjelke, 1973) showed no significant relationship with beer drinking.

Thus, an association between beer drinking and colo-rectal cancers has not been seen consistently. The association could be indirect, possibly indicative of other life style or dietary factors. The evidence for the association is stronger for rectal than colon cancer. If it is causal, it could be partly responsible for that component of rectal cancer that does not behave like colon cancer (Berg and Howell, 1974).

Screening for Colo-rectal Cancer

Screening for colo-rectal cancer has been advocated using sigmoidoscopy and faecal testing for occult blood. Routine sigmoidoscopy has
not proven acceptable to the population, and testing for occult blood
using guaiac-impregnated paper slides (Hemoccult) is still under investigation (Miller, 1978b). Until the controlled trials of the Hemoccult test
in progress in the USA have been reported, screening cannot be advocated in the population generally. However, it should be noted that
even if the trials indicate some mortality reduction following screening,
there will be substantial logistic difficulties that will have to be overcome over acceptance of the test and the costs and potential hazards
of investigating false positives. It seems unlikely, therefore, that screening can make a major impact on mortality from the disease.

Conclusion

At the moment, the greatest potential for the reduction in the toll of
colo-rectal cancer is from primary prevention. There are three main
dietary hypotheses for which supporting data are available in various
strengths from epidemiological studies for both colon and rectal cancer:
a causal association of total and, perhaps particularly, saturated fat;
a protective effect of dietary fibre; and a protective effect of crucifer-
ous vegetables. Several case-control studies now support the dietary
fat hypothesis, particularly the only one so far in which quantitative
estimates of dietary fat consumption have been obtained (Jain *et al.*,
1980). The recent decline in mortality from ischaemic heart disease
(Dwyer and Hetzel, 1980) has been regarded by some as due to
increased consumption of polyunsaturated fat. The lack of any decline
in total fat consumption (Page and Friend, 1978) may explain the lack
of any corresponding decline in colon and rectal cancer mortality.
The apparent differing importance of fat and fibre in different investigations is probably due to differences in the precision in the dietary
methodology used in these studies.

Nevertheless, taking action now to change diet towards that suggested
from the studies taken as a whole is unlikely to be hazardous and will
probably prove beneficial. Indeed, in order to obtain maximum protection from cancer of the colon and rectum it may well be necessary to
combine a high fibre, high vegetable and low fat diet.

References

Armstrong, B. and Doll, R. (1975). Environmental factors and cancer incidence and mortality in different countries, with special reference to dietary practices. *International Journal of Cancer*, 15: 617-31

Berg, J.W. (1975). Can nutrition explain the pattern of international epidemiology of hormone-dependent cancers? *Cancer Research*, 35: 3345-50

────── and Howell, M.A. (1974). The geographic pathology of bowel cancer. *Cancer*, 34: 807-14

────── and Howell, M.A. (1975). Occupation and bowel cancer. *Journal of Toxicology and Environmental Health*, 1: 75-89

Bingham, S., Williams, D.R.R., Cole, T.J. and James, W.P.T. (1979). Dietary fibre and regional large-bowel cancer mortality in Britain. *British Journal of Cancer*, 40: 456-63

Bjelke, E. (1973). Ph.D. thesis, University of Minnesota

────── (1974). Colorectal cancer: clues from epidemiology. In: Bucalossi, P., Veronesi, U. and Cascinelli, N. (eds.), Proceedings 11th International Cancer Congress, Vol. 6, *Excerpta Medica Foundation International Congress Series*, 354: 324-30

────── (1978). Dietary factors and the epidemiology of cancer of the stomach and large bowel. *Aktuelle Ernahrungsmedizin Klinische Praxis*, Suppl. 2: pp. 10-17

Blot, W.J., Fraumeni, J.F., Stone, B.J. and McKay, F.W. (1976). Geographic patterns of large bowel cancer in the United States. *Journal of the National Cancer Institute*, 57: 1225-31

Breslow, N.E. and Enstrom, J.E. (1974). Geographic correlations between cancer mortality rates and alcohol-tobacco consumption in the United States. *Journal of the National Cancer Institute*, 53: 631-9

Bruce, W.R., Correa, P., Lipkin, M., Tannenbaum, S.R. and Wilkins, T.D. (eds.) (1981). *Gastrointestinal Cancer: Endogenous Factors*. Banbury report 7, Cold Spring Harbor Laboratory, Cold Spring Habor, New York

Dales, L.G., Friedman, G.D., Ury, H.K., Grossman, S., and Williams, S.R. (1979). A case-control study of relationships of diet and other traits to colorectal cancer in American blacks. *American Journal of Epidemiology*, 109: 132-44

Dean, G., MacLennan, R., McLoughlin, H. and Shelley, E. (1979). The causes of death of blue-collar workers at a Dublin brewery, 1954-1974. *British Journal of Cancer*, 40: 581-9

deJong, U.W., Day, N.E., Muir, C.S., Barclay, T.H.C., Bras, G., Foster, F.H. *et al.* (1972). The distribution of cancer within the large bowel. *International Journal of Cancer*, 10: 463-77

Doll, R. and Peto, R. (1981). The causes of cancer. Quantitative estimates of available risks of cancer in the United States today. *Journal of the National Cancer Institute*, 66: 1191-308

Dwyer, T. and Hetzel, B.S. (1980). A comparison of trends of coronary heart disease mortality in Australia, USA and England and Wales with reference to three major risk factors − hypertension, cigarette smoking and diet. *International Journal of Epidemiology*, 9: 65-71

Dyer, A.R., Stamler, J., Paul, O., Shekelle, R.B., Schoenberger, J.A., Berkson, D.M. *et al.* (1981). Serum cholesterol and risk of death from cancer and other causes in three Chicago epidemiologic studies. *Journal of Chronic Diseases*, 34: 249-60

Ederer, F., Leren, P., Turpeinen, O. and Frantz, I.D. (1971). Cancer among men on cholesterol lowering diets. Experience from five clinical trials. *Lancet*, 2: 203-6

Enstrom, J.E. (1975). Colorectal cancer and consumption of beef and fat. *British Journal of Cancer*, 32: 432-9
—— (1977). Colorectal cancer and beer drinking. *British Journal of Cancer*, 35: 674-83
—— (1980). Health and dietary practices and cancer mortality among California Mormons. In: Cairns, J., Lyon, J.L. and Skolnick, M., (eds.), *Cancer Incidence in Defined Populations*, Banbury Report 4, Cold Spring Harbor Laboratory, Cold Spring Harbor, New York, pp. 69-90
Finegold, S.M., Flora, D.J., Attebery, H.R. and Sutter, V.L. (1975). Fecal bacteriology of colonic polyp patients and control patients. *Cancer Research*, 35: 3407-17
Fraumeni, J.F., Jr., Lloyd, J.W., Smith, E.M. and Wagoner, J.K. (1969). Cancer mortality among nuns: role of marital status in etiology of neoplastic disease in women. *Journal of the National Cancer Institute*, 42: 455-68
Garcia-Palmieri, M.R., Sorlie, P.D., Costas, R. and Havlik, R.J. (1981). An apparent inverse relationship between serum cholesterol and cancer mortality in Puerto Rico. *American Journal of Epidemiology*, 114: 29-40
Graham, S., Dayal, H., Swanson, M., Mittleman, A. and Wilkinson, G. (1978). Diet in the epidemiology of cancer of the colon and rectum. *Journal of the National Cancer Institute*, 61: 709-14
Haenszel, W. (1961). Cancer mortality among the foreign-born in the United States. *Journal of the National Cancer Institute*, 26: 37-132
—— and Dawson, E.A. (1965). A note on mortality from cancer of the colon and rectum in the United States. *Cancer*, 18: 265-72
—— Berg, J.W., Segi, M., Kurihara, M. and Locke, F.B. (1973). Large bowel cancer in Hawaiian Japanese. *Journal of the National Cancer Institute*, 51: 1765-79
—— Correa, P., and Cuello, C. (1975). Social class differences among patients with large-bowel cancer in Cali, Columbia. *Journal of the National Cancer Institute*, 54: 1031-5
—— Locke, F.B. and Segi, M. (1980). A case-control study of large bowel cancer in Japan. *Journal of the National Cancer Institute*, 64: 17-22
Higginson, J. (1966). Etiological factors in gastro-intestinal cancer in man. *Journal of the National Cancer Institute*, 37: 527-45
Hill, M.J., Crowther, J.S., Drasar, B.S., Hawksworth, G., Aries, V. and Williams, R.E.O. (1971). Bacteria and aetiology of cancer of the large bowel. *Lancet*, 1: 95-100
—— Morson, B.C. and Bussey, H.J.R. (1978). Aetiology of adenoma-carcinoma sequence in large bowel. *Lancet*, 1: 245-7
Irving, D. and Drasar, B.S. (1973). Fibre and cancer of the colon. *British Journal of Cancer*, 28: 462-3
Jain, M., Cook, G.M., Davis, F.G., Grace, M.G., Howe, G.R. and Miller, A.B. (1980). A case-control study of diet and colo-rectal cancer. *International Journal of Cancer*, 26: 757-68
Jansson, B., Jacobs, M.M. and Griffin, A.C. (1978). Gastrointestinal cancer: Epidemiology and experimental studies. *Advances in Experimental Medicine and Biology*, 91: 305-22
Jensen, O.M. (1979). Cancer morbidity and causes of death among Danish brewery workers. *International Journal of Cancer*, 23: 454-63
Kark, J.D., Smith, A.H. and Hames, C.G. (1980). The relationship of serum cholesterol to the incidence of cancer in Evans County, Georgia. *Journal of Chronic Diseases*, 33: 311-22
Knox, E.G. (1977). Foods and diseases. *British Journal of Preventive and Social Medicine*, 31: 71-80

Kolonel, L.N., Hankin, J.H., Lee, J., Chu, S.Y., Nomura, A.M.Y. and Hinds, M.W. (1981). Nutrient intakes in realtion to cancer incidence in Hawaii. *British Journal of Cancer*, 44: 332-9

Kozarevic, Dj., McGee, D., Vojvodic, N., Gordon, T., Racic, Z., Zukel, W. *et al.* (1981). Serum cholesterol and mortality. The Yugoslavia cardiovascular disease study. *American Journal of Epidemiology*, 114: 21-8

Lee, J.A.H. (1976). Recent trends in large bowel cancer in Japan compared to United States and England and Wales. *International Journal of Epidemiology*, 5: 187-94

Lin, D.S. and Connor, W.E. (1980). The long term effects of dietary cholesterol upon the plasma lipids, lipoproteins, cholesterol absorption, and the sterol balance in man: the demonstration of feedback inhibition of cholesterol biosynthesis and increased bile acid excretion. *Journal of Lipid Research*, 21: 1042-52

Linos, D.A., Beard, C.M., O'Fallon, W.M., Dockerty, M.B., Beart, R.W. and Kurland, L.T. (1981). Cholecystectomy and carcinoma of the colon. *Lancet*, 2: 379-81

Lipworth, L.L. and Rice, C.A. (1979). Correlations in mortality data involving cancers of the colo-rectum and esophagus. *Cancer*, 43: 1927-33

Lui, K., Moss, D., Persky, V., Stamler, J., Garside, D. and Soltero, I. (1979). Dietary cholesterol, fat and fibre, and colon cancer mortality. An analysis of international data. *Lancet*, 2: 782-5

Lynch, H.T., Guirgis, H., Lynch, J., Brodkey, F.D. and Magee, H. (1975). Cancer of the colon: socio-economic variables in a community. *American Journal of Epidemiology*, 102: 119-27

—— Albana, W.A., Danes, B.S., Lynch, J. and Lynch, P.M. (1981). Precursor conditions and monitoring of high-risk colon cancer patients. In: Stroehlein, J.R. and Romsdahl, M.M. (eds.), *Gastrointestinal Cancer*, Raven Press, New York, pp. 297-325

Lyon, J.L. and Sorenson, A.W. (1978). Colon cancer in a low-risk population. *American Journal of Clinical Nutrition*, 31: S227-30

—— Gardner, J.W. and West, D.W. (1980). Cancer risk and life-style: Cancer among Mormons from 1967-1975. In: Cairns, J., Lyon, J.L. and Skolnick, M. (eds.), *Cancer Incidence in Defined Populations*, Banbury Report 4, Cold Spring Harbor Laboratory, Cold Spring Harbor, New York, pp. 3-27

MacLennan, R., Jensen, O.M., Mosbech, J. and Vuori, H. (1978). Diet, transit time, stool weight, and colon cancer in two Scandinavian populations. *American Journal of Clinical Nutrition*, 31: S239-42

Malhotra, S.L. (1977). Dietary factors in a study of cancer colon from cancer registry, with special reference to the role of saliva, milk and fermented milk products and vegetable fibre. *Medical Hypotheses*, 3: 122-6

Markman, M. (1982). Cholecystectomy and carcinoma of the colon. *Lancet*, 2: 47

Martinez, I., Torres, R., Frias, Z., Colon, J.R. and Fernandez, M. (1979). Factors associated with adenocarcinomas of the large bowel in Puerto Rico. In: Birch, J.M. (ed.), *Advances in Medical Oncology, Research and Education*, Vol. 3, Epidemiology, Pergamon Press, Oxford and New York, pp. 45-52

McMichael, A.J., Potter, J.D. and Hetzel, B.S. (1979). Time trends in colo-rectal cancer mortality in relation to food and alcohol consumption. United States, United Kingdom, Australia and New Zealand. *International Journal of Epidemiology*, 8: 295-303

—— and Potter, J.D. (1980). Reproduction, endogenous and exogenous sex hormones, and colon-cancer: A review and hypothesis. *Journal of the National Cancer Institute*, 65: 1201-7

—— McCall, M.G., Hartshorne, J.M. and Woodings, T.L. (1980). Patterns of gastro-intestinal cancer in European migrants to Australia: The role of dietary change. *International Journal of Cancer*, 25: 431-7

Miller, A.B. (1978a). Asbestos fibre dust and gastro-intestinal malignancies. Review of literature with regard to a cause–effect relationship. *Journal of Chronic Diseases*, 31: 23-33

—— (1978b). *Screening in Cancer*. UICC Technical Report Series – Volume 40. International Union Against Cancer, Geneva, pp. 306-33

—— (1982). Risk factors from geographic epidemiology for gastro-intestinal cancer. *Cancer*, 50: 2533-40

—— Barclay, T.H.C., Choi, N.W., Grace, M.G., Wall, C., Plante, M. *et al.* (1980). A study of cancer, parity and age at first pregnancy. *Journal of Chronic Diseases*, 33: 595-605

Miller, S.R., Tartter, P.I., Papatestas, A.E., Slater, G. and Aufses, A.H. (1981). Serum cholesterol and human colon cancer. *Journal of the National Cancer Institute*, 67: 297-300

Modan, B., Barrell, V., Lubin, F., Modan, M., Greenberg, R.A. and Graham, S. (1975). Low-fibre intake as an etiologic factor in cancer of the colon. *Journal of the National Cancer Institute*, 55: 15-18

Page, L. and Friend, B. (1978). The changing United States diet. *Bioscience*, 28: 192-7

Pearce, M.L. and Dayton, S. (1971). Incidence of cancer in men on a diet high in polyunsaturated fat. *Lancet*, 1: 464-7

Pernu, J. (1960). An epidemiological study of cancer of the digestive organs and respiratory system. *Annales Medicinae Interae Fenniae*, Suppl. 33: 1-117

Peterson, B., Trall, E. and Sternby, N.H. (1981). Low cholesterol level as risk factor for non-coronary death in middle-aged men. *Journal of the American Medical Association*, 245: 2056-60

Phillips, R.L. (1975). Role of life-style and dietary habits in risk of cancer among Seventh-Day Adventists. *Cancer Research*, 35: 3513-22

—— Kuzma, J.W. and Lotz, T.M. (1980). Cancer mortality among comparable members versus nonmembers of the Seventh Day Adventist Church. In: Cairns, J., Lyon, J.L. and Skolnick, M. (eds.), *Cancer Incidence in Defined Populations*, Banbury Report 4, Cold Spring Harbor Laboratory, Cold Spring Harbor, New York, pp. 93-102

Reddy, B.S. and Wynder, E.L. (1973). Large-bowel carcinogenesis: fecal constituents of populations with diverse incidence rates of colon cancer. *Journal of the National Cancer Institute*, 50: 1437-42

—— Hedges, A.R., Laakso, K. and Wynder, E.L. (1978). Metabolic epidemiology of large bowel cancer. Fecal bulk and constituents of high-risk North American and low-risk Finnish population. *Cancer*, 42: 2832-8

Rose, G., Blackburn, H., Keys, A., Taylor, H.L., Kannel, W.B., Paul, O. *et al.* (1974). Colon cancer and blood-cholesterol. *Lancet*, 1: 181-3

—— and Shipley, M.J. (1980). Plasma lipids and mortality: a source of error. *Lancet*, 1: 523-6

Schmidt, W. and Popham, R.E. (1981). The role of drinking and smoking in mortality from cancer and other causes in male alcoholics. *Cancer*, 47: 1031-41

Schottenfeld, D. and Winawer, S.J. (1982). Large intestine. In: Schottenfeld, D. and Fraumeni, J.F., Jr. (eds.), *Cancer Epidemiology and Prevention*, Saunders, Philadelphia, ch. 40, pp. 703-27

Stemmermann, G.N., Mandel, M. and Mower, H.F. (1979). Colon cancer: its precursors and companions in Hawaii Japanese. *National Cancer Institute Monograph*, 53: 175-9

—— Nomura, A.M.Y., Heilbrun, L.K., Pollack, E.S. and Kagan, A. (1981). Serum cholesterol and colon cancer incidence in Hawaiian Japanese men. *Journal of the National Cancer Institute*, 67: 1179-82

Stocks, P. (1957). Cancer incidence in North Wales and Liverpool region in relation to habits and environment. *British Empire Cancer Campaign 35th Annual Report*, Supplement to Part II, Cancer Research Campaign, London

Teppo, L., Pukkala, E., Hakama, M., Hakulinen, T., Herva, A. and Saxen, E. (1980). Way of life and cancer incidence in Finland. *Scandinavian Journal of Social Medicine*. Suppl. 19: 32-6

Vernick, L.J. and Kuller, L.H. (1981). Cholecystectomy and right-sided colon cancer: an epidemiological study. *Lancet*, 2: 381-3

—— and Kuller, L.H. (1982). A case-control study of cholecystectomy and right-side colon cancer. *American Journal of Epidemiology*, 116: 86-101

Weiss, N.S., Daling, J.R. and Chow, W.H. (1981). Incidence of cancer of the large bowel in women in relation to reproductive and hormonal factors. *Journal of the National Cancer Institute*, 67: 57-60

Williams, R.R., Sorlie, P.D., Feinleib, M., McNamara, P.M., Kannel, W.B. and Dawber, T.R. (1981). Cancer incidence by levels of cholesterol. *Journal of the American Medical Association*, 245: 247-52

Wynder, E.L. and Shigematsu, T. (1967). Environmental factors in cancer of the colon and rectum. *Cancer*, 20: 1520-61

10 CANCER OF THE UTERINE CERVIX
M. Hakama

Introduction

Cervical cancer is one of the most common cancers among females. The range of the age-adjusted (world standard population) incidence rates varies from 5 to 60 per 100,000 women-years between different countries (Waterhouse *et al.*, 1976). In the Nordic countries cervical cancer occupied second or third place among cancerous diseases in the early 1960s (Ringertz, 1971). Rapid changes in the risk of cervical cancer have occurred since then in several populations.

Cervical cancer has a relatively favourable prognosis and therefore mortality rates are generally less than one-half of the incidence rates. The good prognosis and low mean age at diagnosis give rise to a rather high prevalence (patients ever diagnosed as having this cancer and still alive) of the disease (Table 10.1).

Table 10.1: Incidence (1966-1970), Mortality (1966-1970) per 100,000 Woman-years and Prevalence (31 December 1970) per 100,000 Women of Invasive Cervical Cancer in Finland, given as rate, adjusted for age to the world standard population, and as a proportion of all cases

Indicator	Rate	Proportion
Incidence	13.6	7.4
Mortality	5.5	5.1
Prevalence	113.6	13.9

Source: Teppo *et al.*, 1975.

The great majority of cervical cancers are squamous-cell carcinomas. The remainder, approximately 10 per cent, include adenocarcinomas, sarcomas, etc. Incidence data usually refer to all types of cervical cancer while consideration of risk factors and natural history mainly concern squamous-cell carcinomas. There is some evidence that adenocarcinoma of the uterine cervix is epidemiologically different from squamous-cell carcinoma and is closer to adenocarcinoma of the endometrium.

It is assumed that cervical cancer progresses through pre-invasive stages, dysplasia and carcinoma *in situ*, and that the duration of cervical intra-epithelial neoplasia is several years, and possibly even longer. The figures for the occurrence of cervical cancer include the invasive cases only. However, when evaluating the effect of risk factors, the cases sometimes also include pre-invasive lesions.

Time Trends and Geographical Variation

Cervical cancer mortality rates have shown a decreasing trend in several populations (Segi, 1979). In addition to the true occurrence of the disease the changes in mortality are also attributable to clinical efficacy, but comparison of the age-adjusted incidence rates based on different volumes of *Cancer Incidence in Five Continents* (Doll *et al.*, 1970; Waterhouse *et al.*, 1976) reveals that there has also been about a 2-3 per cent annual decrease in the incidence rates as well. Figure 10.1 shows the correlation between the incidence rates reported in the second volume (around 1965) and third volume (around 1970) of *Cancer Incidence in Five Continents*.

Incidence rates for cervical cancer increase rapidly up to the age of menopause, after which there is a levelling-off. The decrease in incidence has mainly affected the younger age groups, and so the rapid increase in rates by age has moved upwards to older age groups. In Finland the decrease in incidence was 70 per cent or more in the 35-50 years age group over a period of 20 years (Figure 10.2), whereas very small changes occurred in the older age groups.

The greatest geographical differences are reported between the female populations in South American countries (highest) and Israel (lowest). High rates are also found among the United States of America (USA) non-white population, the Jamaican population, and some populations in Africa and Central Europe (Waterhouse *et al.*, 1976). In Israel, the United Kingdom, the USA (white) and Hungary the rates of cervical cancer are low.

Both time trends and geographical differences agree with the observation of a relationship between the risk of cervical cancer and low socioeconomic status. Clemmesen and Nielsen (1951) grouped Copenhagen's subdistricts into five classes according to economic status and found a social gradient unfavourable for the poor. The risk in the poorest areas was about three times as high as that in the richest class.

Figure 10.1: Age-adjusted Incidence Rates (per 100,000 woman-years) for Cervical Cancer around 1965 and around 1970

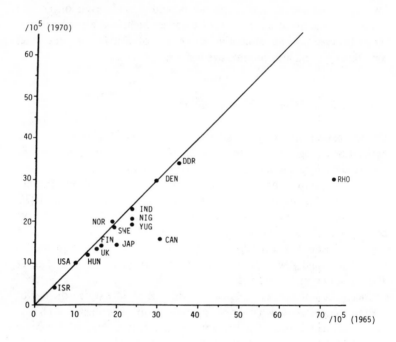

Key: Nigeria, Ibadan (NIG); Rhodesia, Bulawayo (RHO); Canada, Quebec (CAN); USA, Connecticut (USA); India, Bombay (IND); Israel, Jews (ISR); Japan, Miyagi (JAP); Denmark (DEN); Finland (FIN); German Democratic Republic (DDR); Hungary, Szabolcs-Szatmar (HUN); Norway (NOR); Sweden (SWE); UK, Birmingham (UK) and Yugoslavia (YUG).

Source: Doll *et al.*, 1970; Waterhouse *et al.*, 1976.

Socioeconomic status either describes the general or macro-environment or is related to the individual's personal characteristics, i.e. to the micro-environment. It is likely that the latter is a determinant of the high risk of cervical cancer. In Finland the risk of cervical cancer was also highest among females with low socioeconomic status and little education. When geographical areas were examined those areas with a high risk of cervical cancer had a large proportion of the population in the upper social classes and many indicators of a high standard of living. Thus, indicators for the macro-environment were the opposite of those for the micro-environment (Hakama *et al.*, 1982).

Figure 10.2: Age-specific Incidence Rates of Cervical Cancer in Finland, 1953-57 and 1973-77

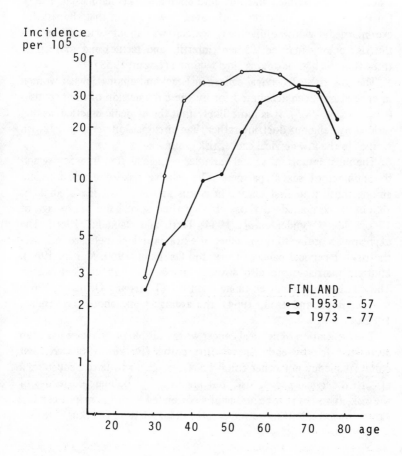

Source: Finnish Cancer Registry

Reproductive and Sexual Determinants

Reproduction and sexual habits are strongly influenced by sociocultural habits and socioeconomic position. There is a correlation between early sexual experience and low social status, and it is likely that the differences in the risk of cervical cancer by socioeconomic status are largely accounted for by sexual habits.

One of the classic results in cancer epidemiology was published by Rigoni Stern in 1842. He found that cervical cancer was common among married women and very rare among nuns (Clemmesen, 1965). On the basis of population death rates, it was shown that the risk for ever-married (widowed/divorced) women was about twice as high as the risk among married women (infertile and fertile) and more than three times as high as among single women (Logan, 1953).

The low risk of cervical cancer in Israel and among Jewish women in general has been accounted for by the circumcision of their spouses (Clemmesen, 1965). It is more likely that the hygienic practices as prescribed by religious doctrine rather than circumcision *per se* put Jewish women in the low cervical cancer risk groups.

The most important sexual variables are age at first intercourse and the number of sexual partners. The relative risk of cervical cancer among those who first engage in coitus at the age of less than 17 is about 2.5 compared to those starting their sexual life at the age of 17 or older (Wynder *et al.*, 1954; Terris and Oalmann, 1960). The exposure according to the number of extramarital partners also increases the risk of cervical cancer (Terris and Oalmann, 1960; Martin, 1967). Multiple marriages are also strongly associated with cervical cancer. The relative risks reported range from 4.7 (Terris and Oalmann, 1960) to 1.7 (Boyd and Doll, 1964), the average being about 2.6 (Hulka, 1982).

The association of cervical cancer with multiple pregnancies has been accounted for by early age at first coitus (Rotkin, 1967). Neither coital frequency nor other coital practices appear to have a substantial effect on cervical cancer risk, but are likely to be mere correlates of the risk. It seems that sexual habits correlated with the risk of cervical cancer are a result of more and earlier sexual relations (Rotkin, 1981).

Contraception

The effect of any contraceptive method on the risk of cervical cancer seems to be limited. Rotkin (1967) found a significantly higher use of diaphragm, jelly and rhythm methods among controls than among patients with cervical cancer, whereas Martin (1967) reported a higher proportion of sheath contraception among the control women. These studies antedate the frequent use of intrauterine devices and oral contraceptives. A review by Rotkin (1973) suggested that a barrier method protects against cervical cancer.

Steroid hormones have been commonly used for contraceptive purposes during the last two decades. Oral contraceptives and intrauterine devices have been subjected to frequent epidemiological studies, with inconsistent results (Hulka, 1982; Report of a WHO Scientific Group, 1978). Vessey *et al.*, (1976) reported no higher risk of cervical intraepithelial lesions among oral contraceptive users than among the users of intrauterine devices. It can be concluded that the effect of oral contraceptives, if any, is only one of promotion (Hulka, 1982).

Elimination of confounding factors is difficult and therefore many of the results are not easy to interpret. Because a long latent period is assumed from the first exposure to the diagnosis of epithelial tumours, and because both oral contraceptives and intrauterine devices are used relatively early in life — which is also likely to be the most vulnerable time — it is possible that not enough evidence has accumulated and cases potentially related to contraception have not yet appeared.

Viral (HSV-2) Hypothesis

All the observations on the risk factors of cervical cancer support the hypothesis of a transmissible agent being involved in its aetiology. A great deal has been written about herpes simplex virus type 2 (HSV-2) and other micro-organisms and gynaecological cancer (Aurelian *et al.*, 1981; Melnick *et al.*, 1974; Nahmias and Sawanabori, 1978). Furthermore, a close relationship between the presence of antibodies to HSV-2 and cervical cancer or preinvasive cervical lesions has been demonstrated. However, several limitations prevent interpretation of a causal relationship from these data.

The accuracy of the assay methods for detecting infection with HSV-2 is likely to vary. Seroepidemiological neutralising techniques have resulted in the prevalence of positive antibody findings from 15 to 100 per cent among the cervical cancer patients and from 7 to 77 per cent among the controls (Rawls and Adam, 1977). The relative risk of cervical cancer among women with antibodies to HSV-2 compared to those without antibodies varied, according to different studies, from less than unity to more than 10 (Melnick *et al.*, 1974), with an average of about 5.

The virological methods of detecting virus-associated antibodies have yielded consistently different results from those above (Aurelian *et al.*, 1981). Cervical cancer patients are positive for antibody against at least two viral antigens designated VP 143 and AG-4 (an antigen that is immunologically identical to ICP 10, an early viral protein) (Aurelian *et al.*, 1981). In different studies the percentage of subjects with antibodies to early viral antigens ranged from 44 to 93 per cent among the cases and from 0 to 40 per cent among controls. As a rule, greater differences were found between cases and controls than by neutralising techniques (Table 10.2). The median relative risk in these studies was 18.

Table 10.2: Relative Risks of Cervical Cancer in Women with Antibodies to Early Viral Antigens

Study population	Antigen	Relative risk
Maryland	AG-4	42
Texas	VP 143	20
Pennsylvania	AG-4	9
Tokyo I	AG-4	18
Tokyo II	AG-4	15
Australia	AG-4	17

Source: Aurelian *et al.*, 1981 (amended data).

Different interpretations have been derived from these results (Aurelian *et al.*, 1981; Rotkin, 1981). The three alternatives are that (1) HSV-2 is an aetiological factor in cervical cancer; (2) cervical cancer patients are susceptible to HSV-2 infection; or (3) HSV-2 is a mere correlate of cervical cancer, indicating another causative factor which is also related to sexual habits.

Cohort studies have shown an increased risk of preclinical cervical lesions associated with HSV-2 infection (Nahmias *et al.*, 1973). The available results combined with other evidence make it unlikely – but not impossible – that HSV-2 infection follows carcinoma or a preinvasive lesion.

The assessment of confounding due to sexual and reproductive factors is incomplete in most studies that show an association between HSV-2 and cervical cancer. Most of the studies are small and do not allow cross-classification by several risk factors, and attempts with multivariate methods have been infrequent. In a recent study Graham *et al.* (1982) showed a more than three times higher risk of cervical cancer among women radio-immuno-assay-positive for HSV-2 than among HSV-2 negative women. The effect in terms of relative risk was similar for those with at most one sex partner and for those with at least two sex partners. On the other hand, the increase in risk due to increase in the number of sex partners disappeared after adjusting for HSV-2 infection.

The strength of the association, the high prevalence of the exposure, overall consistency of the results and similarities in the literature indicate that HSV-2 infection is an important risk indicator of cervical cancer. Assuming that the assay techniques are sufficiently reliable, that the relative risk is about 20 and that 20 per cent of the population (controls) are infected, the proportion of cervical cancer cases associated with HSV-2 out of all cases of cervical cancer in the population (the population attributable risk per cent) would be about 80 per cent. If the true relative risk is only five, the population attributable risk per cent would still be close to 50. On the other hand, the observed relative risks and the probable multiple aetiology of epithelial cancer in general indicate that HSV-2 is not the only risk factor and infection will only seldom result in a malignant growth. With future improvements in assay techniques (Rawls and Adam, 1977), the estimates of the importance of HSV-2 infection as a risk factor of cervical cancer are likely to change.

Even though the observation is well in agreement with the viral hypothesis, its credibility has been challenged (Rawls and Adam 1977; Rotkin, 1981).

Other Infections

Several other sexually transmissible agents have been proposed to be high risk factors for cervical cancer. These include chlamydia, mycoplasma and cytomegalovirus (Alexander, 1973). Dysplasia and cervical cancer were reported to be associated with condylomata (Syrjänen, 1980) and there was a correlation between trichomonas vaginalis and cervical cancer and preinvasive lesions in a large mass screening programme (Kauraniemi *et al.*, 1978). The high risk of syphilis among cervical cancer patients was first reported at the beginning of this century (Clemmesen, 1965). There is not enough evidence to be able to assess the role of these other venereal diseases in the risk of cervical cancer.

Strong support for the involvement of an infectious agent in the aetiology of cervical cancer is provided by the effect of the sexual habits of husbands on the risk of cervical cancer of their wives. Buckley *et al.* (1981) studied the number of sexual partners of the husbands of patients with dysplasia or cervical cancer. These patients claimed in a previous study to have had only one sexual partner, their husbands. The husbands of the patients were compared with the husbands of a control group of women with one sexual partner and matched for age and age at first intercourse. They found that the number of sexual partners of the husband was a strong risk factor with a relative risk of 7.8 for 15 or more partners outside marriage.

In short, it seems that these findings are not in agreement with the hypothesis that a transmissible agent is only a correlate of aetiological factors. Because of the probable multiple aetiology and the conceptual importance of the infectious aetiology of an epithelial cancer, many authors will be hesitant to accept cervical cancer as a communicable disease, even if it is clearly the most credible explanation of the multitude of epidemiological and other observations.

Smoking

Several epidemiological studies have shown an association between cigarette smoking and cervical cancer (Winkelstein, 1977). The association was interpreted to be due to the strong correlation between smoking and sexual habits, but an adjustment for socioeconomic status and sexual habits is not likely to remove the association (Buckley et al., 1981; Clarke et al., 1982). Winkelstein (1977) suggested that smoking is causally related to cervical cancer. This hypothesis is supported by the dose-response relationship (Buckley et al., 1981; Clarke et al., 1982), by the morphological similarities and by similarities in the risks of cervical cancer with well-established tobacco-related cancers (Winkelstein, 1977), and by biological plausibility (Petrakis et al., 1978).

Natural History of Cervical Cancer

Screening programmes practised all over the world have shed light on the natural history of cervical cancer. Cervical cancer is regarded as the most typical example of cancerous disease with a preclinical phase detectable for a long time (Dunn, 1953). Incidence rates of severe dysplasias seem to be at a maximum at very young ages, whereas carcinoma *in situ* lesions have the highest incidence at the age of about 35 and invasive cervical cancer shows an increasing trend in incidence up to the age of 50, after which the age-specific rates become stable (Hakama and Räsänen-Virtanen 1976; Waterhouse *et al.*, 1976). Many studies have shown a difference of five years or more between the mean ages of women with pre-invasive lesions and invasive cervical cancer. However, differences depend on the intensity of screening by age.

Some of the pre-invasive lesions are not likely to progress to invasive cancer. Epidemiological estimates from Canada (Fidler *et al.*, 1968) and Finland (Hakama and Räsänen-Virtanen, 1976) indicate that about 30 to 40 per cent of pre-invasive lesions subjected to surgical treatment would have progressed to invasive cancer if left untreated. Histological classification has a poor reproducibility (Hulme *et al.*, 1968) and it is likely that there is a great deal of variation between cytopathologists and countries. On the other hand, some cervical cancers have a very short preclinical phase, and in general there are no satisfactory estimates of the distribution of the length of the preclinical phase.

There is epidemiological (Ashley, 1966; Hakama and Penttinen, 1981) and clinical (Hakama and West, 1980) evidence in favour of the hypothesis that the rate of growth of the tumour and the age of the patient are correlated in cervical cancer. It is likely that a tumour detected at a young age grows more slowly (and will be easier to diagnose at the pre-invasive or localised stage) than tumours diagnosed at older ages. Hence, age differences at diagnosis between carcinomas *in situ*, localised and non-localised cancers are likely to indicate differences in the biological behaviour of the disease by age rather than advancement in the time of diagnosis, i.e. differences in patient and/or doctor delay.

Efficacy of Screening Programmes

Even if the natural history of cervical cancer is likely to be incompletely understood, this does not necessarily affect the efficacy of the screening programmes themselves. It has been rather conclusively demonstrated that screening for cervical cancer affects the incidence and mortality of the disease, especially in the younger age groups (Miller, 1978).

There are likely to be differences in the efficacy of the screening programmes. The programmes that have an organisation of their own, use personal letters of invitation and are conducted free of charge seem to have a substantial effect on the risk. Such organised programmes are carried out in several of the Nordic countries (Hakama, 1982). In

Finland, Iceland and Sweden these programmes cover the entire female population at the age of high risk of the disease, and since the mid-1960s every woman is screened at two-three (Iceland) to five (Finland) year intervals. In Denmark about 40 per cent of the population is covered by organised screening, and in Norway the coverage is about 5 per cent. At the same time smears are frequently taken during routine gynaecological examinations in all the Nordic countries. The time trends of incidence of cervical cancer showed a strong correlation with the intensity of the organised screening programmes (Hakama, 1982). It was predicted that the organised screening programme for cervical cancer in Finland will result in a reduction of about 60 per cent in the incidence of frankly invasive cancer among the total female population (Hakama and Räsänen-Virtanen, 1976). The observed time trends seem to confirm this estimate.

Survival

Nationwide, population-based survival figures of cervical cancer are known from Denmark, Finland and Norway (Cutler, 1964; Cancer Registry of Norway, 1980; Hakulinen *et al.*, 1981) and regional population-based survival statistics have been published, e.g. in Connecticut, in Birmingham and in South Wales (Cutler, 1964; Hakama and West, 1980; Waterhouse, 1974).

The relative (corrected for normal mortality) five-year survival rates around 1970 were about 100 per cent for the carcinoma *in situ* patients, more than 80 per cent for those with localised carcinoma, and 30-40 per cent for patients with a non-localised carcinoma. There is a substantial variation in the ratio of the number of localised to non-localised tumours (from one-third to two-thirds of all invasive cases being localised). This tends to make comparison of the overall survival meaningless.

For all the cervical cancer patients diagnosed in Finland in 1953-74, the mean expected length of life at the time of diagnosis was 13 years and the general population at the same age had an expected length of life of 24 years. Hence the average patient lost 45 per cent of her remaining life span, the loss being 39 per cent for the localised and 69 per cent for the non-localised cases (Hakulinen *et al.*, 1981).

After five to ten years of follow-up, patients with most epithelial tumours again have a normal expected life span. Cervical cancer seems to be an exception and there is a small but persistent excess risk of death for more than 20 years after the diagnosis (Hakulinen *et al.*, 1981).

Conclusion

In many populations cervical cancer has been and still is one of the most common female cancers. Whether caused by a viral infection or otherwise related to marital, reproductive and sexual habits, cervical cancer is closely related to sexual mores. Therefore, it is likely that without improvement in socioeconomic conditions (hygiene) and preventive measures (screening) there would be an increase in the risk of cervical cancer with time. The overall decrease in the incidence of cervical cancer is supportive evidence in favour of the efficacy of these measures.

References

Alexander, E.R. (1973). Possible aetiologies of cancer of the cervix other than herpesvirus. *Cancer Research*, 33: 1485-96

Ashley, D.J. (1966). The biological status of carcinoma *in situ* of the uterine cervix. *British Journal of Obstetrics and Gynaecology*, 73: 372-81

Aurelian, L., Kessler, I.I., Rosenshein, N.B. and Barbour, G. (1981). Viruses and gynecologic cancers: Herpesvirus protein (ICP 0/AG-4), a cervical tumor antigen that fulfils the criteria for a marker of carcinogenicity. *Cancer*, 48: 455-71

Boyd, J.D. and Doll, R. (1964). A study of the aetiology of carcinoma of the cervix uteri. *British Journal of Cancer*, 18: 419-34

Buckley, J.D., Harris, R.W.C., Doll, R., Vessey, M.P. and Williams, P.T. (1981). Case-control study of the husbands of women with dysplasia or carcinoma of the cervix uteri. *Lancet*, 2: 1010-14

Cancer Registry of Norway (1980). *Survival of Cancer Patients. Cases Diagnosed in Norway 1968-1975*. Oslo

Clarke, E.A., Morgan, R.W. and Newman, A.M. (1982). Smoking as a risk factor in cancer of the cervix: Additional evidence from a case-control study. *American Journal of Epidemiology*, 115: 59-66

Clemmesen, J. (1965). Statistical studies in the aetiology of malignant neoplasms. *Acta Pathologica et Microbiologica Scandinavica*, Suppl. 174, ch. 26, pp. 277-330

────── and Nielsen, A. (1951). The social distribution of cancer in Copenhagen 1943 to 1947. *British Journal of Cancer*, 5: 159-71

Cutler, S.J. (ed.) (1964). *International Symposium on End Results of Cancer Therapy*. National Cancer Institute Monographs No. 15, pp. 51-103

Doll, R., Muir, C. and Waterhouse, J. (eds.) (1970). *Cancer Incidence in Five Continents*. Vol. II. International Union Against Cancer, Springer Verlag, Berlin

Dunn, J.E. (1953). The relationship between carcinoma *in situ* and invasive cervical carcinoma. *Cancer*, 6: 873-86

Fidler, H.K., Boyes, D.A. and Worth, A.J. (1968). Cervical cancer detection in British Columbia. *Journal of Obstetrics and Gynaecology of the British Commonwealth*, 75: 392-404

Graham, S., Rawls, W. Swanson, M. and McCurtis, J. (1982). Sex partners and herpes simplex virus type 2 in the epidemiology of cancer of the cervix. *American Journal of Epidemiology*, 115: 729-35

Hakama, M. (1982). Trends in the incidence of cervical cancer in the Nordic countries. In: Magnus, K. (ed.), *Trends in Cancer Incidence*, Hemisphere, Washington, ch. 6, pp. 279-92

—— and Räsänen-Virtanen, U. (1976). Effect of a mass screening program on the risk of cervical cancer. *American Journal of Epidemiology*, 103: 512-17

—— and West, R. (1980). Cervical cancer in Finland and South Wales: implications of end results data on the natural history. *Journal of Epidemiology and Community Health*, 34: 14-18

—— and Penttinen, J. (1981). Epidemiological evidence for two components of cervical cancer. *British Journal of Obstetrics and Gynaecology*, 88: 209-14

—— Hakulinen, T., Pukkala, E., Saxen, E. and Teppo, L. (1982). Risk indicators of breast and cervical cancer on ecological and individual levels. *American Journal of Epidemiology*, 116: 990-1000

Hakulinen, T., Pukkala, E., Hakama, M., Lehtonen, M., Saxen, E. and Teppo, L. (1981). Survival of cancer patients in Finland in 1953-1974. *Annals of Clinical Research*, 13 (Suppl. 31): pp. 50-2

Hulka, B.S. (1982). Risk factors for cervical cancer. *Journal of Chronic Diseases*, 35: 3-11

Hulme, G.W., Eisenberg, H.S. and Campbell, P.C. (1968). Carcinoma *in situ* of the cervix in Connecticut: A review 1949-1962. *American Journal of Obstetrics and Gynecology*, 102: 415-25

Kauraniemi, T., Räsänen-Virtanen, U. and Hakama, M. (1978). Risk of cervical cancer among an electrocoagulated population. *American Journal of Obstetrics and Gynecology*, 131: 533-8

Logan, W.P.D. (1953) Marriage and childbearing in relation to cancer of the breast and uterus. *Lancet*, 265: 1199-202

Martin, C.E. (1967). Marital and coital factors in cervical cancer. *American Journal of Public Health*, 57: 803-14

Melnick, J.L., Adam, E. and Rawls, W.E. (1974). The causative role of herpesvirus type 2 in cervical cancer. *Cancer*, 34: 1375-87

Miller, A.B. (ed.) (1978). *Screening in Cancer*. UICC Technical Report series No. 40, UICC, Geneva

Nahmias, A.J., Naib, Z.M. and Josey, W.E. (1973). Prospective studies of the association of genital herpes simplex infection and cervical anaplasia. *Cancer Research*, 33: 1491-7

—— and Sawanabori, S. (1978). The genital herpes cervical cancer hypothesis – 10 years later. *Progress in Experimental Tumor Research*, 21: 117-39

Petrakis, N.L., Gruenke, L.D., Beeler, T.C., Gastagnoli, N., Jr. and Graig, J.C. (1978). Nicotine in breast fluid of non-lactating women. *Science*, 199: 303-5

Rawls, W.E. and Adam, E. (1977). Herpes simplex viruses and human malignancies. In: Hiatt, H.H., Watson, J.T. and Winston, J.T. (eds.), *Origins of Human Cancer Book B. Mechanism of Carcinogenesis*, Cold Spring Harbor conferences on cell proliferation, Vol. 4, Cold Spring Harbor, New York, pp. 1133-55

Report of a WHO Scientific Group (1978). *Steroid Contraception and the Risk of Neoplasia*. Technical Report Series 619, World Health Organization, Geneva

Ringertz, N. (ed.) (1971). Cancer incidence in Finland, Iceland, Norway and

Sweden. A comparative study. *Acta Pathologica et Microbiologica Scandinavica*, Section A, Suppl. 224

Rotkin, I.D. (1967). Epidemiology of cancer of the cervix. III. Sexual characteristics of a cervical cancer population. *American Journal of Public Health*, 57: 815-29

—— (1973). A comparison review of key epidemiological studies in cervical cancer related to current searches for transmissible agents. *Cancer Research*, 33: 1353-67

—— (1981). Etiology and epidemiology of cervical cancer. In: Dallenbach-Hellweg, G. (ed.), *Cervical Cancer*, Springer Verlag, Berlin, Heidelberg, New York, ch. 2, pp. 81-110

Segi, M. (1979). *Age-adjusted Death Rates for Cancer for Selected Sites (A-classification) in 51 Countries in 1974*. Segi Institute of Cancer Epidemiology, Nagoya, p. 4

Syrjänen, K. (1980). Condylomatous lesions in dysplastic and neoplastic epithelioma of the uterine cervix. *Surgery, Gynecology and Obstetrics*, 150: 272-6

Teppo, L., Hakama, M., Hakulinen, T., Lehtonen, M. and Saxen, E. (1975). Cancer in Finland 1953-70: Incidence, mortality, prevalence. *Acta Pathologica et Microbiologica Scandinavica*, Section A, Suppl. 252, pp. 38-41

Terris, M. and Oalmann, M.C. (1960). Carcinoma of the cervix: an epidemiological study. *Journal of the American Medical Association*, 174: 155-9

Vessey, M., Doll, R., Peto, R., Johnson, B. and Wiggins, P. (1976). A long term follow-up study of women using different methods of contraception – an interim report. *Journal of Biosocial Sciences*, 8: 373-427

Waterhouse, J.A.H. (1974). *Cancer Handbook of Epidemiology and Prognosis*. Churchill Livingstone, Edinburgh, pp. 144-5

Waterhouse, J., Muir, C., Correa, P. and Powell, J. (eds.) (1976). *Cancer Incidence in Five Continents*. Vol. III, IARC Scientific Publications No. 15, International Agency for Research on Cancer, Lyon

Winkelstein, W. (1977). Smoking and cancer of the uterine cervix: Hypothesis. *American Journal of Epidemiology*, 106: 257-9

Wynder, E.L., Cornfield, J., Schroff, P.D. and Doraiswami, K.R. (1954). A study of environmental factors in carcinoma of the cervix. *American Journal of Obstetrics and Gynecology*, 68: 1016-52

11 CANCER OF THE UTERINE BODY, OVARY AND VAGINA

J.G. Stolk and J. de Graaff

Cancer of the Uterine Body

Introduction

In the Western world endometrial carcinoma is one of the most common malignancies in the female pelvis. In the United States of America (USA) it is more common than carcinoma of the ovary and cervix combined while in some other countries it is as common as cervical carcinoma. Whether or not this situation is due to a real increase in the incidence of endometrial carcinoma or to a decline in cervical carcinoma is still undecided.

Incidence

The worldwide annual incidence of endometrial cancer has been reported as 20 per 100,000 females (Lauritzen, 1977). It is, however, doubtful if it is possible to present reliable figures on the international incidence of this condition for a number of reasons. First, there appears to be wide variation in the proportion of tumours which are histologically confirmed, even in countries with excellent medical care. Secondly, the primary diagnosis of invasive carcinoma is not infrequently reclassified to benign adenomatous hyperplasia after review by an independent pathologist (Mack and Casagrande, 1981); and thirdly, in reports on incidence rates a substantial number of other neoplasms, such as sarcomas of the uterine body, are included with the classification of 'unspecified' neoplasm of the uterus.

    The general consensus is that during the last few decades there has probably been an increase in the incidence of endometrial carcinoma in various countries but it is not easy to substantiate this. Reports from Japan, the Netherlands, Norway and the USA suggest an increase in these countries (Masabuchi *et al.*, 1975; de Graaff and Stolte, 1976; Gusberg, 1976; Weiss *et al.*, 1976). In the USA the incidence rate nearly doubled from 1970 through 1974 and thereafter the incidence rate dropped significantly between 1975 and 1977. Although it is widely recognised that the spectacular rise and fall in frequency coincides with the use of conjugated oestrogens by American women over 50 years of age (Quint, 1975), other factors must also be considered.

It should be emphasised that a similar increase in the incidence rates in the last two decades has also been observed in countries where replacement therapy with oestrogens has not been practised on a large scale (Creasman and Weed, 1981). Several factors could have contributed to the increase in the incidence of endometrial carcinoma (Greenblatt and Stoddard, 1978). These include: (1) more cases detected due to an increase in the frequency of medical examination; (2) more women reaching the critical age for the development of endometrial carcinoma due to a general increase in life expectancy; (3) better diagnostic tools and broadening of criteria for diagnosis; (4) environmental and unknown factors including the use of sequential contraceptive therapy and of conjugated oestrogens.

Age-adjusted Incidence and Socioeconomic Status

The age-specific rates of endometrial cancer show a rapidly increasing incidence from age 40 years to a peak in the postmenopausal period (Mack, 1977; Waterhouse *et al.*, 1976). Impressive variations in age-adjusted incidence have been reported among various ethnic groups internationally. The rates are particularly high in white populations and highest on the Pacific coast of North America. They are lowest in Africa and the rates in Europe are intermediate in value. The socioeconomic status appears to be of significance (Mack and Casagrande, 1981). In white women in Los Angeles county of high socioeconomic status the age-adjusted incidence rate of endometrial carcinoma is almost double that of women of low socioeconomic status. An increase in risk for women of high social status in the USA has also been reported by other authors (Cramer *et al.*, 1974; Mack, 1978).

Mortality

Any attempt to draw conclusions from mortality rates of endometrial cancer meets with substantial problems. There may be considerable variation between countries in the extent to which uterine cancers are classified as malignancies of the cervix, of the corpus or of the uterus 'unspecified' (Clarke, 1978). For example, in the Netherlands (Netherlands CBS, 1980) the mortality from malignant neoplasm of the cervix is reported separately from that due to malignant neoplasms of corpus uteri and uterus 'unspecified'. The age-adjusted mortality due to malignant neoplasm of the corpus uteri and uterus 'unspecified' per 100,000 females has fallen from a rate of 6.5 in 1969 to just over 5.0 in 1978 while mortality by age from these conditions has been increasing steadily.

The five-year survival of the cases treated from 1969 through 1972 has been reported by Kottmeier (1979). The histological grade and the clinical stage of the tumour are both important factors for survival and poorly differentiated (grade 3) tumours have the worst prognosis. Mortality rates have benefited from the recently improved methods for early detection of endometrial carcinoma. The tumour is now usually detected at an earlier stage and is more likely to be confined to the endometrium with only limited invasion of the myometrium.

Aetiology

Endometrial cancer belongs to the group of 'hormone-dependent' tumours. Hormone receptors for oestrogens (ER) and progesterone (PgR) in the cytoplasm and the nuclei are detected in the well-differentiated carcinomas while anaplastic tumours appear to lose the ability to synthesise hormone receptors. The premalignant conditions of endometrial carcinoma (the various stages of atypical adenomatous hyperplasia) have a high concentration of oestrogen receptors. Therefore it is not surprising that changes in the hormonal pattern of the patient may contribute to malignancy in the endometrium.

Familial Cancer. The familial history of patients with endometrial cancer shows a greater than expected frequency of this cancer in first-degree relatives. It is known that breast cancer and endometrial cancer are often associated both in individuals and in families (Lynch *et al.*, 1976) but the relative contributions of genetic and environmental factors have not been clearly elucidated (Mack and Casagrande, 1981). Among populations in which breast cancer and ovarian cancer are common there is also a high frequency of endometrial carcinoma (Fox, 1976).

Parity. Women of high parity appear to have relatively low risk for endometrial cancer and the highest risk seems to be with nulliparous women (Elwood *et al.*, 1977; MacMahon, 1974).

Late Menopause. Those with early menarche and late menopause are considered to be at higher risk than women who reach menarche late and finish their menstrual life before the age of 50 years.

Obesity. Obese women certainly represent an unfavourable group with regard to endometrial cancer and of all the endocrine disturbances that have been connected with endometrial cancer, only obesity has been shown to be associated with an increased risk of developing this condition. Frick *et al.* (1973) reported the association of abnormal carbohydrate tolerance, and furthermore 25 per cent of patients with endometrial carcinoma are found to have hypertension or arterio-sclerotic heart disease (Creasman and Weed, 1981). The associations with diabetes mellitus and hypertension are probably mediated through obesity. None of these conditions has, however, been shown to have any influence on malignant growth of the endometrium. The long accepted hypothesis that there is an underlying endocrine or metabolic disease in patients with endometrial carcinoma has yet to be substan-tiated. The exception to this is the condition of unopposed output of excessive endogenous oestrogens, but in non-obese women who are in the early postmenopausal years the presence of an endometrial carci-noma appears not to be related to metabolic disturbance (Lucas and Yen, 1979).

Oestrogens. The relationship between oestrogens and the development of first hyperplastic and later on malignant changes in the endometrium has been supported by clinical and laboratory studies. Exogenous oestrogens are able to produce tumours in experimental animals in hormone-sensitive tissues (Richardson and MacLaughlin, 1978). Patients with oestrogen-producing tumours of the ovary and patients with the polycystic ovarian syndrome show a higher incidence of endometrial carcinoma. An increase in the use of oestrogens among patients with endometrial cancer has been observed. This applies to the use of conju-gated oestrogens as replacement therapy for postmenopausal patients and to the use of oral sequential contraceptives by women under the age of 40 years (Smith *et al.*, 1975; Silverberg *et al.*, 1977).

Both studies and experiments have led to the formulation of the hypothesis of 'unopposed oestrogen action' (Kistner, 1966; Gusberg, 1976). Briefly this hypothesis states that oestrogens, by accelerating the role of cell proliferation and possible additional effects, generate abnormal cells. In most women these effects of oestrogens are opposed by progestagens and then no abnormalities will occur (King, 1978).

The Woman at Risk for Endometrial Cancer

It has been suggested that many of the factors associated with the development of endometrial carcinoma, such as exposure to exogenous oestrogens, obesity and diminished parity, are intensified in the Western world on a large scale (Gusberg and Frick, 1981; Cohen, 1981a). The woman who is over 50 years old, obese, nulliparous, in high socio-economic status and taking oestrogens continuously and unopposed by progesterone, is considered to be at risk (MacMahon, 1974).

It seems clear that oestrogens – endogenous and exogenous, synthetic or natural – can all lead to hyperplasia and endometrial cancer in some women (Jones, 1982).

After the menopause the principal sources of oestrogen are considered to be the extraglandular conversion of circulating androstenedione to oestrone and of testosterone to oestradiol, both in the subcutaneous fat. The quantity of available fat and the age of the woman determine the percentage of androstenedione conversion. The older woman even without marked obesity has a three- to four-fold greater capability for extraglandular oestrogen production than a young woman of similar body weight (Hemsell *et al.*, 1974).

Preventive Measures and Screening

An ever growing number of women in the Western world reach the age of real risk without their uterus. In the Netherlands the percentage of women who have undergone hysterectomy before the age of 60 years is estimated at more than 30 per cent. In the USA this percentage was estimated in the mid-1960s as approximately 50 per cent of women by the age of 65. It is presumed that subsequent birth cohorts will have experienced higher cumulative hysterectomy rates as they pass through a given age (Lyon and Gardner, 1977). It is regrettable that the rates of uterine cancer are expressed per population unit and have no reference to the rates per intact uterus. Screening of women at high risk, especially those who take oestrogens, is advocated on an individual basis. Diagnosis of premalignant conditions such as atypical hyperplastic changes could be made by endometrial suction and curettage. No attempt has been made for the organisation of large-scale population screening with regard to costs and effectiveness.

The indications for and the risks from long-term postmenopausal oestrogen replacement therapy are still under discussion. It is clear that both the beneficial effects of long-term conjugated oestrogen therapy and the risks must be considered individually before a decision can be taken. The protective effect of oestrogens against osteoporotic fractures in women in whom both ovaries have been removed certainly acts as a positive argument for replacement therapy (Cohen, 1981b). The apparent increase of both endometrial and breast cancer incidences after prolonged and high dosage of oestrogens are considerations on the risk side. If oestrogen therapy is considered necessary, the risk should be minimised by prescribing the lowest dose that will control symptoms while administration should be cyclic (three weeks on and one week off). Moreover, it should be borne in mind that the oestrogen-associated endometrial cancers in general are the well-differentiated types with an excellent prognosis (Underwood *et al.*, 1979). Additionally it must be emphasised that 99 per cent of the postmenopausal oestrogen users never acquire endometrial cancer (Weiss, 1978).

Ovarian Cancer

Introduction

Ovarian cancer is now the leading cause of death from gynaecological neoplasia in many countries. Among the six most common malignancies of women (breast, colon, corpus uteri, cervix uteri, lung and ovary) only lung cancer has a poorer prognosis (Axtell *et al.*, 1976). The median survival for all stages of ovarian cancer is about 18 months. This result is in particular caused by the great difficulty of diagnosing ovarian cancer in its early stages; in 60 to 70 per cent the cancer has extended beyond the true pelvis at the time of diagnosis.

Ovarian cancer is an intriguing tumour because of its wide variation in histogenesis. The most common types (80 per cent) are those originating from the epithelial surface of the ovary. Classification, adopted by the World Health Organization, is based on the current concepts of the embryology of the female urogenital tract.

Incidence and Mortality

The incidence rates vary internationally by a factor of four or more, with northern Europe at high and Asia at low risk. The incidence rate in Finland is approximately 13.0 per 100,000 women (of all ages) while in Sweden it is 21.0 per 100,000 women (Waterhouse *et al.*, 1976). In the past decades there has been a rising trend in the incidence rates in most industrialised countries.

In Western Europe and North America it is now the sixth leading cancer in women. There seems to be a clear relationship with environmental factors such as race, geographical area and socioeconomic classes. In Japan the incidence of ovarian cancer is lower than in the USA. But among the first generation Japanese women in the USA, ovarian cancer appears more commonly than in Japan. Black women in the USA have about one-third less ovarian cancer than white women, but in South Africa whites and blacks experience very similar rates. A relationship between ovarian cancer and socioeconomic class with the highest rate in the more affluent classes is suggested but in most studies it is clear that this correlation is weak (Mack and Casagrande, 1981).

The annual age-adjusted incidence rate for ovarian cancer in the Netherlands is unknown because there is no central cancer registration. However, the cause of death is registered in the Netherlands Central Bureau of Statistics and from these statistics the mortality rate which has not altered appreciably over the past ten years can be calculated. The five-year survival for ovarian malignancy is about 35 per cent in spite of improvements in chemotherapy and radiotherapy in the last three decades.

The age-specific incidence rates for ovarian cancer are very low in the younger age groups under 20 years (0.5 per 100,000 women less than 20 years old) and rise steadily up to the age of 80. The greatest number of women with ovarian cancer are in the age group 50-60 years.

In the Netherlands the percentage of women who died of ovarian cancer is unaltered during the last ten years compared with the total female population in the same period. The mortality rate in other countries in Western Europe, the USA and Canada is only slightly increased in parallel with the increase in the incidence of ovarian cancer (Doll *et al.*, 1970; Waterhouse *et al.*, 1976). In the Netherlands ovarian cancer causes 14 per cent of cancer deaths in women.

Aetiological Factors

The ovary is complex in its embryology, histology, steroidogenesis and potential for malignancy. The process of steroidogenesis can be influenced by endocrine and environmental factors; pregnancy and diet influence this. Ovarian cancer is not a single entity, but it is often composed of a combination of several types that may vary in their biological behaviour. Approximately 80-90 per cent of ovarian cancers originate from the epithelial surface (pelvic mesothelium) of the ovary. These are serous, mucinous, mesonephroid and endometrioid carcinomas. The ovarian stroma is specialised and may be stimulated by the growth of a variety of tumours. The stroma also produces steroids.

Wynder *et al.* (1969) reported in their epidemiological study a higher proportion of nulliparity in the ovarian cancer group compared with the control group. Subsequently more studies were published, suggesting a high ovarian cancer risk among women of low parity (Annegers *et al.*, 1979; Demopoulos *et al.*, 1979; McGowan *et al.*, 1979). As in endometrial cancer, pregnancy is also protective against ovarian cancer, possibly by temporary inhibition of ovulation. It is speculated that regularly occurring ovulation injures the ovarian surface epithelium, predisposing it to malignant changes (Fathalla, 1971). Newhouse *et al.* (1977) have suggested that use of oral contraceptives may be associated with a lower incidence of ovarian cancer based on their case-control studies. However, Willett *et al.* (1981) reported from a case-control study of married nurses under 55 years of age that there is no link between the use of oral contraceptives and reduced risk of ovarian cancer but they found an association between nulliparity and an increased risk of this cancer. This result lends credence to the concept that ovarian dysfunction is a common cause of both ovarian cancer and infertility.

Another view about the origin of ovarian epithelial cancers is that a carcinogen could come into contact with the surface epithelium through the vagina, uterus and fallopian tubes (Parmley and Woodruff, 1974). The patency of the fallopian tube could make the female pelvic mesothelium more accessible to carcinogenic or cocarcinogenic substances. Agents introduced into the vagina could be responsible for pelvic mesothelial proliferation. Such agents could be: talc from the doctor's gloves, asbestos, nitrosamines or viral material introduced by intercourse.

Women at Risk

Ovarian cancers very rarely occur prior to the onset of menstruation and increase rapidly after the age of 40, with a maximum some years after the menopause, so the function and dysfunction (e.g. resulting in nulliparity) of the ovaries is related to risk. Demographic factors also play a part as evidenced by higher rates among Japanese women in the USA compared with those in Japan. There may be a relationship with dietary habits (e.g. overconsumption of fat) or with other environmental influences not yet identified. A review of family histories has not demonstrated a familial tendency to ovarian cancer but there are reports on selected families in whom there is a high incidence of this cancer. Women with breast cancer have a greater risk of subsequently developing a separate primary cancer of the ovary (Lynch and Krush, 1971).

Survival Evaluation

The stage of ovarian cancer at presentation is the single most important prognostic factor but histological classification and the grade of differentiation of the tumour are also important as is the amount of residual disease at the time other therapy is instituted following surgery. At diagnosis only 30 to 40 per cent of patients have localised disease amenable to complete surgical resection. Ovarian cancer with metastases beyond the true pelvis (stage III) is the most common presentation and the five-year survival figures range from 0 to 10 per cent, regardless of whether surgery, radiotherapy or single-agent chemotherapy has been used. When the tumour is localised in the true pelvis (stages I and II), the five-year survival rate is much better and ranges from 50 to 90 per cent (Kottmeier, 1979). In all stages, surgery alone is frequently non-curative, except in those few patients with a well-differentiated stage I tumour. In advanced ovarian cancer, aggressive tumour reduction followed by effective chemotherapy can improve the survival rate from 10 to 25 per cent.

Preventive Action

The problem with ovarian cancer is the great difficulty of early diagnosis. In 60 to 70 per cent of the patients the tumour has extended beyond the true pelvis (stages III and IV) at the time of diagnosis.

In order to diagnose ovarian cancer earlier, routine pelvic examinations, cervical cytology, biochemical assays of tumour markers and routine laparoscopy have been recommended (Stolk *et al.*, 1980). All these methods, however, have failed to improve the detection rate. The chance of detecting an ovarian tumour during routine pelvic examination in an asymptomatic woman is only 1 in 10,000. Moreover, every gynaecologist knows that in a number of patients it is impossible to feel any abnormality, notwithstanding the existence of a widespread cancer. A diagnostic sign of early cancer of the ovary in the postmenopausal woman is ovarian enlargement to the size of a premenopausal ovary: the postmenopausal ovary syndrome. Normal ovaries of postmenopausal women are about 2 cm in diameter or less and if the diameter is 3 cm or more, one has to remove the ovaries before they become malignant (Barber, 1978).

Yearly about 550 women per 100,000 of 20 years of age and over have a hysterectomy in the Netherlands. From studies throughout the world it is possible to calculate the chances of developing ovarian cancer if the ovaries are retained or removed during an elective hysterectomy. It certainly must be recommended to remove the ovaries during an elective hysterectomy in those patients who are considered to be at risk of developing ovarian cancer.

Carcinoma of the Vagina

Introduction

Invasive cancer of the vagina forms only a small part of the malignancies of the female genital tract. The majority of the vaginal cancers comprise squamous cell carcinomas occurring in older women. In recent years, however, vaginal cancer has drawn worldwide attention by the occurrence of clear cell adenocarcinoma of the vagina in young women after exposure to diethylstilboestrol (DES).

The inclusion of cytological screening of vagina and cervix in the last decades has revealed more cases of intraepithelial carcinoma of the vagina. This lesion may be part of a multifocal widespread disease involving the whole area of cervix, vagina, vulva and peritoneum.

The diagnosis of primary invasive carcinoma may present difficulties. Secondary malignant tumours from cancer of the adjacent organs extending into the vagina are more common than the primary lesions and this possibility must be ruled out prior to the diagnosis of primary carcinoma.

Incidence

The WHO report on cancer incidence (Waterhouse *et al.*, 1976) does not include data on vaginal cancer. The average annual incidence rate per 100,000 women of all ages has been calculated for squamous cell carcinoma as approximately 0.9 (Wade-Evans, 1976; Wharton *et al.*, 1981). Vaginal carcinoma is the second rarest gynaecological tumour, accounting for 1 to 2 per cent of all gynaecological malignances. Only cancer of the fallopian tube is seen less frequently than carcinoma of the vagina. In the FIGO annual report the ratio of vaginal cancer to carcinoma of the cervix was 1:31 for the years 1969-1972 inclusive (Kottmeier, 1979). The literature survey up to 1971 records that 1,847 cases have been reported (Palmer and Biback, 1954; Daw, 1971). More than 95 per cent of the cases were of squamous cell carcinoma type. Prior to 1970, adenocarcinoma of the vagina was seldom seen and specifically clear cell carcinoma in women below the age of 25 was extremely rare. However, in recent years adenocarcinoma of the vagina is diagnosed more frequently at all ages with a predominance of the clear cell type in younger and of the mucine producing papillary adenocarcinoma in older women.

The clear cell carcinoma of the vagina in young women has been associated with exposure to DES during pregnancy in the 1940s and 1950s. On 1 June 1980 in the USA, 429 cases of adenocarcinoma of the vagina and cervix had been reported to the special registry for this purpose (Herbst, 1981). From these cases 220 were due to DES-exposure. In the Netherlands DES medication was initiated in the 1950s, ten years later than in the USA, and this fact might be responsible for the differences in incidence between the two countries. In the USA a rise and fall in the incidence curve was observed before and after 1975 while in the Netherlands two-thirds of the clear cell carcinomas were registered after 1976. On 1 January 1982, 22 young women had been registered in the Netherlands with adenocarcinoma of the vagina and cervix; 16 of these patients had a positive DES history. It has been calculated from available statistics that the risk of clear cell carcinoma in a DES-exposed female is about 0.14 to 14 per 1,000 by 24 years.

Mortality

The five-year survival rate for the patients reviewed prior to 1971 was reported to be 23 per cent (Palmer and Biback, 1954; Daw, 1971). The FIGO annual reports for 1973 and 1979 mention that 34 and 37.3 per cent, respectively, of the vaginal carcinoma patients were alive five years later (Kottmeier, 1979). The five-year survival rate for clear cell carcinomas of the vagina in young women is 85 per cent, which is a more favourable result in comparison with the survival rate for other types of vaginal and cervical cancer (Sandberg, 1981).

Age

The age of the patients in whom a squamous cell carcinoma occurs varies from 30 to 90 years, with a mean age of 60 at diagnosis (Park and Parmley, 1978) and with the highest incidence occurring in the sixth and seventh decades of life (Wharton *et al.*, 1981). The youngest DES-exposed patient with a clear cell carcinoma in the USA was seven years old at the time of diagnosis and the oldest was 31 years of age with a mean age of 18.9 years (Herbst, 1981). To date the youngest patient in the Netherlands with vaginal cancer after DES-exposure was 15 years and the oldest 25, with a mean age of 19.

Aetiology

Several predisposing factors are thought to have a stimulating effect on the development of squamous cell carcinoma of the vagina: a human papillomavirus may be involved and patients on chemotherapy and immunosuppressive therapy show a higher incidence. Intraepithelial carcinoma of the vagina is reported to occur in increasing numbers after hysterectomy and after pelvic irradiation therapy for cervical cancer.

Synthetic oestrogens are believed to have an initiating effect in clear cell carcinomas in young women. DES has been used since 1938 as a highly effective inexpensive oral oestrogen. It was introduced to treat habitual and threatened abortion in the late 1940s and was given to pregnant women in high doses. Although DES-exposure *in utero* could be traced in the majority of young women with clear cell carcinoma, this tumour may also occur in non-DES-exposed women.

Screening Examinations

Systematic and meticulous colposcopic visualisation of the entire vaginal wall and cervix in all patients with a history of DES-exposure and in other patients at risk is necessary and cytological examination is essential. Recurrent prophylactic examinations for the early detection of carcinoma in all DES-exposed women are recommended.

References

Annegers, J.F., Strom, H., Decker, D.G., Dockerty, M.B. and O'Fallon, W.M. (1979). Ovarian cancer, incidence and case-control study. *Cancer*, 43: 723-9

Axtell, L.M., Asire, A.J. and Myers, M.H. (1976). *Cancer Patient Survival*. Report 5 DHEW, Publication no. (NIH), 77-992

Barber, H.R.K. (1978). The postmenopausal palpable ovary syndrome (PMPO). In: Barber, H.R.K. (ed.), *Ovarian Carcinoma. Etiology, Diagnosis and Treatment*, Masson, New York, ch. 15, p. 175

Clarke, M. (1978). Cancer of the endometrium-epidemiology. In: Brush, M.G., King, R.J.B. and Taylor, R.W. (eds.), *Endometrial Cancer*, Baillière Tindall, London, ch. 1, p. 3

Cohen, C.J. (1981a). Advanced (FIGO stages III & IV) and recurrent carcinoma of endometrium. In: Coppleson, M. (ed.), *Gynecologic Oncology*, Churchill Livingstone, London/New York, ch. 45, p. 578

—— (1981b). Osteoporosis versus endometrial carcinoma: are estrogens the cure or the cause of lethal disease? In: Ballon, S.C. (ed.), *Gynecologic Oncology. Controversies in Cancer Treatment*, Hall Med. Publishers, Boston, pp. 199-207

Cramer, D.W., Cutler, S.J. and Christine, B. (1974). Trends in the incidence of endometrial cancer in the United States. *Gynecologic Oncology*, 2: 130-43

Creasman, W.T. and Weed, J.C., Jr. (1981). Carcinoma of endometrium (FIGO stages I & II): clinical features and management. In: Coppleson, M. (ed.), *Gynecologic Oncology*, Churchill Livingstone, London/New York, ch. 44, p. 562

Daw, E. (1971). Primary carcinoma of the vagina. *Journal of Obstetrics and Gynaecology of the British Commonwealth*, 78: 853-6

de Graaff, J. and Stolte, L.A.M. (1976). Trends in incidence rates of cervical and endometrial cancer. *European Journal of Obstetrics and Gynecology*, 6: 265-9

Demopoulos, R.I., Seltzer, V., Dubin, N. and Gutman, E. (1979). The association of parity and marital status with the development of ovarian carcinoma:

clinical implications. *Obstetrics and Gynecology*, 54: 150-5

Doll, R., Muir, C. and Waterhouse, J. (eds.) (1970). *Cancer Incidence in Five Continents*, Volume II, International Union Against Cancer, Springer Verlag, Berlin, pp. 29-33

Elwood, J.M., Cole, P., Rothman, K.J. and Kaplan, S.D. (1977). Epidemiology of endometrial cancer. *Journal of the National Cancer Institute*, 59: 1055-60

Fathalla, M.F. (1971). Incessant ovulation – a factor in ovarian neoplasm? *Lancet*, 1: 163

Fox, H. (1976). The aetiology and pathology of endometrial cancer. In: Langley, F.A. (ed.), *Cancer of the Vulva, Vagina and Uterus. Clinics in Obstetrics and Gynaecology*, vol. 3, no. 2, Saunders, London/Philadelphia/Toronto, ch. 9, p. 371

Frick, H.C., Munnel, E.W., Richart, R.M., Berger, A.P. and Lawry, M.F. (1973). Carcinoma of the endometrium. *American Journal of Obstetrics and Gynecology*, 115: 663-76

Greenblatt, R.B. and Stoddard, L.D. (1978). The estrogen-cancer controversy. *Journal of the American Geriatric Society*, 26: 1-8

Gusberg, S.B. (1976). The individual at high risk for endometrial carcinoma. *American Journal of Obstetrics and Gynecology*, 126: 535-42

—— and Frick, H.C., II (eds.) (1978). *Corscaden's Gynecologic Cancer*, 5th edn., Williams and Wilkins, Baltimore, ch. 10, pp. 265-300

Hemsell, D.L., Grodin, J.M., Brenner, P.F., Süteri, P.K. and MacDonald, P.C. (1974). Plasma precursors of estrogen. II. Correlation of the extent of conversion of plasma androstenedione to estrone with age. *Journal of Clinical Endocrinology and Metabolism*, 38: 476-9

Herbst, A.L. (1981). The epidemiology of vaginal and cervical clear cell adenocarcinoma. In: Herbst, A.L. and Bern, H.A. (eds.), *Developmental Effects of Diethylstilbestrol (DES) in Pregnancy*, Thieme Stratton Inc., New York, ch. 5, p. 63

Jones, H.W., III (1982). Endometrial carcinoma. In: Jones, G.S. and Jones, H.W., Jr. (eds.), *Gynecology*, Williams and Wilkins, Baltimore/London, ch. 15, p. 230

King, R.J.B. (1978). Are oestrogens carcinogens? In: Williams, D.C. and Briggs, M.G. (eds.), *Some Implications of Steroid Hormones in Cancer*, Heinemann, London, pp. 62-9

Kistner, R.W. (1966). Carcinoma of the endometrium – a preventable disease? *American Journal of Obstetrics and Gynecology*, 95: 1011-24

Kottmeier, H.L. (ed.) (1979). *Annual Report on the Results of Treatment in Gynaecologic Cancer*, 17th volume, 1969 to 1972, inclusive, International Federation of Gynecology and Obstetrics, pp. 45, 154, 155-86

Lauritzen, C. (1977). Oestrogens and endometrial cancer: A point of view. In: Greenblatt, R.B. and Studd, J. (eds.), *The Menopause. Clinics in Obstetrics and Gynecology*, vol. 4, no. 1, Saunders, London/Philadelphia/Toronto, ch. 8, p. 162

Lucas, W.E. and Yen, S.S.C. (1979). A study of endocrine and metabolic variables in postmenopausal women with endometrial carcinoma. *American Journal of Obstetrics and Gynecology*, 134: 180-6

Lynch, H.T. and Krush, A.J. (1971). Carcinoma of the breast and ovary in three families. *Surgery, Gynecology and Obstetrics*, 133: 644-8

—— Krush, A.J., Thomas, R.J. and Lynch, J. (1976). Cancer family syndrome. In: Lynch, H.T. (ed.), *Cancer Genetics*, Thomas, Springfield, Ill., ch. 19, pp. 355-87

Lyon, J.L. and Gardner, J.W. (1977). The rising frequency of hysterectomy: its effect on uterine cancer rates. *American Journal of Epidemiology*, 105: 439-43

Mack, T.M. (1977). Cancer Surveillance Program in Los Angeles County. *National Cancer Institute Monographs*, 47: 99-101
—— (1978). Exogenous oestrogens and endometrial carcinoma; studies, criticisms and current status. In: Brush, M.G., King, R.J.B. and Taylor, R.W. (eds.), *Endometrial Cancer*, Baillière Tindall, London, ch. 3, p. 17
—— and Casagrande, J.T. (1981). Epidemiology of gynecologic cancer. II. Endometrium, ovary, vagina, vulva. In: Coppleson, M. (ed.), *Gynecologic Oncology*, Churchill Livingstone, London/New York, ch. 3, p. 19
MacMahon, B. (1974). Risk factors for endometrial cancer. *Gynecologic Oncology*, 2: 122-9
Masabuchi, K., Nemoto, H., Masubuchi, S., Jr., Fujimoto, I. and Uchino, S. (1975). Increasing incidence of endometrial carcinoma in Japan. *Gynecologic Oncology*, 3: 335-46
McGowan, L., Parent, L., Lednar, W. and Norris, H.J. (1979). The woman at risk for developing ovarian cancer. *Gynecologic Oncology*, 7: 325-44
Netherlands Central Bureau of Statistics; Department of Health Statistics (1980). *Atlas of Cancer Mortality in The Netherlands 1969-1978*. Staatsuitgeverij, The Hague, ch. 18, p. 69
Newhouse, M.L., Pearson, R.M., Fullerton, J.M., Boesen, E.A.M. and Shannon, H.S. (1977). A case control study of carcinoma of the ovary. *British Journal of Preventive and Social Medicine*, 31: 148-53
Palmer, J.B. and Biback, S.M. (1954). Primary cancer of the vagina. *American Journal of Obstetrics and Gynecology*, 67: 377-97
Park, R.C. and Parmley, T.H. (1978). Vaginal Cancer. In: McGowan, L. (ed.), *Gynecologic Oncology*, Appleton-Century-Crofts, New York, ch. 8, p. 174
Parmley, T.H. and Woodruff, J.D. (1974). The ovarian mesothelioma. *American Journal of Obstetrics and Gynecology*, 120: 234-41
Quint, B.C. (1975). Changing patterns in endometrial carcinoma. *American Journal of Obstetrics and Gynecology*, 122: 498-501
Richardson, G.S. and MacLaughlin, D.T. (1978). Hormonal biology of endometrial cancer. *UICC Technical Reports*, vol. 42, Geneva
Sandberg, E.C. (1981). DES exposure in utero: what are the effects? Perspective. In: Ballon, S.C. (ed.), *Gynecologic Oncology. Controversies in Cancer Treatment*, Hall, Boston, ch. 4, p. 83
Silverberg, S.G., Makowski, E.L. and Roche, W.D. (1977). Endometrial carcinoma in women under 40 years of age. *Cancer*, 39: 592-8
Smith, D.C., Prentice, R., Thompson, D.J. and Herrmann, W.L. (1975). Association of exogenous estrogen and endometrial carcinoma. *New England Journal of Medicine*, 293: 1164-7
Stolk, J.G., Baak, J.P.A., Van der Putten, H.W. and Kurver, P.H.J. (1980). Premalignancy of the ovary. In: Sakamoto, S., Tojo, S. and Nakayama, T. (eds.), *Gynecology and Obstetrics*, Proceedings of the IX World Congress, Tokyo, 1979, Excerpta Medica, Amsterdam/Oxford/Princeton, pp. 291-5
Underwood, P.B., Miller, M.C., Kreutner, A., Joyner, C.A. and Lutz, M.H. (1979). Endometrial carcinoma: the effect of estrogens. *Gynecologic Oncology*, 8: 60-73
Wade-Evans, T. (1976). The aetiology and pathology of cancer of the vagina. In: Langley, F.A. (ed.), *Cancer of the Vulva, Vagina and Uterus. Clinics in Obstetrics and Gynaecology*, vol. 3, no. 2, Saunders, London/Philadelphia/Toronto, ch. 3, p. 229
Waterhouse, J., Muir, C., Correa, P. and Powell, J. (eds.) (1976). *Cancer Incidence in Five Continents*, Vol. III, IARC Scientific Publications no. 15, World Health Organisation, International Agency for Research on Cancer, Lyon, pp. 514-15
Weiss, N.S. (1978). Noncontraceptive estrogens and abnormalities of endometrial

proliferation. *Annals of Internal Medicine*, 88: 410-12

——— Szekely, D.R. and Austin, D.F. (1976). Increasing incidence of endometrial cancer in the United States. *New England Journal of Medicine*, 294:
1259-62

Wharton, J.T., Fletcher, G.H. and Delclos, L. (1981). Invasive tumors of vagina:
clinical features and management. In: Coppleson, M. (ed.), *Gynecologic
Oncology*, Churchill Livingstone, London/New York, ch. 27, p. 345

Willett, W.C., Bain, C., Hennekes, C.H., Rosner, B. and Speizer, F.E. (1981).
Oral contraceptives and risk of ovarian cancer. *Cancer*, 48: 1684-7

Wynder, E.L., Dodo, H. and Barber, H.R.K. (1969). Epidemiology of cancer of
the ovary. *Cancer*, 23: 352-60

12 CANCER OF THE BREAST

B. Herity

Introduction

Carcinoma of the breast is the most commonly occurring cancer in women in industrialised countries and mortality from the disease has been increasing steadily from the beginning of this century. It is a disease which has been recognised from antiquity (Shimkin, 1977) and Ramazzini in 1713 records its high incidence in nuns, probably the first recorded association of breast cancer with nulliparity.

When cancer of the breast is reported as a cause of death the diagnosis is usually reliable, but there is probably some under-reporting in older age groups and among patients surviving a considerable time following therapy (Logan, 1975). It is a disease which is responsible for substantial premature morbidity and mortality among women, and treatment methods have not improved overall survival in recent years. It is important then to identify aetiological factors which may be influenced by preventive approaches and to continue to pursue methods of early detection of the disease.

Mortality and Incidence

Mortality

Breast cancer accounts for one-fifth of all female deaths from cancer and approximately one-twenty-fifth of deaths from all causes. It is the second most important cause of death in women aged 25-34 years, the leading cause in women aged 35-54, and second only to cardiovascular disease at older ages (Logan, 1975). Mortality and incidence rates vary greatly in different areas of the world and these differences have been present for many years. Figure 12.1 shows age-standardised mortality rates for various countries for 1973-5 and annual mortality rates from breast cancer in 24 countries for 1973-5 are shown in Figure 12.2. In most of these countries, including Ireland, mortality rates increased over this period but in the United States, Canada, Australia, the Netherlands, Great Britain and Japan very little change was seen.

191

Figure 12.1: Average Annual Mortality Rates for Breast Cancer per 100,000 Females. Mortality rates for breast cancer for 1973-5, age adjusted to the total population of the United States in 1950.

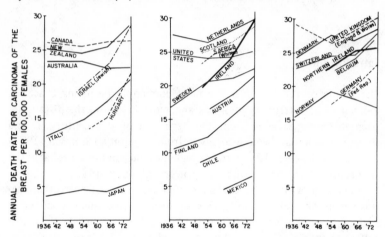

Source: From Haagensen *et al.*, 1981, with kind permission. Calculated from data published in *World Health Statistics Annual*, WHO, Geneva, Volume 1, 1977, and Volume 1, 1973-6.

Incidence

Incidence rates for breast cancer are 4-6 times higher in North America, Western Europe, Australia and New Zealand than they are in most countries of Asia and Africa; central and southern Europe and South America have intermediate rates (Doll *et al.*, 1970). In addition age-specific incidence rates vary. In areas of high rates the risk increases throughout life, whereas in areas of low rates, notably Japan, the risk tends to level off at middle age and after about the age of 50 years to decline slightly.

Another feature of breast cancer incidence frequently, though not consistently, observed is a slight fall in the 50-54 age group. (Clemmeson, 1948; de Waard *et al.*, 1964; Wagoner *et al.*, 1967). This phenomenon (sometimes called Clemmeson's Hook) is seen in areas of high incidence of breast cancer and it has been suggested that it results from hormonal changes around the time of the menopause. Differences in age-specific incidence of breast cancer in different areas of the world led de Waard (1969) to postulate that there are essentially two different types of breast cancer, one common in Japan and other low-incidence areas with a peak prior to the menopause associated with imbalance of ovarian

Figure 12.2: Annual Mortality Rates for Breast Carcinoma per 100,000 Females in 24 Countries from 1936-1975, age adjusted to the total population of the United States in 1950.

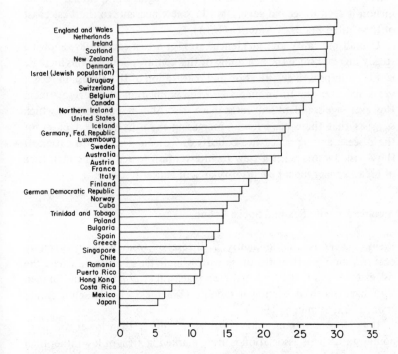

Sources: From Haagensen *et al.*, 1981, with kind permission. Calculated from *World Health Statistics Annual*, WHO, Geneva, 1965, Volume 1, 1977, and Volume 1, 1973-6; *Epidemiological and Vital Statistics Report*, Volume 10, 1957, Volume 12, 1959 and Volume 20, 1967, WHO, Geneva.

hormones, and the other in high-incidence areas where rates increase with age and which is associated with nutritional patterns. However, a study in Iceland (Bjarnason *et al.* 1974) which examined age-specific incidence curves in that country, where the pattern has changed from the Japanese type in the early years of the century to the Western type in recent years, showed that the shape of the age-specific curves was the same if the analysis was conducted by birth cohort. What had occurred was that incidence had increased in successive birth cohorts. This suggests that there may be only one type of breast cancer but that it is capable of being influenced by an external risk factor such as diet.

Increases in rates in Japanese women lend some support to this theory. There has been an increase detected in women aged 40-49 years, who would have undergone the changes in life style which occurred in Japan following World War II at relatively young ages, and a similar phenomenon is seen in second generation Japanese migrants to the west coast of the United States of America (USA).

Overall mortality and incidence rates for breast cancer have shown a steady increase since the beginning of this century. Some of this increase is due to improved certification and registration of the disease in recent years and also due to an increase in the population of elderly women. However age-standardised rates have also shown an increase which suggests that there has been an increasing exposure to risk factors for the disease among successive cohorts of women. The identification of those risk factors with a view to intervention to reduce the incidence of breast cancer must be a priority area of cancer research.

Association with Sex and Social Group

Breast cancer is predominantly a disease of women but may rarely occur in men, particularly those with Klinefelter's syndrome where the risk is 66 times that of normal men (Jackson *et al.*, 1965) and in men who have received oestrogen therapy (Lilienfeld, 1963; Schottenfeld *et al.*, 1963; Symmers, 1968).

It is more common among women of higher than lower socioeconomic status. This association is more marked in areas of low rather than high risk for breast cancer and in an international study (MacMahon *et al.*, 1970b) was not substantially altered by adjusting for age at first birth.

Aetiology

Genetic Factors

It has been well recognised that female relatives of women with breast cancer have two to three times the rate of breast cancer of the general population (Macklin, 1959; Lilienfeld, 1963; Papadrianos *et al.*, 1967). Anderson (1976) has reported that first-degree relatives of patients with bilateral disease have three times the risk of similar relatives with unilateral disease, i.e. 6-9 times the risk of the general population, and also noted that bilateral disease was a feature of familial breast cancer in women under 45 years of age. Twin studies have shown that the concordance rate of breast cancer occurrence in monozygotic twins is about double that in dizygotic twins (Macklin, 1940; Miller, 1971; Knudson *et al.*, 1973).

Li and Fraumeni (1969) reported families in which multiple soft tissue neoplasms occurred with high frequency, as did Lynch and Krush (1971). Cancers of the breast and endometrium have been shown to be significantly associated (Bailar, 1963; Schoenberg *et al.*, 1969; MacMahon and Austin 1969; Vontama *et al.*, 1970; Schottenfeld and Berg, 1971). Associations of breast and ovarian cancer have been reported (Schoenberg *et al.*, 1969; Schottenfeld and Berg, 1971; Lynch and Krush, 1971). Cancer of the colon has also been associated with increased risk of breast cancer (Schoenberg *et al.*, 1969; Schottenfeld *et al.*, 1976). The association of cancer of the breast with acute myeloid leukaemia (Carey *et al.*, 1967) and with salivary gland cancer (Dunn *et al.*, 1972) has been also described.

One explanation of the frequently demonstrated familial aspect of breast cancer is the influence of genetic factors. The possibility that a genetic marker linked to the glutamate-pyruvate transaminase (GPT) locus may have been identified, is mentioned by Miller (1981). Since members of the same family may be exposed to similar environmental risk factors there is likely to be some familial association of breast cancer. Brinton and her colleagues (1982) have studied the interaction of familial and hormonal risk factors in breast cancer, and suggest that familial susceptibility to breast cancer may be mediated through hormonal factors which operate in early life. However, occurrences in high-risk families are rare and contribute little to the overall problem of breast cancer (Lynch *et al.*, 1974).

Reproductive Factors

Age at First Birth and Parity. One of the most consistent observations in studies of breast cancer has been the association between high parity and a reduced risk of developing the disease (Lane-Claypon, 1926; Wainwright, 1931; Gilliam, 1951; Stocks, 1957; Segi *et al.*, 1957; Wynder *et al.*, 1960; Levin *et al.*, 1964; Kaplan and Acheson, 1966). An international collaborative study by MacMahon and his colleagues (1970b) identified a striking relationship between age at first birth and subsequent lifetime risk of breast cancer which was confirmed by Henderson *et al.* (1974) and by Lilienfeld *et al.* (1975). This study of over 4,000 women with breast cancer and almost 13,000 control women in seven areas of the world representative of high, low and intermediate rates of breast cancer, showed that a woman who had her first child under the age of 18 years had only one-third the risk of developing breast cancer of a woman who had a first birth at 35 years of age or older. The risk of a woman who had had her first child at age 30-34 years was similar to that of a nulliparous woman. Births after the first, even if they occurred at a young age, had very little additional protective effect. The association described in earlier studies between total parity and reduced risk of breast cancer resulted from the strong correlation of age at first birth with total parity. Only full-term pregnancy exerted this protection; abortion when it was associated with risk of breast cancer increased rather than decreased the risk.

It has been postulated (MacMahon *et al.*, 1973) that the decade or so after menarche is associated with a high risk of tumour initiation and that the first full-term pregnancy either produces a permanent change in the factors responsible for this risk or affects the breast tissue thus making it less susceptible to malignant transformation. The same authors suggest that the increased risk seen in women whose first birth was at 35 years of age and older compared to nulliparous women (MacMahon *et al.*, 1970b) may be due to a promoting effect of pregnancy on already-initiated tumour cells.

A study by Alderson (1981), which reported a lower mean age for breast cancer in parous compared to non-parous women in England and Wales might reflect an effect of pregnancy on the growth of breast cancer but Miller *et al.* (1980) found in a study of women in Canada that when age at first pregnancy was controlled for, parity had no effect on risk of breast cancer. The available evidence suggests that early age at first birth is the main protective factor and Miller and Bulbrook (1980) suggest that a population which achieved a five-year reduction in age at first delivery might achieve a 30 per cent reduction in incidence of breast cancer.

Lactation. Lactation was believed for many years to be highly protective against breast cancer but MacMahon and his colleagues (1970a) stated 'the support to be found in the literature is not as strong as the popularity of the hypothesis would suggest'. They found that when the confounding effects of socioeconomic status and age at first pregnancy were allowed for no constant effect of lactation was seen. It is generally true that women who start their families at a young age have larger families and more breastfeeding experience than those who are older at first pregnancy; it appears therefore that the association between age at first pregnancy and duration of lactation accounts for the apparent decrease in risk associated with breastfeeding.

Other Endocrine Factors

Age at Menarche and Menopause.   Early age at menarche (<13 years) has been associated with an increase in risk of breast cancer in many case-control studies; in some the difference was small and in a few no difference was seen (MacMahon *et al.*, 1973), but in a study from Ireland (Herity *et al.*, 1975) in which no difference was found difficulty in precise recall of age at menarche was noted. The available evidence is in favour of such an association. Age at puberty has been declining in industrialised countries since the early nineteenth century at a rate of about four months per decade (Haagensen *et al.*, 1981) and is believed to be related to improved nutrition. The weight of evidence also suggests that late age at natural menopause (>50 years) increases the risk of developing breast cancer (Valaoras *et al.*, 1969; Yuasa and MacMahon 1970; Lin *et al.*, 1971; Herity *et al.*, 1975). Trichopoulos *et al.* (1972) found that a woman whose natural menopause occurred at age 55 or older had twice the risk of one whose age at menopause was 45 years or less. The relationship of breast cancer with age at menarche and menopause is supportive evidence that ovarian activity is an important determinant of risk of this disease.

Further evidence of the effect of ovarian activity comes from the risk-lowering effect of surgical menopause. Trichopoulos and his colleagues (1972) studied breast cancer patients reported to the Connecticut Cancer Registry and population controls and found an overall reduction in risk of 40 per cent associated with surgical menopause. The protective effect was greatest for women who had induction of menopause below 35 years but was also in evidence for those who had surgery up to 50 years and persisted beyond age 70. It has been suggested that this effect is limited to women in whom hysterectomy was accompanied by oophorectomy, but in many studies the proportion of women having oophorectomy as part of the operative procedure was unknown. MacMahon and his colleagues (1973) suggest that if the effect is indeed limited to oophorectomised women, the effect of castration must be even greater than that manifested by all women classified as having had a surgical menopause.

Endogenous Hormones.   Attempts to quantify or define the role of endocrine factors in breast cancer have not met with great success. A review by Kirschener (1977) discussed the role of oestrogens, androgens, progesterone, prolactin and thyroid function. Higher levels of oestriol in Japanese than Caucasian women were reported by MacMahon *et al.*

(1971) and by Dickinson *et al.* (1974). However, although the oestriol hypothesis, i.e. that oestriol protected against the effect of the more potent oestrogens oestrone and oestradiol, gained some popularity, more recent studies suggest that it is no longer valid in explaining altered risks of breast cancer either in individuals or populations. Fishman and his colleagues (1978) measured hormone concentrations in high-risk women (premenopausal with a family history of breast cancer) and age-matched low-risk controls and found no statistically significant differences in oestriol, oestrone, oestradiol, prolactin or gonadotrophin levels.

Similarly studies of androgen metabolism have had conflicting results. Altered urinary 17-ketosteroids have been found in some studies (Bulbrook *et al.*, 1960; 1962a; 1962b; Bulbrook and Hayward, 1967; Kumaoka, 1968) but not in another (Wilson *et al.*, 1967). The potential importance of androstenedione, which is the major precursor of oestrone in postmenopausal women, and the rate of metabolism of which is influenced by obesity (MacDonald *et al.*, 1969) and ageing (Longcope, 1971), is not fully understood. Since dietary factors are important in breast cancer further research into this relationship is desirable.

In animal experiments prolactin stimulates breast tumour growth (Pearson *et al.*, 1972), however studies of women with breast cancer showed normal levels (Boyns *et al.*, 1973; Kwa *et al.*, 1974; Mittra *et al.*, 1974; Wilson *et al.*, 1974; Fishman *et al.*, 1978). Neither is there at present any good evidence linking thyroid function with risk of breast cancer. However, the breast is a target organ for many hormones and in spite of failure to identify any obvious abnormal hormonal pattern in women at risk for breast cancer, it is clear that the production and metabolism of hormones must be regarded as a priority research area.

Exogenous Hormones. There has been considerable research into the possibility of a relationship between the use of exogenous hormone preparations and risk of developing breast cancer. Both oral contraceptive usage and hormone replacement therapy have been studied.

Two large cohort studies (Royal College of General Practitioners, 1981; Vessey *et al.*, 1981) and several case-control studies (Boston Collaborative Drug Surveillance Program, 1973; Henderson *et al.*, 1974; Paffenbarger *et al.*, 1977; Sartwell *et al.*, 1977; Kelsey *et al.*, 1978; Ravnihar *et al.*, 1979) have found no significant overall relationship between breast cancer and oral contraceptives. However, in some studies certain subgroups of women were shown to be at increased risk of the disease. The Royal College of General Practitioners' (1981) study has emphasised the need for continuing follow-up of the younger women in the cohort, in whom the risk ratio of 3.33 just failed to reach statistical significance, and Pike and his colleagues (1981) found that young women who had been on a contraceptive pill for more than eight years prior to their first pregnancy had over three times the risk of developing breast cancer before the age of 32 years than matched controls. Paffenbarger *et al.* (1977) also found increased risks in women who had used oral contraceptives at a young age and the same study showed that women with a history of benign breast disease prior to use of oral contraceptives were at increased risk of breast cancer. However, initial analysis of a large ongoing multicentre study (cited in a Morbidity and Mortality Weekly Report, 1982) does not show an increased risk in high-risk women. It is clear that further research is needed into the long-term effects of oral contraceptive usage. Widespread use of oral contraceptives began less than 20 years ago and those women who used them then are only now entering the period of maximal risk of breast cancer. Further research is also needed into the use of oral contraceptives by young women to delay first pregnancy and into their usage by women with a previous history of benign breast disease. The fact that the formulation of oral contraceptives has changed over the years will also have to be taken into account (Miller and Bulbrook, 1980).

A number of case-control studies (Boston Collaborative Drug Surveillance Program, 1973; Craig *et al.*, 1974; Henderson *et al.*, 1974; Casagrande *et al.*, 1976; Sartwell *et al.*, 1977; Ravnihar *et al.*, 1979) have shown no significant association between noncontraceptive oestrogens and breast cancer. In a prospective study (Hoover *et al.*, 1976) no increased risk was seen until 12 years after initial use, after which it approximately doubled; the risk was related to the strength of the preparation used but not to duration of usage. In women who developed benign breast disease following oestrogen usage the risk of breast cancer was increased seven-fold, while those with a prior history of benign breast disease experienced a doubling of the risk. In this study the risk of breast cancer increased with the duration of follow-up, and this finding is consistent with the long latent period associated with development of many cancers. It is clear that research must continue into the association of noncontraceptive oestrogen usage with breast cancer, and it would be prudent to avoid excessive usage of these preparations, in particular in women with a prior history of benign breast disease.

Diet

The marked variation in breast cancer incidence in different areas of the world points to the importance of environmental factors in the aetiology of this disease. Studies of migrant populations, in particular of Japanese immigrants to the west coast of the USA, have shown that acculturation produces substantial changes in incidence and mortality of breast cancer (Buell, 1973).

Evidence that diet is a major environmental risk factor comes from two sources, from laboratory studies of animals and from dietary studies of populations. Carroll (1981) has summarised the evidence in relation to high fat diets and the development of cancers. Many studies have shown that animals on a high fat diet consistently developed tumours more readily than those on a low fat diet and it was found that polyunsaturated fats were more effective in tumour promotion than saturated fats (Gammal *et al.*, 1967; Carroll and Khor, 1971). However, the addition of a small amount of polyunsaturated fat to the saturated fat diet produced an effect comparable to a total unsaturated fat diet (Carroll and Hopkins, 1979). Chan and Cohen (1974) suggest that the effect is mediated through prolactin.

Carroll *et al.* (1968) have shown that in human populations breast cancer mortality correlates best with total fat intake, less well with animal fat intake and not at all with vegetable fat. Armstrong and Doll (1975) also found a strong correlation with total fat consumption and also with Gross National Product (GNP) in that tumour. Hirayama (cited in Miller, 1977) has produced evidence of a sharp increase in morbidity and mortality from breast cancer in Japan seen first in the age group 40-54 and extending later to older age groups. He found a strong correlation with dietary fat and dietary pork intake but with no other nutrient; dietary fat intake has increased greatly in Japan in recent years. Again in Iceland, where Westernisation has brought dietary changes, the incidence of breast cancer has changed from the low-level Japanese-type pattern to a Western-type pattern from 1950 onwards (Bjarnason *et al.*, 1974). Gray *et al.* (1979) found a weak association with dietary fat and animal protein intake which are highly correlated. A case-control study from Canada (Miller *et al.*, 1978) in which dietary intake of nutrients of cases and neighbourhood controls was recorded, showed a weak association with total fat intake but no evidence of a dose-response relationship. However, the difficulty of assessing dietary intake in case-control studies is well known.

Alcoholic beverage consumption in relation to breast cancer has been studied (Williams and Horm, 1977; Rosenberg *et al.*, 1982) and both studies showed a higher consumption of alcoholic beverages by breast cancer patients than controls. In the latter study the relative risk compared with controls with endometrial or ovarian cancer was 1.4 and compared with women with nonmalignant conditions 1.9. However, other dietary correlates of alcohol were not controlled for in this study and the authors suggest that further work is needed to rule out chance or bias as explanations for their findings.

The evidence in relation to weight and height as risk factors in breast cancer is inconclusive. Only in the Netherlands and in Japan (de Waard, 1975; de Waard and Baanders-van Halewjin, 1974) have positive associations been described. In other studies (MacMahon *et al.*, 1970b; Herity *et al.*, 1975; Choi *et al.*, 1978) no effect was seen. De Waard's original hypothesis (de Waard *et al.*, 1964) was that over-nutrition was a major factor for breast cancer in postmenopausal women, whereas endocrine imbalance in relation to ovarian hormones was more important in the premenopausal patient. However, he later (de Waard *et al.*, 1977) modified this hypothesis to suggest that height and lean body mass were more important risk factors, which would point to nutritional factors operating in childhood. Further studies are necessary to eluci-date whether or not nutritional influences are important in early life, if they can operate at any age, or if they operate mainly in the post-menopausal woman.

Miller (1981) reviews the evidence in relation to dietary factors and suggests that approaches to prevention might include attempts to modify total fat intake in adolescence and early adult life, possibly even up to the time of menopause and emphasis on weight reduction in postmenopausal women. He acknowledges that the evidence to support intervention in population groups is still far from complete but suggests that the fact that the dietary modification proposed is also advocated to reduce the frequency of large bowel cancer and cardiovascular disease may justify more positive approaches. The lack of success to date of health education in influencing behavioural changes in popula-tions must suggest that any attempt to alter dietary habits must of necessity be a long-term and difficult task.

Benign Breast Disease

A consistent finding in studies of breast cancer is that women with a prior history of benign breast disease have up to a three-fold increase in risk of developing the disease. Davis and his colleagues (1964) have reviewed the literature up to that year. Differences in histological classification and terminology have made studies difficult to interpret but it is suggested that epithelial hyperplasia is the most significant abnormality (Black *et al.*, 1972). Page and his colleagues (1978) followed up 1,127 women who had biopsies for benign breast disease and found that epithelial proliferative lesions, notably atypical lobular hyperplasia which increased the risk up to six times, were associated with development of breast cancer. Women with cysts, sclerosing adenosis, fibrosis and other non-hyperplastic changes were not at increased risk compared with women in the general population.

It seems clear that histopathological classification of benign breast disease is essential to distinguish those women who are at increased risk of breast cancer from those whose breast condition is not a risk factor for the disease.

Radiation

It is not possible to distinguish radiation-induced breast cancer from a naturally occurring tumour, therefore risk from radiation can only be estimated from epidemiological data comparing incidence in women exposed to this particular risk factor with that in non-exposed women.

MacKenzie (1965) reported an increase in breast malignancies among women who had undergone repeated X-ray examination following treatment for pulmonary tuberculosis by artificial pneumothorax, as did Boice and Monson (1977). In the latter study a risk of 100-400 cases of breast cancer per 100,000 women exposed to 1 gy was estimated. Myrden and Hiltz (1969) reported similar findings from a study in Nova Scotia. Wanebo (1968) reported an excess of breast cancer among female survivors of an atomic bomb explosion who had been exposed to doses of 10 rads or greater compared with those who had received doses of 9 rads or less. An excess of breast cancer among women exposed to radiation from atomic bombs before the age of ten years was recently reported (Tokunaga *et al.*, 1982). Jablon and Kato (1972) similarly described an excess of breast cancer among women who had received a dose of 10 rads or greater. A latent period of 15-30 years or longer was found in all these studies.

In a study by Mettler and his colleagues (1969) an excess of breast cancer was found among women treated with X-rays for post partum mastitis, and Baverstock *et al.* (1981) studied women who worked with paint containing radium in the United Kingdom between 1939 and 1961. They found that those who were under 30 years of age when they started work had a significantly increased risk of dying from breast cancer. However, they noted that their estimated risk of 200-500 deaths per 100,000 women exposed to 1 gy, which agrees with that of Boice and Monson (1977), may be subject to some uncertainty since comparison of age at first pregnancy among the study group with that of the general population was not carried out.

Recently Simon and Silverstone (1976) suggested that the use of mammography may increase the incidence of radiation-induced breast cancer. Improvements in mammographic techniques have reduced the radiation dose to the breast but Mole (1975) in discussing the practical problems in estimating risk from low-level radiation concluded it must be assumed that there is no threshold for carcinogenesis and that the probability of developing cancer increases with increasing dosage.

Other Possible Risk Factors

Reserpine

Routine scanning of hospital inpatient data in Boston in 1972 (Boston Collaborative Drug Surveillance Program, 1974) revealed an association between use of the drug reserpine and a diagnosis of breast cancer. A case-control study in Helsinki (Heinonen *et al.*, 1974) showed similar findings. However, subsequent studies have not confirmed these findings (Lilienfeld *et al.*, 1975; Kodlin and McCarthy, 1978).

Viruses

There is no good evidence that a virus has any role in human breast cancer, despite the identification of the mammary tumour virus in mice (Moore *et al.*, 1971; Fraumeni and Miller, 1971; Tokuchata, 1969).

Primary Prevention

The present state of knowledge of the aetiology of breast cancer does not offer a sound basis for practicable primary preventive measures, although further research into dietary and endocrine factors may in the future identify a group of women who are at high risk of the disease. Survival rates for breast cancer have shown only a minimal increase in recent years; almost 50 per cent of patients still die within five years of diagnosis and not until 20 years following treatment does life-expectancy run parallel to that of the general population (Brinkley and Haybittle, 1975). Since there is a marked difference in survival between cases diagnosed at different stages of the disease it is not surprising that interest has centred on early diagnosis and treatment.

Secondary Prevention

Screening

Screening methods are now limited to X-ray mammography and physical examination performed by doctors, nurses or women themselves. Advances in X-ray techniques have improved the efficiency of mammography which has been shown to be more sensitive and specific than physical examination (Lundgren, 1979) and is at present being used as a single modality in trials in Sweden (Tabar and Gad, 1981) and in the United Kingdom (UK) (Thomas *et al.*, 1981). Physical examination in addition to mammography will increase detection of cancer by 5-10 per cent, but reveals many non-malignant abnormalities which have to be followed up with increased cost both financial and psychological (*Lancet*, 1982). The recommendations of the International Union Against Cancer (UICC) group in relation to exposure to radiation is that when the dose is monitored and kept below 1 rad per examination that it may be used in screening women for whom benefit from early detection has been demonstrated, i.e. those of 50 years and older. The most recent report of the UICC Multidisciplinary Project on Breast Cancer (Miller and Bulbrook, 1982) reviews the evidence in relation to screening for breast cancer as a public health measure. To date much of the published data on screening reports result from clinics which are open to volunteer subjects and are not based on a defined population. The only published trial of screening which included a control group is that of the Health Insurance Plan of Greater New York (the HIP Study) of Shapiro and his colleagues (1971; 1982). The latest results of this study are encouraging; 14 years after entry to the trial the study group of women diagnosed at 50 years or older had significantly fewer deaths from breast cancer than the control group. There was no difference in mortality for women diagnosed younger than 50 years of age.

Further trials of screening are at present underway in the Netherlands (de Waard *et al.*, 1978), Canada (Miller, 1980), Sweden (Tabar and Gad, 1981) and in the UK (UK Trial of Early Detection of Breast Cancer Group, 1981). It is hoped that these trials will add to the evidence already available, particularly in relation to the independent contributions of mammography, physical examination and self examination to improved survival, the extent of possible over-treatment following early diagnosis, the optimum interval between screening tests and whether or not screening women of less than 50 years of age is of benefit (*Lancet*, 1982). Until this information is available the establishment of breast cancer screening services as a public health measure would be premature.

Research into non-radiological methods of screening should continue. So far thermography has been shown to have a low sensitivity and specificity, and ultrasound has not developed sufficiently to identify solid tumours of less than 5 mm or to detect microcalcification (Miller and Bulbrook, 1982). If a nonradiological method of screening for breast cancer becomes feasible an important constraint on repeating screening tests, namely the cumulative effect of low-dosage radiation, would no longer be valid.

Prognosis

The natural history of breast cancer is variable. Some tumours grow rapidly and metastasise early, some grow relatively slowly. It is generally accepted that only about 25-30 per cent of women who present with breast cancer have local disease and that therefore in up to 75 per cent of new breast cancer cases dissemination has already occurred (Mueller and Jeffries, 1975). Even 20 years following treatment a breast cancer patient is still more likely to die of the disease than the normal population (Brinkley and Haybittle, 1975). It is estimated that 80-85 per cent of women with breast cancer die of the disease (Mueller and Jeffries, 1975).

Survival in breast cancer is related to the size of the primary tumour and to the degree of axillary node involvement. Small tumours (< 2 cm diameter) with no nodal involvement have up to 80 per cent, 20-year survival but survival decreases with size of primary tumour, nodal involvement and metastatic spread. The treatment of choice for early disease is generally agreed to be simple mastectomy with radiotherapy to involved axillary nodes, but trials of chemotherapy following primary surgical treatment to patients with axillary node involvement have shown an improvement in disease-free survival rate in premenopausal patients (Bonadonna, 1980). In advanced disease radiotherapy, hormone therapy and cytotoxic drugs are used in a variety of therapeutic regimes.

Hormone Receptors

Hormone deprivation can cause regression of the tumour in about 30 per cent of women with metastatic breast cancer, but selection of patients likely to respond to such therapy cannot be made on either clinical or histological grounds. The effectiveness of a hormone is determined by its circulating concentration and by the responsiveness of the end-organ, and breast cancer is the first disease in which estimation of tissue receptors can be used to predict the effect of therapy (*British Medical Journal*, 1980).

Specific high-affinity binding for oestradiol is found over a wide range of concentrations in extracts from tumours of 60-70 per cent of women with metastatic breast cancer (McGuire, 1978; Allegra *et al.*, 1980). Regression of the tumour with endocrine treatment occurs in about 50 per cent of patients with oestrogen-receptor positive tumours but only in 5-10 per cent of those with oestrogen-receptor negative tumours (McGuire *et al.*, 1975). Concentration of oestrogen-receptor is an important prognostic factor but not the only one since in tumours with relatively high concentrations response rates do not exceed 80 per cent (*British Medical Journal*, 1980).

The British Breast Group and Colleagues (1980) have reported on the current status of oestradiol receptor analyses in relation to the management of breast cancer. They suggest that receptor assays should be included in protocols for future clinical trials in breast cancer whenever possible.

Summary

Breast cancer is a disease which causes major morbidity and mortality among women and although mortality rates are tending to level off in more highly industrialised countries, adoption of the Western life style appears to be increasing the rates of the disease in less highly developed societies. In spite of extensive epidemiological, laboratory and clinical research the underlying causative factors are far from clear and therapeutic measures for the most part improve the quality rather than the quantity of survival following diagnosis. It seems that in many cases of breast cancer the biological nature of the tumour predetermines the progress of the disease.

The evidence available would support the hypothesis that it is a tumour which is primarily hormonally mediated, but the hormonal profile of women who are at high risk of breast cancer is not yet clearly identified. However, external endocrine influences are recognised, some of which may be amenable to intervention, e.g. reproductive practices and use of exogenous hormones. The influence of nutritional factors on hormone levels is also an important area for research. There is some evidence that population screening will reduce mortality for breast cancer by detecting the tumour at an earlier stage, but the cost is excessive with present screening methods.

It is clear that the present state of knowledge of breast cancer does not give grounds for optimism that a substantial reduction in incidence of the disease or an improved response to therapy is likely in the foreseeable future. It is important, therefore, that interdisciplinary research continues to try to identify causal mechanisms in the development of breast cancer which might lead to more effective primary prevention, and also to search for better techniques for early diagnosis and improved therapeutic regimes for established disease.

References

Alderson, M. (1981). Parity and breast cancer. *British Medical Journal*, 283: 9-10

Allegra, J.C., Lippman, M.E., Thomson, E.B., Simon, R., Barlock, A., Green, L. *et al.* (1980). Estrogen receptor status: an important variable in predicting response to endocrine therapy in metastatic breast cancer. *European Journal of Cancer*, 16: 323-31

Anderson, D.E. (1976). Genetic predisposition to breast cancer. In: Stoll, B. (ed.), *Risk Factors in Breast Cancer*, Vol. 2, Heinemann, London, ch. 1, p. 6

Armstrong, B. and Doll, R. (1975). Environmental factors and cancer incidence and mortality in different countries, with special reference to dietary practices. *International Journal of Cancer*, 15: 617-31

Bailar, J.C., III (1963). The incidence of independent tumors among uterine cancer patients. *Cancer*, 16: 842-53

Baverstock, K.F., Papworth, D. and Vennart, J. (1981). Risks of radiation at low dose rates. *Lancet*, 1: 430-3

Bjarnason, O., Day, N., Snaedal, G. and Tulinius, H. (1974). The effect of year of birth on the breast cancer age incidence curve in Iceland. *International Journal of Cancer*, 13: 689-96

Black, M.M., Barclay, T.H., Cutler, S.J., Hankley, B.F. and Asire, A.J. (1972). Association of typical characteristics of benign breast disease lesions with subsequent risk of breast cancer. *Cancer*, 29: 338-43

Boice, J.D. and Monson, R.R. (1977). Breast cancer in women after repeated fluoroscopic examinations of the chest. *Journal of the National Cancer Institute*, 59: 823-32

Bonadonna, G. (1980). Adjuvant chemotherapy of breast cancer. *British Journal of Hospital Medicine*, 23: 40-53

Boston Collaborative Drug Surveillance Program (1973). Oral contraceptives and venous thromboembolic disease surgically confirmed, gall-bladder disease, and breast tumours. *Lancet*, 1: 1399-401

—— (1974). Reserpine and breast cancer. *Lancet*, 2: 669-71

Boyns, A.R., Cole, E.N., Griffiths, K., Roberts, M.M., Buchan, R., Wilson, R.G. *et al.* (1973). Plasma prolactin in breast cancer. *European Journal of Cancer*, 9: 99-108

Brinton, L.A., Hoover, R. and Fraumeni, J.F., Jr. (1982). Interaction of familial and hormonal risk factors for breast cancer. *Journal of the National Cancer Institute*, 69: 817-22

Brinkley, D. and Haybittle, J.L. (1975). The curability of breast cancer. *Lancet*, 2: 95-7

British Breast Cancer Group and Colleagues (1980). Steroid receptor assays in human breast cancer. *Lancet*, 1: 298-300

British Medical Journal (1980). Editorial. Hormone receptors and human breast cancer, 281: 694-5

Buell, P. (1973). Changing incidence of breast cancer in Japanese American women. *Journal of the National Cancer Institute*, 51: 1479-83

Bulbrook, R.D., Greenwood, F.C. and Hayward, J.L. (1960). Selection of breast cancer patients for adrenalectomy or hypophysectomy by determination of 17-hydroxy corticosteroids and aetiocholanotone. *Lancet*, 2: 1154-7

—— Hayward, J.L., Spicer, C.C. and Thomas, B.S. (1962a). A comparison between the urinary steroid excretion of normal women and women with advanced breast cancer. *Lancet*, 2: 1235-7

—— Hayward, J.L. and Spicer, C.C. (1962b). Abnormal excretion of urinary steroids by women with early breast cancer. *Lancet*, 2: 1238-40

—— and Hayward, J.L. (1967). Abnormal urinary steroid excretion and subsequent breast cancer. A prospective study in the island of Guernsey. *Lancet*, 2: 519-21

Carey, R.W., Holland, J.F., Sheehe, P.R. and Graham, S. (1967). Association of cancer of the breast and acute myelocytic leukemia. *Cancer*, 20: 1081-8

Carroll, K.K. (1981). Neutral fats and cancer. *Cancer Research*, 41: 3695-9

—— Gammal, E.B. and Plunkett, E.R. (1968). Dietary fat and mammary cancer. *Canadian Medical Association Journal*, 98: 590-4

—— and Khor, H.T. (1971). Effects of level and type of dietary fat on incidence of mammary tumours induced in female Sprague-Dawley rats by 7, 12-dimethyl benzanthracene. *Lipids*, 6: 415-20

—— and Hopkins, G.J. (1979). Dietary polyunsaturated fat versus saturated fat in relation to mammary carcinogenesis. *Lipids*, 14: 155-8

Casagrande, J., Gerkins, J., Henderson, B.E., Mack, T. and Pike, M.C. (1976). Exogenous oestrogens and breast cancer in women with natural menopause. *Journal of the National Cancer Institute*, 56: 839-41

Chan, P. and Cohen, L.A. (1974). Effect of dietary fat, antiestrogen and anti-prolactin on the development of mammary tumours in rats. *Journal of the National Cancer Institute*, 52: 25-30

Choi, N.W., Howe, G.R., Miller, A.B., Matthews, V., Morgan, R., Munan, L. *et al.* (1978). An epidemiologic study of breast cancer. *American Journal of Epidemiology*, 107: 510-21

Clemmeson, J. (1948). Carcinoma of the breast; results from statistical research. *British Journal of Radiology*, 21: 583-90

Craig, T.J., Comstock, G.W. and Geiser, P.B. (1974). Epidemiologic comparison of breast cancer patients with early and late onset of malignancy and general population controls. *Journal of the National Cancer Institute*, 53: 1577-81

Davis, H.H., Simons, M. and Davis, J.B. (1964). Cystic disease of the breast: relationship to carcinoma. *Cancer*, 17: 957-78
de Waard, F. (1969). The epidemiology of breast cancer; review and prospects. *International Journal of Cancer*, 4: 577-86
────── (1975). Breast cancer incidence and nutritional status with particular reference to body weight and height. *Cancer Research*, 35: 3351-6
────── Baanders-van Halewjin, E.A. and Huixinga, J. (1964). The bimodal age-distribution of patients with mammary carcinoma. *Cancer*, 17: 141-51
────── and Baanders-van Halewjin, E.A. (1974). A prospective study in general practice on breast cancer risk in post-menopausal women. *International Journal of Cancer*, 14: 153-60
────── Cornelis, J.P., Aoki, K. and Yoshida, M. (1977). Breast cancer incidence according to weight and height in two cities of the Netherlands and in the Aichi Prefecture, Japan. *Cancer*, 40: 1269-75
────── Rombach, J.J. and Colette, H.J.A. (1978). The DOM project for breast cancer screening in the city of Utrecht. In: Miller, A.B. (ed.), *Screening in Cancer*, UICC Technical Report, No. 40, Geneva, pp. 183-200
Dickinson, L.E., MacMahon, B., Cole, P. and Brown, J.B. (1974). Oestrogen profiles of Oriental and Caucasian women in Hawaii. *New England Journal of Medicine*, 291: 1211-13
Doll, R., Muir, C. and Waterhouse, J. (eds.) (1970). *Cancer Incidence in Five Continents*, Vol. II, International Union Against Cancer, Springer Verlag, Berlin, Heidelberg and New York, ch. VI, pp. 356-7
Dunn, J.E., Bragg, K.V., Santter, C. (1972). Breast cancer risk following a major salivary gland carcinoma. *Cancer*, 29: 1343-6
Fishman, J., Fukushima, D., O'Connor, J., Rosenfeld, R.S., Lynch, H.T., Lynch, J.F. *et al.* (1978). Plasma hormone profiles of young women at risk for familial breast cancer. *Cancer Research*, 38: 4006-11
Fraumeni, J.F. and Miller, R.W. (1971). Breast cancer from breast feeding. *Lancet*, 2: 1196-7
Gammal, E.B., Carroll, K.K. and Plunkett, E.R. (1967). Effects of dietary fat on mammary carcinogenesis by 7, 12-dimethylbenz(a)anthracene in rats. *Cancer Research*, 27: 1737-42
Gilliam, A.G., (1951). Fertility and cancer of the breast and uterine cervix — comparisons between rates of pregnancy in women with cancer of these and other sites. *Journal of the National Cancer Institute*, 12: 287-304
Gray, G.E., Pike, M.C. and Henderson, B.E. (1979). Breast cancer incidence and mortality rates in different countries in relation to known risk factors and dietary practices. *British Journal of Cancer*, 39: 1-7
Haagensen, C.D., Bodian, C. and Haagensen, D.E. (1981). *Breast Carcinoma, Risk and Detection*, Saunders, Philadelphia, ch. 5, p. 30
Heinonen, O.P., Shapiro, S., Tuonenen, L. and Turunen, M.I. (1974). Reserpine use in relation to breast cancer. *Lancet*, 2: 675-7
Henderson, B.E., Dowell, D., Rosario, I., Keys, C., Hanish, R., Young, M. *et al.* (1974). An epidemiologic study of breast cancer. *Journal of the National Cancer Institute*, 53: 609-14
Herity, B.A., O'Halloran, M.J., Bourke, G.J. and Wilson-Davis, K. (1975). A study of breast cancer in Irish women. *British Journal of Preventive and Social Medicine*, 29: 178-81
Hoover, R., Gray, L.A., Cole, P. and MacMahon, B. (1976). Menopausal estrogens and breast cancer. *New England Journal of Medicine*, 295: 401-5
Jablon, S. and Kato, H. (1972). Studies of the mortality of A-bomb survivors. 5. Radiation dose and mortality, 1950-1970. *Radiation Research*, 50: 649-98
Jackson, A.W., Muldal, S., Ockey, C.H. and O'Connor, P.J. (1965). Carcinoma of

the male breast in association with the Klinefelter syndrome. *British Medical Journal*, 5429: 223-5

Kaplan, S.D. and Acheson, R.M. (1966). A single etiological hypothesis for breast cancer? *Journal of Chronic Disease*, 19: 1221-30

Kelsey, J.L., Holford, T.R., White, C., Mayer, E.S., Kilty, S.E. and Acheson, R.M. (1978). Oral contraceptives and breast disease, an epidemiological study. *American Journal of Epidemiology*, 107, No. 5, 236-44

Kirschener, M.A. (1977). The role of hormones in the etiology of human breast cancer. *Cancer*, 39: 2716-26

Kodlin, D. and McCarthy, N. (1978). Reserpine and breast cancer. *Cancer*, 41: 761-8

Knudson, A.G., Jr., Strong, L.C. and Anderson, D.E. (1973). Heredity and cancer in man. *Progress in Medical Genetics*, 9: 113-58

Kumaoka, S., Sakauchi, N., Abe, O., Kusama, M. and Takatani, O. (1968). Urinary 17 ketosteroid excretion of women with advanced breast cancer. *Journal of Clinical Endocrinology*, 28: 667-72

Kwa, H.G., Engelsman, E., de Jong-Bakken, M. and Cuton, F.J. (1974). Plasma prolactin in human breast cancer. *Lancet*, 1: 433-5

Lancet (1982). Editorial. Screening for breast cancer. 1: 1103-4

Lane-Claypon, J.E. (1926). A further report on cancer of the breast with special reference to its associated antecedent conditions. *Report on Public Health and Medical Subjects*, No. 32, HMSO, London

Levin, M.L., Sheehe, P.R., Graham, S. and Glidewell, O. (1964). Lactation and menstrual function as related to cancer of the breast. *American Journal of Public Health*, 54: 580-7

Li, F.P. and Fraumeni, J.F., Jr. (1969). Soft tissue sarcomas, breast cancer and other neoplasms. A familial syndrome? *Annals of Internal Medicine*, 71: 747-52

Lilienfeld, A.M. (1963). The epidemiology of breast cancer. *Cancer Research*, 23: 1503-13

—— Coombs, J., Bross, I.D.J. and Chamberlain, A. (1975). Marital and reproductive experience in a community-wide epidemiological study of breast cancer. *Johns Hopkins Medical Journal*, 136: 157-62

Lin, T.M., Chen, K.P. and MacMahon, B. (1971). Epidemiologic characteristics of cancer of the breast in Taiwan. *Cancer*, 27: 1497-504

Logan, W.P.D. (1975). Cancer of the breast: no decline in mortality. *WHO Chronicle*, 29: 462-71

Longcope, C. (1971). Metabolic clearance and blood production rates of estrogens in post-menopausal women. *American Journal of Obstetrics and Gynecology*, III. 778-81

Lundgren, B. (1979). Efficiency of single view mammography. *Journal of the National Cancer Institute*, 62: 799-802

Lynch, H.T. and Krush, A.J. (1971). Genetic predictability in breast cancer risk. *Archives of Surgery*, 103: 84-8

—— Guirgis, H., Albert, S. and Brennan, M. (1974). Familial breast cancer in a normal population. *Cancer*, 34: 2080-6

MacDonald, P.C., Grodin, J.M. and Siiteri, P.K. (1969). The utilisation of plasma androstenedione for oestrone production in women. In: Gual, C. (ed.), *Progress in Endocrinology*, Excerpta Medica, International Congress Series, 184, 770-6

MacKenzie, I. (1965). Breast cancer following multiple fluoroscopies. *British Journal of Cancer*, 19: 1-8

Macklin, M.T. (1940). An analysis of tumours in monozygous and dizygous twins. With a report of fifteen unpublished cases. *Journal of Heredity*, 31: 277-90

—— (1959). Comparison of number of breast cancer deaths observed in relatives of breast-cancer patients, and the number expected on the basis of mortality rates. *Journal of the National Cancer Institute*, 22: 929-51

MacMahon, B. and Austin, J.H. (1969). Association of carcinoma of the breast and corpus uteri. *Cancer*, 23: 275-80

—— Lin, T.M., Lowe, C.R., Mirra, A.P., Ravnihar, B., Salber, E.J. *et al.* (1970a). Lactation and cancer of the breast. Summary of an international study. *Bulletin of the World Health Organization*. 42: 185-94

—— Cole, P., Lin, T.M., Lowe, C.R., Mirra, A.P., Ravnihar, B. *et al.* (1970b). Age at first birth and breast cancer risk. *Bulletin of the World Health Organization*, 43: 209-21

—— Cole, P., Brown, J.B., Aoki, K., Lin, T.M., Morgan, R.W. *et al.* (1971). Oestrogen profiles of Asian and North American women. *Lancet*, 2: 900-2

—— Cole, P. and Brown, J. (1973). Etiology of breast cancer; a review. *Journal of the National Cancer Institute*, 50: 21-41

McGuire, W.L. (1978). Hormone receptors: their role in predicting prognosis and response to endocrine therapy. *Seminars in Oncology*, 5, 428-33

—— Carbone, P.P., Sears, M.E. and Escher, G.C. (1975). Estrogen receptors in human breast cancer: an overview. In: McGuire, W.L., Carbone, P.P. and Voltmer, E.P. (eds.), *Estrogen Receptors in Human Breast Cancer*, Raven Press, New York, ch. 1, pp. 1-7

Mettler, F.A., Hempelmann, L.H., Dutton, A.M., Pifer, J.W., Tooyoka, E.T. and Ames, W.R. (1969). Breast neoplasms in women treated with X-rays for postpartum mastitis. *Journal of the National Cancer Institute*, 43: 803-11

Miller, A.B. (1977). Role of nutrition in the etiology of breast cancer. *Cancer*, 39: 2704-8

—— (1980). National breast cancer screening gets underway. *Canadian Medical Association Journal*, 122: 243-4

—— (1981). Breast cancer. *Cancer*, 47: 1109-13

—— Kelly, A., Choi, N.W., Matthews, V., Morgan, R.W., Munan, L. *et al.* (1978). A study of diet and breast cancer. *American Journal of Epidemiology*, 107: 499-509

—— and Bulbrook, R.D. (1980). The epidemiology and etiology of breast cancer. *New England Journal of Medicine*, 30:3: 1246-8

—— Barclay, T.H.C., Choi, N.W., Grace, M.C., Wall, C., Plante, M. *et al.* (1980). A study of cancer, parity and age at first pregnancy. *Journal of Chronic Disease*, 33: 595-605

—— and Bulbrook, R.D. (1982). Screening, detection and diagnosis of breast cancer. *Lancet*, 1: 1109-11

Miller, R.W. (1971). Deaths from childhood leukemia and solid tumors among twins and other sibs in the United States, 1960-67. *Journal of the National Cancer Institute*, 46: 203-9

Mittra, I., Hayward, J.L. and McNeilly, A.S. (1974). Hypothalamic-pituitary-prolactin axis in breast cancer. *Lancet*, 1: 889-91

Mole, R.H. (1975). Ionizing radiation as a carcinogen: practical questions and academic pursuits. *British Journal of Radiology*, 48: 157-69

Moore, D.H., Charney, J., Kramarsky, B., Lasfargues, E.Y., Sarkar, N.H., Brennan, M.J. *et al.* (1971). Search for a human breast cancer virus. *Nature*, 229: 611-14

Morbidity and Mortality Weekly Report (1982). Oral contraceptives and cancer risk, 31, No. 29, pp. 393-4

Mueller, C.B. and Jeffries, W. (1975). Cancer of the breast: its outcome as measured by the rate of dying and causes of deaths. *Annals of Surgery*, 182: 334-41

Myrden, J.A. and Hiltz, J.A. (1969). Breast cancer following multiple fluoroscopies during artificial pneumothorax treatment of pulmonary tuberculosis. *Journal of the Canadian Medical Association*, 100: 1032-4

Paffenbarger, R.S., Jr., Fasal, E., Simmons, M.E. and Kampert, J.B. (1977). Cancer risk as related to oral contraceptives during fertile years. *Cancer*, 39: 1887-91

Page, H.L., Vanderzwaag, R., Rogers, L.W., Williams, L.T., Walker, S.E. and Hartmann, W.H. (1978). Relation between component parts of fibrocystic disease complex and breast cancer. *Journal of the National Cancer Institute*, 61: 1055-60

Papadrianos, E., Haagensen, C.D. and Cooley, E. (1967). Cancer of the breast as a familial disease. *Annals of Surgery*, 165: 10-19

Pearson, O.H., Murray, R.L.M., Mozafforian, G. and Densky, S. (1972). In: Boyars, A.R. and Griffiths, K. (eds.), *Prolactin and Carcinogenesis*, Alpha Omega Alpha Publishing Company, Cardiff, p. 154

Pike, M.C., Henderson, B.E., Casagrande, J.T., Rosario, I. and Gray, G.E. (1981). Oral contraceptive use and early abortion as risk factors for breast cancer in young women. *British Journal of Cancer*, 43: 72-6

Ramazzini, B. (1713). *Diseases of Workers*, translated from the Latin text, *De Mortis Artificum*, by W.C. Wright (1964), Hafner Publishing Company, New York, p. 191

Ravnihar, B., Seigel, D.G. and Lindtner, J. (1979). An epidemiologic study of breast cancer and benign breast disease neoplasias in relation to the oral contraceptive and estrogen use. *European Journal of Cancer*, 15: 395-405

Rosenberg, L., Slowe, D., Shapiro, S., Kaufman, D.W., Helmrich, S.P., Miettinen, O.S. *et al.* (1982). Breast cancer and alcoholic beverage consumption. *Lancet*, 1: 267-71

Royal College of General Practitioners (1981). Breast cancer and oral contraceptives: findings in a Royal College of General Practitioners Study. *British Medical Journal*, 282: 2089-93

Sartwell, P.E., Arthes, F.G. and Tomascia, J.A. (1977). Exogenous hormones, reproductive history and breast cancer. *Journal of the National Cancer Institute*, 59: 1589-92

Schoenberg, B., Greenberg, R.A. and Eisenberg, H. (1969). Occurrence of multiple primary cancers in females. *Journal of the National Cancer Institute*, 43: 15-37

Schottenfeld, D., Lilienfeld, A.M. and Diamond, H. (1963). Some observations on the epidemiology of breast cancer among males. *American Journal of Public Health*, 53: 890-7

―――― and Berg, J. (1971). Incidence of multiple primary cancers. IV. Cancer of the female breast and genital organs. *Journal of the National Cancer Institute*, 46: 161-70

―――― Berg, J.W. and Vitsky, B. (1976). Incidence of multiple primary cancers. II. Index cancers arising in the stomach and lower digestive system. *Journal of the National Cancer Institute*, 43: 77-86

Segi, M., Fukushima, I., Fujisako, S., Kurihara, M., Sarto, S., Asano, K. *et al.* (1957). An epidemiological study of cancer in Japan. *Gann* 48, Supplement 1-63

Shapiro, S., Strax, P. and Venet, L. (1971). Periodic breast cancer screening in reducing mortality from breast cancer. *Journal of the American Medical Association*, 215: 1777-85

―――― Venet, W., Strax, P., Venet, L. and Roeser, R. (1982). Ten to fourteen year effects of breast cancer screening on mortality. *Journal of the National Cancer Institute*, 69: 349-55

Shimkin, M.B. (1977). *Contrary to Nature*, Castle House Publications, Tunbridge Wells, Kent, ch. II, pp. 21, 33; ch. IV, pp. 57, 63-5

Simon, N. and Silverstone, S.M. (1976). Radiation as a cause of breast cancer. *Bulletin of the New York Academy of Medicine*, 52: 741-51

Stocks, P. (1957). The epidemiology of carcinoma of the breast. *Practitioner*, 179: 233-40

Symmers, W. St. C. (1968). Carcinoma of the breast in trans-sexual individuals after surgical and hormonal interference with primary and secondary sex characteristics. *British Medical Journal*, 2: 83-5

Tabar, L. and Gad, A. (1981). Screening for breast cancer – the Swedish trial. *Radiology*, 138: 219-22

Thomas, R.A., Price, J.L. and Boulter, P. (1981). Breast cancer population screening by single view mammography and selective clinical examination – a pilot study. *Clinical Oncology*, 7: 201-4

Tokuchata, G.K. (1969). Morbidity and mortality among offspring of breast cancer mothers. *American Journal of Epidemiology*, 89: 139-50

Tokunaga, M., Land, C.E., Yamamoto, T., Asano, M., Tokuoka, S., Ezaki, H. and Nishimori, I. (1982). 'Breast cancer in Japanese A-bomb survivors' (correspondence), *Lancet*, 2: 924

Trichopoulos, P., MacMahon, B. and Cole, P. (1972). Menopause and breast cancer risk. *Journal of the National Cancer Institute*, 48: 605-13

UK Trial of Early Detection of Breast Cancer Group (1981). Trial of early detection of breast cancer: description of method. *British Journal of Cancer*, 44: 618-27

Valaoras, V.G., MacMahon, B., Trichopoulos, D. and Polychronopoulou, A. (1969). Lactation and reproductive histories of breast cancer patients in greater Athens, 1966-67. *International Journal of Cancer*, 4: 330-53

Vessey, M.P., McPherson, K. and Doll, R. (1981). Breast cancer and oral contraceptives: findings in the Oxford Family Planning Association Contraceptive Study. *British Medical Journal*, 282: 2093-4

Vongtama, V., Kurohara, S.S., Badib, A.O. and Webster, J.H. (1970). Second primary cancers of endometrial carcinoma. *Cancer*, 26: 842-6

Wagoner, J.K., Chiazze, L. and Lloyd, J.W. (1967). Cancer of the breast at menopausal age. *Cancer*, 20: 354-62

Wainwright, J.M. (1931). A comparison of conditions associated with breast cancer in Great Britain and America. *American Journal of Cancer*, 15: 2610-45

Wanebo, C.K., Johnson, K.G., Sato, K. and Thorslund, T.W. (1968). Breast cancer after exposure to the atomic bombing of Hiroshima and Nagasaki. *New England Journal of Medicine*, 279: 667-71

Williams, R.G. and Horm, J.W. (1977). Association of cancer sites with tobacco and alcohol consumption and socioeconomic status of patients: interview study from the Third National Cancer Survey. *Journal of the National Cancer Institute*, 58: 527-47

Wilson, R.E., Crocker, D.W., Fairgrieve, J., Bartholomay, A.F., Emerson, K. and Moore, F.D. (1967). Adrenal structure and function in advanced carcinoma of the breast. II. The relation of steroid excretion to adrenal morphology and the outcome of adrenalectomy with description of a new discriminant function. *Journal of the American Medical Association*, 199: 474-82

Wilson, R.G., Buchan, R., Roberts, M.M., Forest, A.P.M., Boyns, A.R., Cole, E.N. *et al.* (1974). Plasma prolactin and breast cancer, *Cancer*, 33: 1325-7

Wynder, E.L., Bross, I.J. and Hirayama, T. (1960). A study of the epidemiology of cancer of the breast. *Cancer*, 13: 559-601

Yuasa, S. and MacMahon, B. (1970). Lactation and reproductive histories of breast cancer patients in Tokyo, Japan. *Bulletin of the World Health Organization*, 42: 195-204

13 LYMPHORETICULAR MALIGNANCIES

N.J. Vianna and D. Straus

Introduction

During the past decade lymphoma and leukaemia research has been in a rapid state of flux largely due to a growing knowledge in the field of immunology. Perhaps this is best exemplified in the changes that have occurred in classifying these disorders. During the 1950s non-Hodgkin's lymphomas were divided into three groups: reticulum cell sarcoma, lymphosarcoma and follicular lymphomas. In the latter part of the 1950s Rappaport et al. (1956) classified these disorders as lymphocytic, histiocytic, or mixtures of the two. In addition, they suggested that these disorders be further subtyped as to whether they were nodular or diffuse. With the rapid advances being made in immunological research, it became apparent that the human immune system could be divided into three components – the thymic system (T) involved primarily with cell mediated immunity, the bursal (B) system which mediates humoral immunity, and the histiocyte-macrophage system. These observations prompted the development of additional classifications of the malignant lymphomas and lymphatic leukaemias which attempted to classify each type according to its immunological cell origin (Lukes and Collins, 1974). B cell disorders include some acute and most chronic lymphatic leukaemias, most non-Hodgkin's lymphomas and Burkitt's lymphoma (Cooper, 1981). T cell tumours include some acute and chronic lymphomas, Sezary syndrome and mycosis fungoides (Cooper, 1981). Acute lymphoblastic leukaemia, generally accepted in the past as a single entity, is currently considered to consist of at least three different types of disorder (Bernard et al., 1979). Even within this categorisation there is evidence to suggest a possible heterogeny. Using a T cell subset specific heteroantisera to phenotype T cell lymphoblastic malignancies, Nadler et al. (1980) found that lymphoblastic lymphoma and T cell acute lymphoblastic leukaemia are probably not a single disease process.

It is beyond the scope of this review to go into further detail about the classification of lymphatic malignancies. These brief comments do serve, however, to indicate the complexities that arise when one considers possible aetiological factors for these disorders. At present

214

many malignant lymphomas are viewed as the uncontrolled clonal proliferation of different types of immune cells at various stages of their differentiation (Lukes and Collins, 1974; Parker, 1981). Perhaps this is best exemplified with Hodgkin's disease. The Rye classification (Lukes *et al.*, 1966a, b; Lukes and Butler, 1966) has been almost universally accepted for this disorder, but to date we do not know the neoplastic cell of origin (Forbes, 1979). The varied histological features of this lymphoma may well be the result of different types of immune cell reactions. Since all of the immune systems interact, the ultimate system of classifying these disorders may not depend on the specific cell type involved but rather upon a characterisation of the type of interaction that occurs. This review will summarise three major issues: the current knowledge of the epidemiological patterns for these disorders in various parts of the world, possible aetiological factors and recent advances in diagnosis and treatment.

Epidemiological Patterns

Perhaps the strongest evidence suggesting that environmental factors are important in the aetiology of many lymphomas is the marked variation in overall incidence and age distribution in various countries. Certain lymphomas and closely related disorders occur in localised geographical areas where they may be truly characterised as endemic. In contrast, the more common types of lymphomas (e.g. Hodgkin's disease, non-Hodgkin's lymphomas) are widespread in their distribution. But even within this latter group there is a great variability with regard to factors such as age, sex and socioeconomic status.

Endemic Lymphomas and Sarcomas

Table 13.1 lists the characteristics of certain important endemic lymphomas and sarcomas. Burkitt's lymphoma is the most common childhood neoplasm observed in sections of East Africa (Burkitt, 1958; 1962). While this disorder does occur in the United States of America (USA) and other developed countries, it manifests an older age distribution and lymph nodes and bone marrow are more frequently involved in American cases than in Africa where jaw involvement is more common (Levine *et al.*, 1982; Ziegler, 1981). American Burkitt's lymphoma does, however, resemble the African type with regard to time-space clustering, male predominance and excellent response to chemotherapy (Levine *et al.*, 1982). Throughout the world the target

Table 13.1: Characteristics of Certain Endemic Lymphomas and Sarcomas

	Burkitt's lymphoma	Mediterranean intestinal lymphoma	T-cell leukaemia lymphoma	Kaposi's sarcoma
Geographic location	Tropical Africa, New Guinea	East coast of the Mediterranean Sea (poorly developed countries)	Japan (Kyusha, South Shikoka, South Kit Peninsula)	Equatorial Africa, Eastern-central Europe
Age	Children	Young adults	Adults	Adults, black children
M:F sex ratio	Greater than 2:1	Close to unity	Close to unity	Greater than 10:1
Familial predisposition	Yes	—	Yes	Rare
Possible causal agent	Epstein-Barr virus	Chronic infection	Virus-filariasis	Cytomegalic virus

cell for this disorder is the B lymphocyte, and available evidence suggests that a strong association exists between this tumour and the Epstein-Barr virus (EBV) in some areas of the world (Ziegler, 1981). It has also been suggested that the geographical localisation of Burkitt's lymphoma might be related to the frequency of malarial infection in certain parts of the world (Burkitt, 1969; O'Conor, 1970). It has been shown that antigenic stimulation by malaria produces a large number of immunocompetent stem cells that are highly sensitive to malignant transformation by the EBV (Schwartz, 1980). Evidence supporting this possible association is the similarity in geographical distribution and also the time trends of the incidence of Burkitt's lymphoma and malaria (Epstein *et al.*, 1964). Since 1960 antimalarial drugs have become available in Africa and New Guinea and dichlorodiphenyltrichloroethane (DDT) has been used to control malaria. Subsequent studies have demonstrated that the incidence of Burkitt's lymphoma actually decreased in these areas (Morrow *et al.*, 1976). However, further research will be required to establish a causal relationship between malaria and this lymphoma.

The intestinal lymphoma syndrome occurs primarily in poorly developed countries along the east coast of the Mediterranean Sea (Ramot and Many, 1972). It is most prevalent in children and available evidence suggests that chronic immunological stimulation from infection is essential in the development of this tumour. While the tumour is rare in well developed countries, it occurs in children and young adults and there appears to be a strong association with prior coeliac disease (Vianna, 1977). The intestinal site most commonly affected is the midjejunum. In contrast, in poorly developed countries the terminal ileum, duodenum and proximal jejunum are the more common sites. As is true with Burkitt's lymphoma, Mediterranean intestinal lymphoma is a B cell tumour.

Adult T cell leukaemia-lymphoma occurs primarily in coastal areas of Japan which are warm in winter and humid in the summer (Tajima *et al.*, 1981). Most patients develop this disorder after the age of 40, by which time the thymus is remarkably involuted. Interestingly, a recent article by Catovsky *et al.* (1982) describes this disorder among six blacks age 21 to 55 years in the United Kingdom. Five of these individuals were born in the West Indies and one in Guyana. To date, there appear to be no confirmed cases of this disorder among children, an age group characterised by rapid T cell division. Furthermore, all of the cases described outside of Japan have occurred among blacks (Catovsky *et al.*, 1982). Further study is clearly indicated to explain this important observation.

Kaposi's sarcoma appears to be associated with an increased incidence of lymphoreticular neoplasms (Safai *et al.*, 1980). This disorder is a multicentric process which manifests as multiple vascular tumours which are composed of proliferating connective tissue and capillary vessels (Safai and Good, 1981). This disease is endemic in Equatorial Africa and is also found in Eastern-central Europe, Italy and North America (Davis, 1968). In Uganda it accounts for 9 per cent of all cancers (Öettle, 1963), whereas in the United States the annual incidence is between 0.02 and 0.06 per 100,000 population (Rothman, 1962). Recently there have been several reports documenting an increased incidence of Kaposi's sarcoma in homosexuals (Durack, 1981; *Lancet*, 1981). Most of the patients are males less than 50 years of age from urban areas such as New York City, Los Angeles and San Francisco. In addition, patients have had concomitant opportunistic infections with such organisms as pneumocystis, cryptococcus, candida and cytomegalovirus (CMV).

Similar, albeit poorly defined, situations have been described in other areas. In Egypt there is a high frequency of malignant lymphomas found in individuals under 20 years of age and it has been suggested that chronic bilharziasis might be an important factor (El-Gazayerli *et al.*, 1962). Certain South American countries appear to have a high frequency of splenic and nasal lymphoma. In Peru and Columbia nasal lymphoma is frequently observed in patients with a history of chronic rhinitis (Weiss, 1954). Lymphoma of the spleen has been described in females with a history of chronic schistosomiasis infection in Brazil (Andrade and Waldeck, 1971). All of these observations would tend to support the concept that environmental agents are of potential importance in the aetiology of many malignant lymphomas. Further detailed investigation will be required to determine if these kinds of associations are causal or indirect; but it seems possible in many instances that environmental agents might exert their major influence by altering man's immune system in a fashion that predisposes to malignant lymphomas.

The Major Lymphomas. Figures 13.1 and 13.2 illustrate the average age-specific incidence rates for males and females diagnosed with the three major types of lymphomas in New York State. The age distributions depicted are characteristic for most industrialised countries throughout the world. In contrast to the other lymphomas, Hodgkin's disease manifests a bimodal age-specific incidence curve for each sex

Figure 13.1: Average Age-specific Incidence Rates for Males Diagnosed with Lymphoma in New York State (excluding New York City), 1974-1978

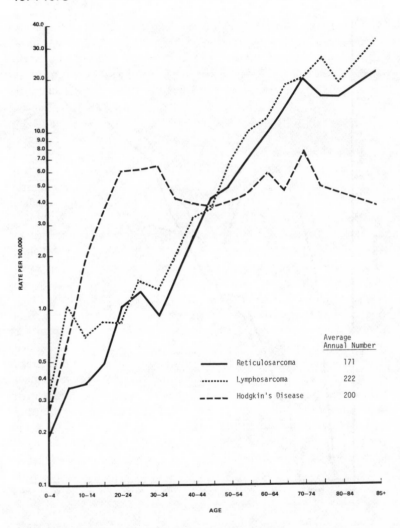

with peaks in the young adult and elderly age groups (Figures 13.1 and 13.2). This type of curve has also been described in Great Britain, Israel, Denmark and the Netherlands, while in Asian countries, such as Japan, the first age peak is absent (MacMahon, 1966). At present there is no acceptable explanation for this difference, although it has been

Figure 13.2: Average Age-specific Incidence Rates for Females Diagnosed with Lymphoma in New York State (excluding New York City), 1974-1978

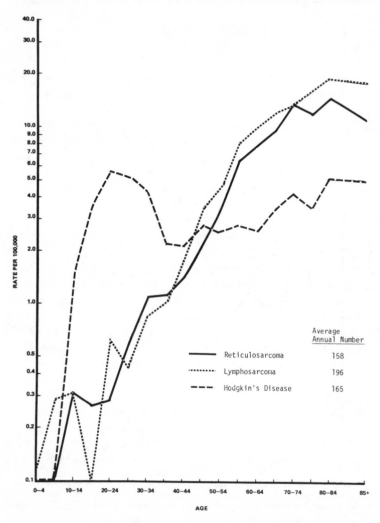

suggested that this lymphoma might be a different disease in the young and the old (MacMahon, 1966).

Correa and O'Conor (1971) have identified three different patterns of Hodgkin's disease and related each to the degree of urbanisation in various countries. The classical young adult–elderly bimodal curve has already been referred to. Another pattern is characterised by a high incidence rate in children, especially males, intermediate incidence rates in the third decade and the second peak in the elderly. This pattern seems to characterise developing countries such as Central America, Peru and Columbia (Correa and O'Conor, 1971). And an intermediate pattern, characterised by high rates in both children and young adults, has been observed in developing areas such as Puerto Rico. Further analyses have indicated that a reciprocal relationship exists between the average annual incidence rates for Hodgkin's disease in children and each of the other two age groups (young adults and the elderly) (Correa and O'Conor, 1971; Vianna and Polan, 1978). These observations strongly suggest that environmental factors, particularly during the early years of life, might be important determinants of the type of epidemiological pattern observed for this lymphoma in a given country. The possibility that family factors, such as sibship size and birth order, might play an important role in the different international patterns observed will be discussed later.

In general, the risk of lymphosarcoma and reticulum cell sarcoma increases with age (Figures 13.1 and 13.2). At least one investigation, however (Grundy *et al.*, 1973), suggests that there might be a distinct childhood peak for lymphosarcoma. This is interesting in view of the fact that lymphosarcoma is frequently associated with an acute lymphatic leukaemic stage (Gendelman *et al.*, 1969), whereas this is quite unusual for reticulum cell sarcoma. Acute lymphatic leukaemia of childhood has a distinct age peak at three to four years of age (Court Brown and Doll, 1961). Rates for this disorder actually decrease from this point through the age of 30 and then gradually increase with advanced age. In contrast, the chronic form of lymphatic leukaemia is primarily a disease of the elderly (MacMahon, 1966). It is doubtful if chronic lymphatic leukaemia ever occurs in children.

The incidence of most lymphoreticular diseases with the possible exception of multiple myeloma appears to be lower for blacks in the USA than whites (MacMahon, 1966). Incidence rates for Hodgkin's disease are low in Japan, but available evidence suggests that they may be high for Jews (MacMahon, 1966). Examination of Figures 13.1 and 13.2 reveals that males are at greater risk for each of the major lymphomas than females. Although acute lymphatic leukaemia used to be viewed as primarily a disease of white children, rates for blacks in the four years and under age group have approached those for whites (Slocumb and MacMahon, 1963). Finally, little is known about the influence of socioeconomic status on the frequency of most lymphoreticular malignancies, but available evidence suggests that high socioeconomic status might be a risk factor for Hodgkin's disease (MacMahon, 1966).

Aetiological Considerations. The occurrence of endemic lymphomas and the great variability in epidemiological patterns of some of the major lymphomas in different countries strongly suggests that environmental factors may be of great importance in the aetiology of many lymphoreticular malignancies. Many of these factors appear to alter man's immune system. There is also some compelling information implicating certain genetically related conditions (Burnet and Holmes, 1964; Mellors, 1966).

Environmental Factors. The strongest evidence that alterations of man's immune system can be associated with an increased risk of certain lymphomas comes from transplant studies. Hoover and Fraumeni (1973) studied over 6,000 renal transplant recipients and found that the risk of lymphoma was approximately 35 times that of normal. The vast majority of lymphomas were classified as reticulum cell sarcomas, and the risk of developing this specific type of disorder was estimated to be 350 times greater than expected. A significant excess of lymphomas, categorised as either reticulum cell or unclassified, has been observed among cardiac transplant patients (Anderson *et al.*, 1978). Of great interest are the facts that a significant majority of the lymphomas arose in patients who underwent cardiac transplantation for idiopathic cardiomyopathy and the sites of occurrence were the central nervous system and lungs. Patients with coronary artery disease who underwent this operative procedure did not seem to be at increased risk for the subsequent development of a malignant lymphoma. Interestingly, Anderson *et al.* (1978) also found a defect in mitogen-induced suppressor activity in patients with idiopathic cardiomyopathy. Several additional features of the transplant–lymphoma syndrome are noteworthy. The occurrence of Hodgkin's disease in transplant patients is exceedingly rare (Penn, 1981). Post-transplant lymphomas tend to occur at a relatively young age, and the induction period is relatively short (mean 47 months, range 1 to 187 months) (Penn, 1981). In addition to lymphomas the frequency of Kaposi's sarcoma was surprisingly high in transplant patients (Penn, 1981). This might be an exceedingly important observation in view of the evidence suggesting an association between this malignancy, certain other lymphomas and possibly cytomegalovirus infection (Giraldo *et al.*, 1972a, b; 1978;

1980). Finally, while there is limited information regarding the origin of the lymphomas in this setting, evidence suggests that six lymphomas were of host origin and one arose from donor cells.

It has long been thought that infectious agents, primarily viruses, might play an aetiological role in certain lymphoreticular malignancies. This is particularly true of childhood lymphatic leukaemia. Stewart *et al.* (1958) were among the first to suggest that some association might exist between childhood cancer and viral infection during pregnancy. Certain studies have found that the offspring of mothers with an influenza-like illness during pregnancy had a significantly greater frequency of acute leukaemia (Fedrick and Alberman, 1972; Hakulinen *et al.*, 1973). Other investigations have implicated varicella in the aetiology of childhood lymphatic leukaemia. Adelstein and Donovan (1972) found two deaths from this disorder among 270 children of mothers with chickenpox during pregnancy. Similar observations were made by Bithell *et al.* (1973). Vianna and Polan (1976) have suggested that maternal infection with varicella during various trimesters of pregnancy might be related to the age at which acute lymphatic leukaemia develops in different childhood age groups. These hypotheses are worthy of further investigation, particularly in view of the heterogeneous nature of this type of leukaemia.

In recent years, there has been a growing body of evidence suggesting that viral and other infectious agents might be important in the pathogenesis of certain lymphomas. Since its discovery, EBV has been implicated in a wide variety of disorders, including infectious mononucleosis (Niederman, 1956; Henle *et al.*, 1968), Burkitt's lymphoma (Epstein *et al.*, 1965), certain other B cell malignant lymphomas (Purtilo *et al.*, 1979), and nasopharyngeal cancer (Henle *et al.*, 1970). While the evidence implicating EBV in the aetiology of infectious mononucleosis is compelling, it remains unclear whether this agent causes certain malignant disorders or merely colonises neoplastic cells (Schwartz, 1980). In contrast to other herpes viruses, such as CMV, which stimulate a wide variety of cells, EBV is a polyclonal stimulator of B lymphocytes (Pattengale *et al.*, 1973). While it is beyond the scope of this review to examine the biological aspects of EBV in further detail, African patients with Burkitt's lymphoma have been found to have significantly elevated antibody titres to a variety of EBV determined antigens (Levine *et al.*, 1982). Eighty to 90 per cent of these tumours contain multiple markers of the EBV-DNA genome. In nonendemic areas such as the USA, EBV is found in 15 to 20 per cent of cases (Levine *et al.*, 1982). The reason(s) for this apparent discrepancy are currently unknown.

The recent case reports are of interest which suggest that diffuse polyclonal B cell lymphomas might result from primary infection with EBV in certain patients. The four-year-old female patient presented by Robinson *et al.* (1980) is particularly noteworthy since she had all of the classical features of infectious mononucleosis and subsequently developed a rapidly fatal lymphoplasmacytic neoplasia. The amazing feature in this patient was that her malignant lymphoproliferative response occurred despite the fact that her antiviral immune response was normal. Other atypical syndromes have been associated with primary EBV infection. Provisor *et al.* (1975) described three male children with infectious mononucleosis complicated by agammaglobu-linaemia. There have also been reports of fatal lymphoproliferative x-linked recessive syndromes that were probably associated with EBV infection (Purtilo *et al.*, 1979). These observations prompted Schwartz (1980) to suggest that EBV might not be inherently oncogenic. However, this agent might function in certain patients as an initiator of an abnormal thymic-bursal cell response. For example, the development of agammaglobulinaemia in patients with infectious mononucleosis might be viewed as an excessive response by suppressor T cells. This hypothesis gains some support from the fact that cell-mediated immunity can be depressed in infectious mononucleosis (Mangi *et al.*, 1974). It seems plausible that the outcome of primary EBV infection in certain patients, presumably those with some genetic defect, might be an excessive proliferation of B lymphocytes which ultimately results in a malignant lymphoma.

Other viruses, particularly CMV, can produce several immuno-suppressive effects in man. Carney *et al.* (1981) have demonstrated that CMV infection can reverse the normal ratio of T helper to T suppressor cells. In addition, patients with CMV mononucleosis seem to have a diminished response to certain mitogens (Rinaldo *et al.*, 1980). The studies of Giraldo *et al.* (1972b; 1975; 1978) suggest that CMV infection might play a role in the aetiology of Kaposi's sarcoma. The clustering of this multicentric vascular neoplasm (Öettle, 1963; Lothe, 1963) and the more recent reports of its excessive frequency among certain homosexuals does suggest an infectious aetiology. Unfortunately, CMV is ubiquitous and particularly common among homosexual men (Drew *et al.*, 1981). This would argue that other factors, possibly cultural, might be important. Durack (1981) has suggested that the so called 'recreational' drugs (e.g. alkyl nitrites, marijuana) might explain the apparently recent occurrence of Kaposi's sarcoma outbreaks in homosexual men. The incidence of this disorder has been reported to be approximately ten times higher than that seen in the white population in the same geographical area (Öettle, 1962). Thus, genetic factors might also be of aetiological importance. Another potentially important consideration is the high incidence of lymphomas and leukaemias in patients with Kaposi's sarcoma (Rothman, 1962; Moertel and Hagedorn, 1957). Safai *et al.* (1980) studied 92 patients with this disorder and found a 20-fold increase in the incidence of lymphoreticular neoplasms. This association is undoubtedly a reflection of the fact that altered immunity plays a fundamental role in the aetiology of all these disorders.

Infectious agents are also thought to be important in other lymphomas. Mediterranean intestinal lymphoma, a B cell disorder, is thought to be endemic along the eastern coast of the Mediterranean Sea because of the high frequency of intestinal parasitism and some form of chronic antigenic stimulation. Adult T cell leukaemia-lymphoma is endemic in the coastal and rural areas of southwestern Japan (Tajima *et al.*, 1981). This unique observation has led to the search for environmental factors, especially infectious agents, which might have a similar geographical distribution. One candidate at the present time is filariasis. The filarial worm can produce a wide range of lymphoreticular disorders and interestingly most of the adults in Japan who develped this disorder lived in endemic areas for filariasis during their childhood (Tajima *et al.*, 1981). Since filariasis has become very rare in those districts where adult T cell leukaemia-lymphoma is currently endemic, it will be important to monitor the future time trends of this lymphoreticular disorder.

Two fundamental characteristics which most of the endemic lymphomas share are that they occur primarily in non-industrialised areas and various infectious agents appear to be implicated. The distribution of some of these agents is universal (e.g. EBV, CMV). But other agents (e.g. parasitic diseases) which have been associated with lymphoreticular malignancies are most prevalent in poorly developed countries. It is now well established that many infections of this type can impair the immune system. In certain experimental animals malaria can depress the humoral response and possible cellular immunity (Jayawardena, 1981). Polyclonal activation of B cells has also been documented in malaria and other protozoan infections. *Schistosoma mansoni* appears to be able to cause immunosuppression in man (Colley, 1976). This might partially explain the unusually high occurrence of follicular lymphoma of the spleen in countries such as Brazil (Andrade and

Abreu, 1971).

In industrialised communities it seems possible that certain chemicals might play a similar role to that of infectious disorders. Experimental studies in animals and epidemiological observations in man support this possibility. Immunological dysfunction has been observed in lower animals exposed to various compounds including halogenated aromatic hydrocarbons such as 2, 3, 7, 8 tetrachlorodibenzo-p-dioxin (Vos *et al.*, 1973), polychlorinated biphenyl and hexachlorobenzene (Loose *et al.*, 1977). Chemically-induced alteration of host resistance to bacterial (Thigpen *et al.*, 1975) and viral infection (Friend and Trainer, 1970), and protozoan infestation (Loose *et al.*, 1978) has been demonstrated in several species. In addition, humoral and cell-mediated immunity (Loose *et al.*, 1977) can be altered in rodents following chronic exposure to low levels of certain chemicals.

In man several chemicals and/or occupations with potential exposure to toxic agents might be important in the aetiology of certain malignant lymphomas. The preliminary results of a proportionate mortality study by Nicholson and Selikoff (1978) suggested that an excess of leukaemias and lymphomas might have occurred among styrene-polystyrene polymerisation workers. Workers in the plant manufactured these compounds, during certain periods, from benzene and ethyl-benzene. These results support the hypothesis that benzene workers might be at increased risk for malignant lymphomas (Vianna and Polan, 1979; Olin, 1978) and occupational exposure to wood might predispose to Hodgkin's disease (Milham and Hesser, 1967). These observations are of interest particularly in light of the more recent evidence which suggest that in certain animals 2-4 dichlorophenoxy acetic acid (Edling, 1981) and in man exposure to herbicides (Olsson and Brandt, 1981) and phenoxyacetic acids (Hardell, 1979) might be a predisposing factor to malignant lymphomas. Aluminium reduction workers appear to have an excess mortality due to leukaemias and lymphomas (Milham, 1979). Chemists in the United States (Li *et al.*, 1969), Sweden (Olin, 1978) and Great Britain (Searle and Waterhouse, 1978) also appear to have increased mortality due to malignant lymphomas. Others have failed to confirm these results (Benn *et al.*, 1979). At present all of these observations must be viewed as preliminary. They do, however, merit further investigation in view of the different epidemiological patterns observed for certain lymphomas in industrialised and poorly developed countries. Furthermore, the evidence should be recalled that hydantoin drugs (Hyman and Sommers, 1966) and other pharmaceutical agents such as amphetamines (Boston Collaborative Drug Surveillance

Program, 1974) might be important in the aetiology of certain malignant lymphomas. Still other factors such as trauma (Bichel, 1979; Weh and Andrieu, 1979), burns (Panke *et al.*, 1978), chronic osteomyelitis (Posnett *et al.*, 1979; Laurent *et al.*, 1980) and heroin addiction (Dworsky and Henderson, 1974) might play some role in the pathogenesis of these disorders.

If certain infectious agents predispose to certain lymphoreticular malignancies, it would seem possible that other infections might have an antagonistic effect on the course of these disorders. There have been several reports of remission of Hodgkin's disease after measles infection (Hernandez, 1949; Zygiert, 1971; Taqi *et al.*, 1981). Post-transfusion hepatitis has been associated with beneficial effects in patients with acute myelogenous leukaemia (Barton and Conrad, 1979), and more recently with leukaemic reticuloendotheliosis (Brody *et al.*, 1981). Various infectious disorders, including acute appendicitis (Einhorn, 1961), staphylococcus, streptococcus, varicella and feline leukopenia (Bierman *et al.*, 1953), appear to influence favourably the course of acute lymphatic leukaemia of childhood. All of these observations are based on case reports, and accordingly the possibility that they represent chance associations cannot be excluded. However, these descriptive observations are quite intriguing since they lend support to the concept that certain infectious diseases might be associated with specific lymphoreticular malignancies through their ability to alter the host's immune response. Perhaps an analogous situation exists among those patients who develop multiple haematological malignancies. The immunological response to one malignancy might in fact suppress the course of another. This might be particularly true with regard to myeloproliferative and lymphoproliferative disorders in the same patient. Several case reports suggest that an antagonistic response exists between the two processes (Vianna and Essman, 1971; Iland *et al.*, 1980).

In contrast to Burkitt's lymphoma and other endemic lymphomas, Hodgkin's disease has been well recognised for over a century and many of its epidemiological features have been well defined. Despite this Hodgkin's disease remains one of the most mystifying lymphoreticular disorders, largely due to its heterogeneous, clinical, histological and epidemiological patterns. While certain epidemiological evidence is consistent with the hypothesis that this disorder might be two or more entities (MacMahon, 1966), it is now generally accepted that this lymphoma is a single entity which is strongly influenced by sociological and immunological factors. The well-documented geographical differences in the age distribution of this lymphoma in developing and industrialised communities has already been presented (Correa and O'Conor, 1971). There is also a variability in the morphological expression of this disorder in different areas. In poorly developed countries, the high incidence of childhood Hodgkin's disease is associated with a high frequency of the mixed cellularity Rye subtype (Correa and O'Conor, 1971). In the USA and other well-developed countries, the young adult incidence peak is accompanied by an excess of nodular sclerosis (Correa and O'Conor, 1971). Interestingly the epidemiological and histological pattern observed among blacks in New York State closely resembles that observed in developing countries (Vianna *et al.*, 1977).

One of the truly unique features of Hodgkin's disease is the fact that a significant negative correlation has been observed between the average annual incidence rates for childhood and each of the two older age groups (i.e. young adults and the elderly) in American and European countries (Correa and O'Conor, 1971; Vianna and Polan, 1978). Available evidence also suggests that family factors such as high birth order (5 and greater) might be associated with a significant reduction in the risk for this disorder (Vianna and Polan, 1978). Taken collectively the above observations support the hypothesis that Hodgkin's disease might be a neoplasia arising from some environmental factor presumably infectious in nature. Family factors such as birth order might have a major influence on the time of primary exposure (Vianna and Polan, 1978), and the age of initial exposure can be viewed as a fundamental determinant with the outcome of infection (immunity *vs.* clinical disease). In many countries there is an inverse association between the frequency of reproduction and economic development. In contrast to affluent communities, poorly developed countries are generally characterised by large sibship. The high incidence of childhood Hodgkin's disease in these areas may reflect early exposure which primarily results in natural immunity. This would be analogous to the situation in many infectious diseases where higher birth orders are associated with a greater probability of contracting infection at an early age from an older sibling (Fox *et al.*, 1970). In addition, the risk of clinical disease arising from infection is generally low if exposure occurs early in life. It is interesting that the risk ratios for Hodgkin's disease are lower for male adults who have experienced various common contagious diseases in childhood (Paffenbarger *et al.*, 1977). In addition, a case-control study conducted by Abramson *et al.* (1980) suggested that susceptible people living in certain sections of Israel had an enhanced risk of Hodgkin's disease. These authors suggest that Israeli-born adults might have little prior exposure to some unknown oncogenic virus and hence little immunity.

How might the above concepts relate to the numerous Hodgkin's disease aggregates that have been described? Epidemiological studies in generally affluent communities (Vianna *et al.*, 1972; Vianna and Polan, 1973; Schimpff *et al.*, 1975; Zack *et al.*, 1977) have suggested that horizontal transmission, primarily through an asymptomatic carrier state, might occur in settings that tend to promote close repetitive contact (e.g. schools). When elderly patients have been involved in a presumed chain of contacts, it was usually in association with an asymptomatic young adult. In contrast, when a similar investigation was conducted in the city of Boston (Grufferman *et al.*, 1979), no significant excess of cases was observed. These apparently conflicting results might be explained by the fact that in urbanised areas such as cities, there is a high population density and early exposure results in a high level of asymptomatic infection and natural immunity. This concept is supported by the more recent study of Gutensohn and Cole (1980). These investigators conducted a case-control study in the Boston Metropolitan area regarding childhood factors affecting the age of exposure to infectious agents. Hodgkin's disease patients were more likely than controls to come from small families of higher socio-economic status and the relative risk for this disease increased with birth order. Persons of low socioeconomic status had a significantly lower relative risk of Hodgkin's disease than upper- and middle-class persons.

If natural immunity is an important factor in the epidemiological patterns of Hodgkin's disease as suggested by international studies and community aggregates, it would seem that the agent involved is probably viral. With few exceptions viral diseases produce a more persistent immunity than bacterial infections. In addition, the aetiological agent(s) is (are) probably ubiquitous, since natural immunity usually influences disease occurrence only when the infectious agent is frequently encountered and confers a relatively durable immunity. The evidence that prior tonsillectomy increases the risk of developing Hodgkin's disease further supports this concept. During the past decade it has become well established that the tonsils are immunocompetent organs (Ogra, 1971) which protect man from a wide variety of pathogens, primarily viral disorders such as poliomyelitis. Interestingly, prior tonsillectomy seems to be a risk factor for Hodgkin's disease not only in well-developed cities such as in New York (Vianna *et al.*, 1971; 1974a; 1980) and

Boston (Gutensohn *et al.*, 1975) but also in lesser developed countries such as Brazil (Kirchhoff *et al.*, 1980) where this operative procedure is undoubtedly less common.

The results of family studies also point to the likelihood that Hodgkin's disease is due to infection. Early studies (Devore and Doan, 1957; Razis *et al.*, 1959) indicated that the two major patterns were sib-sib and parent-child. A subsequent investigation (Vianna *et al.*, 1974) suggested that the time interval between diagnoses for first-degree blood relatives living in the same household was significantly shorter than that for patients of a similar relationship but living apart. There also appears to be an increased incidence of this disease in siblings of the same sex (Grufferman *et al.*, 1977).

It is clear that some commonly encountered environmental factors, probably viral in nature (is) are of aetiological importance in this lymphoma. As we have seen, similar conclusions have been reached with Burkitt's lymphoma and Kaposi's sarcoma. However, unlike these disorders, Hodgkin's disease remains a disorder looking for a candidate virus. Various agents such as EBV and poliovirus (Vianna *et al.*, 1971; Vianna, 1975; Gutensohn and Cole, 1980) have been considered, primarily because of the epidemiological characteristics of this disease. But compelling virological and serological evidence is lacking.

Genetic Factors. Various congenital immunodeficiency diseases appear to be associated with lymphoreticular disorders in man. Some of these are congenital x-linked immunodeficiency, common variable immunodeficiency, severe combined system immunodeficiency, the Wiskott-Aldrich syndrome, ataxia telangiectasia and various immunoglobulin deficiencies (Spector *et al.*, 1978). Chromosomal disorders have also been associated with certain congenital immunodeficiency disorders and lymphoproliferative malignancies. For example, translocation involving the long arm (q) of chromosome 14 has been observed in ataxia telangiectasia (McCaw *et al.*, 1975), Burkitt's lymphoma (Zech *et al.*, 1976), occasional cases of Hodgkin's and other lymphomas (Reeves, 1973), acute lymphoblastic leukaemia (Garson and Milligan, 1974), chronic T cell leukaemia (Finan *et al.*, 1978), B cell leukaemia (Roth *et al.*, 1979) and more recently Sezary syndrome (Shah-Reddy *et al.*, 1982). Cytogenetic abnormalities of chromosome 18 might also be common in certain lymphomas (Reeves, 1973). Certain histocompatibility antigens might also play a role in the aetiology of certain malignant lymphomas. Susceptibility to the Gross virus which can induce murine leukaemia appears to be influenced by genes located on the H-2 locus (Lilly, 1968). Several studies have suggested that an association might exist between various cross-reacting HLA antigens and Hodgkin's disease (Forbes and Morris, 1970; Falk and Osoba, 1971) and other lymphomas (Rege *et al.*, 1972). The ultimate significance of all of these observations remains to be established.

Recent Advances in Diagnosis and Treatment

The outlook for patients with many types of malignant lymphoma has vastly improved in recent years. This has partly been the result of more accurate staging. The staging classification proposed by the Ann Arbor Conference (Carbone *et al.*, 1971) has been widely adopted for Hodgkin's disease and, with some modifications (Musshoff and Schmidt-Vellmer, 1975; Weingard *et al.*, 1982; Straus *et al.*, 1982), has also been found to correlate with the prognosis for patients with non-Hodgkin's lymphoma. Although bone marrow aspiration and biopsy demonstrates tumour involvement in less than 5 per cent of patients with Hodgkin's disease, it may be found in over 40 per cent of patients with some types on non-Hodgkin's lymphomas (Vinciguerra and Silver, 1973; Rosenberg, 1975). The yield of the procedure may be increased by 10-20 per cent if bilateral posterior iliac crest bone marrow biopsies are performed (Brunning *et al.*, 1975). Bipedal lymphangiography (Lee *et al.*, 1964) provided a means to assess lymphoma involvement of retroperitoneal nodes with an accuracy exceeding 80 per cent in experienced hands. Abdominal and pelvic computerised tomography is probably less accurate than lymphangiography for assessing retroperitoneal node involvement but may detect disease in the mesenteric and coeliac axis nodes which are generally not visualised by lymphangiography (Castellino, 1982). This is particularly important for non-Hodgkin's lymphoma, since these are common sites of involvement. Radionuclide tumour scanning with Gallium-67 citrate is an adjunctive test and is particularly useful for following selected patients for disease activity while undergoing treatment (Johnston *et al.*, 1977). Liver-spleen scanning with ^{99m}Tc-labelled sulphur colloid is most useful for assessing spleen size (Milder *et al.*, 1973). Liver biopsy under laparoscopic visualisation may detect liver involvement in approximately 5 per cent of patients with Hodgkin's disease and in a higher proportion of patients with non-Hodgkin's lymphoma (Rosenberg *et al.*, 1971; Bagley *et al.*, 1973; Coleman *et al.*, 1976). Staging laparotomy with splenectomy and liver and retroperitoneal node biopsies is used when a major treatment decision depends on the outcome (Rosenberg *et al.*, 1971). This is particularly important for patients with clinical stage I or II Hodgkin's disease when radiotherapy is used as a single treatment modality, since 20-25 per cent of patients will become pathological stage III because of occult disease in the spleen or high abdominal nodes (Glatstein *et al.*, 1969; Kaplan *et al.*, 1973a). It does not appear to be necessary when clinical stage I and II Hodgkin's disease patients are treated with the combined modalities of radiotherapy and chemotherapy, since chemotherapy seems to eradicate occult disease in the abdomen (Koziner *et al.*, 1981).

Advances in treatment have been particularly dramatic for patients with Hodgkin's disease. The major contributions to the improvement in the prognosis of patients with early stage Hodgkin's disease were the determination of a tumouricidal dose of radiotherapy for Hodgkin's disease and the administration of this dose with megavoltage beam equipment to 'extended' fields including involved and adjacent nodal areas at high risk for relapse (Peters, 1950; Kaplan, 1966a, b). Disease-free survival was increased with the use of extended field as compared with involved field radiotherapy in a national Hodgkin's disease trial (Hutchinson, 1976), although overall survival was similar. Disease-free survival for extended field radiotherapy for pathological (laparotomy) stage I and II patients has varied between 52 per cent (Koziner, 1982b) and 77 per cent (Hoppe *et al.*, 1982a). A 97 per cent disease-free survival has been achieved with the use of combined modality treatment with involved field radiotherapy and MOPP chemotherapy (nitrogen mustard, vincristine, procarbazine and prednisone) at a median follow-up time of 42 months (Koziner, 1982b). Although overall survival has not been increased with combined modality treatment thus far, it remains to be determined what proportion of patients relapsing after radiotherapy alone can be successfully 'salvaged' into a second long-term unmaintained remission (Portlock *et al.*, 1978; Koziner *et al.*, 1981). Patients who are not successfully 'salvaged' will probably eventually die of Hodgkin's disease.

Some groups have identified subgroups of stage II, those with direct extensions into the lung (Wiernik and Slawson, 1982), those with large mediastinal masses (Mauch *et al.*, 1978), and those with B symptoms (Koziner *et al.*, 1981) which seem to do better with combined modality treatment than with radiotherapy alone. Substaging has also identified patients with stage IIIA disease who seem to fare better with chemotherapy (Stein *et al.*, 1982) than with extended field radiotherapy.

These are patients with low para-aortic and pelvic lymph node involvement. The Stanford group has reported excellent disease-free survival results for stage II with lung extension, IIB and IIIA disease using radical extended field and total nodal irradiation alone (Hoppe *et al.*, 1982a, 1982b).

For patients with advanced stage Hodgkin's disease (stages III and IV), the use of MOPP by DeVita and co-workers (1970; 1980) represented a dramatic improvement over previous treatment with 80 per cent of patients achieving a complete remission and approximately two-thirds of these remaining in unmaintained remission at ten years. Bonadonna *et al.* (1975) developed a drug combination potentially non-cross-resistant with MOPP: doxorubicin (Adriamycin®), bleomycin, vinblastine and dacarbazine (ABVD). The use of this regimen in alternation with MOPP with or without adjunctive radiotherapy has resulted in approximately a 90 per cent complete remission rate (Straus *et al.*, 1981; Santoro *et al.*, 1982). In the Memorial Hospital experience with alternating cycles of MOPP and ABVD in combination with low-dose radiotherapy, 84 per cent of the complete responders are remaining disease-free at a median follow-up time of four years (Young *et al.*, 1982).

An improvement in the prognosis of patients with non-Hodgkin's lymphomas has also been made in recent years. Disease-free survival has exceeded 50 per cent for patients with stage I non-Hodgkin's lymphoma with radiotherapy alone (Lipton and Lee, 1971; Sweet *et al.*, 1981) or chemotherapy alone (Miller and Jones, 1979), although the numbers of patients are small and follow-up time short in many of the published series.

For more advanced stages, combination chemotherapy has also improved survival. The results of treatment of childhood non-Hodgkin's lymphoma with intensive chemotherapy designed originally for acute lymphoblastic leukaemia have been particularly dramatic with a 75 per cent disease-free survival rate at a median follow-up time of 3½ years (Wollner, 1982). Improved survival has also been achieved for adults with lymphoblastic lymphoma with a similar approach (Koziner *et al.*, 1978). Survival has also been improved for adults with large cell lymphomas ('histiocytic' and 'mixed lymphocytic histiocytic' by the Rappaport classification). Complete remission rates of 40-70 per cent have been reported for patients with diffuse histiocytic lymphoma with a number of drug combinations with long-term survival rates of 30-60 per cent (DeVita *et al.*, 1975; McKelvey *et al.*, 1976; Schein *et al.*, 1976; Cadman *et al.*, 1977a; Koziner, 1982a; Fisher *et al.*, 1982). This represents a dramatic improvement over long-term survival rates for single-agent chemotherapy and palliative radiotherapy (Jones *et al.*, 1973; Straus *et al.*, 1982). The potential for cure of the diffuse small cell lymphomas ('poorly-differentiated lymphocytic') seems to be less (Canellos *et al.*, 1982) than for the large cell lymphomas. Some groups are showing an early survival advantage with chemotherapy with the addition of non-specific immunotherapy, in some series for patients with 'favourable-histology' nodular non-Hodgkin's lymphomas (Diggs *et al.*, 1981; Kempin *et al.*, 1981; Jones *et al.*, 1979). Although some patients may be cured, particularly those with the nodular histiocytic (Osborne *et al.*, 1980) and mixed types (Anderson *et al.*, 1977), the long-term survival of most patients with nodular lymphomas may not be affected by current intensive treatment modalities (Portlock and Rosenberg, 1979).

The improved results with intensive treatment have been associated with some long-term toxicity. This includes radiation pulmonary pneumonitis (Kaplan and Stewart, 1973b) and pericarditis (Cohn *et al.*, 1967). Both intensive radiotherapy and chemotherapy have carcinogenic potential (Cadman *et al.*, 1977b; Nelson *et al.*, 1981). The former is more associated with solid tumours and the latter with leukaemia. The combination of chemotherapy and radiotherapy may further increase the risk of leukaemia (Coleman *et al.*, 1977). Combination chemotherapy may produce sterility (Chapman *et al.*, 1979a, b). Future research in the treatment of malignant lymphoma will be directed toward decreased toxicity as well as improved treatment results.

References

Abramson, J.H., Goldblum, N., Avitzur, M., Pridan, H., Sacks, M.I. and Peritz, E. (1980). Clustering of Hodgkin's disease in Israel: a case-control study. *International Journal of Epidemiology*, 9: 137-44

Adelstein, A.M. and Donovan, J.W. (1972). Malignant disease in children whose mothers had chickenpox, mumps or rubella in pregnancy. *British Medical Journal*, 4: 629-31

Anderson, J.L., Fowles, R.E., Bieber, C.P. and Stinson, E.B. (1978). Idiopathic cardiomyopathy, age, and suppressor-cell dysfunction as risk determinants of lymphoma after cardiac transplantation. *Lancet*, 2: 1174-7

Anderson, T., Bender, R.A., Fisher, R.I., DeVita, V.T., Chabner, B.A., Berard, C.W. *et al.* (1977). Combination chemotherapy in non-Hodgkin's lymphoma: Results of long-term follow-up. *Cancer Treatment Reports*, 61: 1057-66

Andrade, Z. and Abreu, W.N. (1971). Follicular lymphoma of the spleen in patients with hepatosplenic schistosomiasis mansoni. *American Journal of Tropical Medicine and Hygiene*, 20: 237-43

Bagley, C.M., Jr., Thomas, L.B., Johnson, R.E., Chretien, P.B. and DeVita, V.T. (1973). Diagnosis of liver involvement by lymphoma: Results in 96 consecutive peritoneoscopies. *Cancer*, 31: 840-7

Barton, J.C. and Conrad, M.E. (1979). Beneficial effects of hepatitis in patients with acute myelogenous leukemia. *Annals of Internal Medicine*, 90: 188-90

Benn, R.T., Mangood, A. and Smith, A. (1979). Hodgkin's disease and occupational exposure to chemicals. *British Medical Journal*, 2: 1143

Bernard, A., Boumsell, L., Bayle, C., Richard, Y., Coppin, H., Penit, C. *et al.* (1979). Subsets of malignant lymphomas in children related to the cell phenotype. *Blood*, 54: 1058-68

Bichel, J. (1979). Trauma and Hodgkin's disease. *Acta Medica Scandinavica*, 205: 347-9

Bierman, H.R., Crile, D.M., Dod, K.S., Kelly, K.H., Petrakis, N.L., White, L.P. *et al.* (1953). Remissions in leukemia of childhood following acute infectious disease. *Cancer*, 6: 591-605

Bithell, J.F., Draper, G.J. and Borbach, P.D. (1973). Association between malignant disease in children and maternal virus infections. *British Medical Journal*, 1: 706-8

Bonadonna, G., Zucali, R., Monfardini, S., DeLena, M. and Uslenghi, C. (1975). Combination chemotherapy of Hodgkin's disease with adriamycin, bleomycin, vinblastine, and imidazole carboximide versus MOPP. *Cancer*, 36: 252-9

Boston Collaborative Drug Surveillance Program (1974). Amphetamines and malignant lymphoma. *Journal of the American Medical Association*, 229: 1462-3

Brody, S.A., Russell, W.G., Krantz, S.B. and Graber, S.E. (1981). Beneficial effect of hepatitis in leukemic reticuloendotheliosis. *Archives of Internal Medicine*, 141: 1080-1

Brunning, R.D., Bloomfield, C.D., McKenna, R.W. and Peterson, L. (1975). Bilateral trephine bone marrow biopsies in lymphoma and other neoplastic disorders. *Annals of Internal Medicine*, 82: 365-6

Burkitt, D. (1958). A sarcoma involving the jaws in African children. *British Journal of Surgery*, 46: 218-23

—— (1962). A 'Tumour Safari' in East and Central Africa. *British Journal of Cancer*, 26: 379-86

—— (1969). Etiology of Burkitt's lymphoma – an alternative hypothesis to a vectored virus. *Journal of the National Cancer Institute*, 42: 19-28

Burnet, F.M. and Holmes, M.C. (1964). Thymic changes in the mouse strain NZB in relation to the autoimmune state. *Journal of Pathology and Bacteriology*, 88: 229-41

Cadman, E., Farber, L., Berd, D. and Bertino, J. (1977a). Combination therapy for diffuse histiocytic lymphoma that includes antimetabolites. *Cancer Treatment Reports*, 61: 1109-16

—— Capizzi, R.L. and Bertino, J. (1977b). Acute non-lymphocytic leukemia. A delayed complication of Hodgkin's disease therapy: Analysis of 109 cases. *Cancer*, 40: 1280-96

Canellos, G., Skarin, A., Rosenthal, D., Anderson, K., Leonard, R.D., Pinkus, G. *et al.* (1982). High-dose methotrexate combination chemotherapy (M-BACOD) of advanced favorable and intermediate prognosis histology non-Hodgkin's lymphoma (NHL). *Proceedings of the American Association of Clinical Oncology*, 1: 159 (abstract)

Carbone, P.P., Kaplan, J.S., Musshoff, K., Smithers, D.W. and Tubiana, M. (1971). Report of the committee on Hodgkin's disease staging classification. *Cancer Research*, 31: 1860-1

Carney, W.P., Rubin, R.H., Hoffman, R.A., Hansen, W.P., Healey, K. and Hirsch,

M.S. (1981). Analysis of T lymphocyte subsets in cytomegalovirus mononucleosis. *Journal of Immunology*, 126: 2114-16

Castellino, R.A. (1982). Imaging techniques for staging abdominal Hodgkin's disease. *Cancer Treatment Reports*, 66: 697-700

Catovsky, D., Rose, M., Goolden, A.W.G., White, J.M., Bourikas, G., Brownell, A.I. *et al.* (1982). Adult T-cell lymphoma-leukemia in blacks from the West Indies. *Lancet*, 1: 639-43

Chapman, R., Sutcliffe, S.B., Rees, L., Edwards, C.R.W. and Malpas, J. (1979a). Cyclical combination chemotherapy and gonadal function: Retrospective male study. *Lancet*, 1: 285-9

―――― Sutcliffe, S.B. and Malpas, J.S. (1979b). Cytotoxic-induced ovarian failure in women with Hodgkin's disease. I. Hormone function. *Journal of American Medical Association*, 242: 1877-81

Cohn, K.E., Stewart, J.R., Fajardo, L.F. and Hancock, E.W. (1967). Heart disease following radiation. *Medicine*, 46: 281-98

Coleman, C.N., Williams, C.J., Flint, A., Glatstein, E.J., Rosenberg, S.A. and Kaplan, H.S. (1977). Hematologic neoplasia in patients treated for Hodgkin's disease. *New England Journal of Medicine*, 297: 1249-52

Coleman, M., Lightdale, C.J., Vinciguerra, V.P., Degnan, T.J., Goldstein, M., Horwitz, T. *et al.* (1976). Peritoneoscopy in Hodgkin's disease: Confirmation of results by laparotomy. *Journal of the American Medical Association*, 236: 2634-6

Colley, D.G. (1976). Adoptive suppression of granuloma formation. *Journal of Experimental Medicine*, 143: 696-700

Cooper, M.D. (1981). Immunologic analysis of lymphoid tumors. *New England Journal of Medicine*, 302: 964-5

Correa, P. and O'Conor, G.T. (1971). Epidemiologic patterns of Hodgkin's disease. *International Journal of Cancer*, 8: 192-201

Court Brown, W.M. and Doll, R. (1961). Leukaemia in childhood and young adult life: trends in mortality in relation to aetiology. *British Medical Journal*, 1: 981-8

Davis, J. (1968). Kaposi's sarcoma. Present concept of clinical course and treatment. *New York State Journal of Medicine*, 68: 2067-73

DeVita, V.T., Serpick, A.A. and Carbone, P.P. (1970). Combination chemotherapy in the treatment of advanced Hodgkin's disease. *Annals of Internal Medicine*, 73: 881-95

―――― Canellos, G.P., Chabner, B., Schein, P., Hubbard, S.P. and Young, R.C. (1975). Advanced diffuse histiocytic lymphoma, a potentially curable disease. Results with combination chemotherapy. *Lancet*, 1: 248-50

―――― Simon, R.M., Hubbard, S.M., Young, R.C., Berard, C.W., Moxley, J.H. *et al.* (1980). Curability of advanced Hodgkin's disease with chemotherapy. Long-term follow-up of MOPP-treated patients at the National Cancer Institute. *Annals of Internal Medicine*, 92: 587-95

Devore, J.W. and Doan, C.A. (1957). A study of the Hodgkin's syndrome. XII. Hereditary and epidemiologic aspects. *Annals of Internal Medicine*, 47: 300-8

Diggs, C.H., Wiernik, P.H. and Ostrow, S.S. (1981). Modular lymphoma. Prolongation of survival by complete remission. *Cancer Clinical Trials*, 4: 107-11

Drew, W.L., Mintz, L., Miner, R.D., Sands, M. and Ketterer, B. (1981). Prevalence of cytomegalovirus infection in homosexual men. *Journal of Infectious Diseases*, 143: 188-92

Durack, D.T. (1981). Opportunistic infections and Kaposi's sarcoma in homosexual men. *New England Journal of Medicine*, 305: 1465-7

Dworsky, R.L. and Henderson, B.E. (1974). Hodgkin's disease clustering in families and communities. *Cancer Research*, 34: 1161-3

Edling, C. (1981). Yrkesmedicinska kliniken, Regionsjukhuset, Linkoping, Sweden. *Lakartiolningen*, 78: 2861-2

Einhorn, M. (1961). Temporary remission in acute leukemia after an attack of 'acute appendicitis'. *Journal of the American Medical Association*, 175: 1006-8

El-Gazayerli, M., Khalil, H. and Abdel, A. (1962). Observations on some bilharzial reactions. *Alexandria Medical Journal*, 8: 434

Epstein, M.A., Achong, B.G. and Barr, Y.M. (1964). Virus particles in cultured lymphoblasts from Burkitt's lymphoma. *Lancet*, 1: 702-3

—— Barr, Y.M. and Achong, B.G. (1965). Studies with Burkitt's lymphoma. *Wistar Institute Symposium Monograph*, 4: 69

Falk, J. and Osoba, D. (1971). HL-A antigens and survival in Hodgkin's disease. *Lancet*, 2: 1118-20

Fedrick, J. and Alberman, E.D. (1972). Reported influenza in pregnancy and subsequent cancer in the child. *British Medical Journal*, 2: 485-8

Finan, J., Daniele, R. and Rowlands, D., Jr. (1978). Cytogenetics of chronic T cell leukemia, including two patients with a 14+ translocation. *Virchows Archiv. Abteilung B. Cell Pathology*, 29: 121

Fisher, R.I., DeVita, V.T., Hubbard, S.M., Jaffe, E.S., Cossrnan, J., Wesley, R. *et al.* (1982). Improved survival of diffuse aggressive lymphomas following treatment with proMACE-MOPP chemotherapy. *Proceedings of the American Society of Clinical Oncology*, 1: 161 (abstract)

Forbes, I.J. (1979). Recent advances in the study of the lymphoproliferative diseases. *Australian and New Zealand Journal of Medicine*, 9: 320-2

Forbes, J.F. and Morris, P.J. (1970). Leucocyte antigens in Hodgkin's disease. *Lancet*, 2: 849-51

Fox, J.P., Hall, C.E. and Elveback, L.R. (1970). *Epidemiology: Man and Disease.* Collier-Macmillan, London, ch. 9, p. 200

Friend, M. and Trainer, D.O. (1970). Polychlorinated biphenyl: Interaction with duck hepatitis virus. *Science*, 170: 1314-6

Garson, O.M. and Milligan, W.J. (1974). Acute leukemia associated with an abnormal genotype. *Scandinavian Journal of Haematology*, 12: 256-62

Gendelman, S., Rizzo, F. and Mones, R.J. (1969). Central nervous system complications of leukemic conversion of the lymphomas. *Cancer*, 24: 676-82

Giraldo, G., Beth, E. and Haguenaw, F. (1972a). Herpes-type virus particles in tissue culture of Kaposi's sarcoma from different geographic regions. *Journal of National Cancer Institute*, 49: 1509-26

—— Beth, E., Coeur, P., Vogel, C.L. and Dhru, D.S. (1972b). Kaposi's sarcoma: a new model in the search for viruses associated with human malignancies. *Journal of National Cancer Institute*, 49: 1495-507

—— Beth, E., Kourilsky, F.M., Henle, W., Henle, G., Mike, V. *et al.* (1975). Antibody patterns to herpesviruses in Kaposi's sarcoma: serologic association of European Kaposi's sarcoma with cytomegalovirus. *International Journal of Cancer*, 15: 839-48

—— Beth, E., Henle, W., Henle, G., Mike, V., Safai, B. *et al.* (1978). Antibody patterns to herpesviruses in Kaposi's sarcoma. II. Serologic association of American Kaposi's sarcoma with cytomegalovirus. *International Journal of Cancer*, 22: 126-31

—— Beth, E. and Huang, E.S. (1980). Kaposi's sarcoma and its relationship to cytomegalovirus (CMV). III. CMV DNA and CMV early antigens in Kaposi's sarcoma. *International Journal of Cancer*, 26: 23-9

Glatstein, E., Guernsay, J.M., Rosenberg, S.A. and Kaplan, H.S. (1969). The value of laparotomy and splenectomy in the staging of Hodgkin's disease. *Cancer*, 24: 708-18

238   Lymphoreticular Malignancies

Grufferman, S., Cole, P., Smith, P.C. and Lukes, R.J. (1977). Hodgkin's disease in siblings. *New England Journal of Medicine*, 296: 248-50
—— Cole, P. and Levitan, T.R. (1979). Evidence against transmission of Hodgkin's disease in high schools. *New England Journal of Medicine*, 300: 1006-11
Grundy, G.W., Creagen, E.T. and Fraumeni, J.F. (1973). Non-Hodgkin's lymphoma in childhood epidemiologic features. *Journal of the National Cancer Institute*, 51: 767-76
Gutensohn, N., Li, F., Johnson, R.E. and Cole, P. (1975). Hodgkin's disease, tonsillectomy and family size. *New England Journal of Medicine*, 292: 22-5
—— and Cole, P. (1980). Childhood social environment and Hodgkin's disease. *New England Journal of Medicine*, 304: 135-40
Hakulinen, T., Hovi, L., Karkinen-Jaaskelainen, M., Penttinen, K., and Saxen, L. (1973). Association between influenza during pregnancy and childhood leukaemia. *British Medical Journal*, 4: 265-7
Hardell, L. (1979). Malignant lymphoma of histiocytic type and exposure to phenoxyacetic acids or chlorophenols. *Lancet*, 1: 55-6
Henle, G., Henle, W. and Diehl, V. (1968). Relation of Burkitt's tumor associated herpes-type virus to infectious mononucleosis. *Proceedings of National Academy of Science*, 59: 94-101
Henle, W., Henle, G., Ho, H., Burtin, P., Cachin, Y., Clifford, P. *et al.* (1970). Antibodies to Epstein-Barr virus in nasopharyngeal carcinoma, other head and neck neoplasms and control groups. *Journal of National Cancer Institute*, 44: 225-31
Hernandez, S.A. (1949). Observation de un caso de enfermedad de Hodgkin con regresion de los sitomas e infartos ganglionares, post-sarampion. *Arch Cubanos Cancer*, 8: 26-31
Hoover, R. and Fraumeni, J.F., Jr. (1973). Risk of cancer in renal-transplant recipients. *Lancet*, 2: 55-7
Hoppe, R.T., Coleman, C.N., Cox, R.S., Rosenberg, S.A. and Kaplan, H.S. (1982a). The management of stage I-II Hodgkin's disease with irradiation alone or combined modality therapy: The Stanford experience. *Blood*, 59: 455-65
—— Cox, R.S., Rosenberg, S.A. and Kaplan, H.S. (1982b). Prognostic factors in pathologic stage III Hodgkin's disease. *Cancer Treatment Reports*, 66: 743-9
Hutchison, G.B. (1976). Survival and complications of radiotherapy following involved and extended field therapy of Hodgkin's disease stages I and II: A collaborative effort. *Cancer*, 38: 288-325
Hyman, G. and Sommers, S. (1966). The development of Hodgkin's disease and lymphoma during anticonvulsant therapy. *Blood*, 28: 416-27
Iland, H., Chan, W. and Vincent, P.C. (1980). Myeloproliferative and lymphoproliferative disorders in the same patient. *Australian and New Zealand Journal of Medicine*, 10: 650-3
Jayawardena, A.N. (1981). Immune responses in malaria. In: Mansfield, J.M. (ed.), *Parasitic Diseases*, Marcel Dekker, New York, p. 85
Johnston, G.S., Go, M.F., Benua, R.S., Larson, S.M., Andrews, G.A. and Hubner, K.F. (1977). Gallium-67 citrate imaging in Hodgkin's disease: Final report of cooperative group. *Journal of Nuclear Medicine*, 18: 692-8
Jones, S.E., Fulks, Z., Bull, M., Kaden, M.E., Dorfman, R.F., Kaplan, H.S. *et al.* (1973). Non-Hodgkin's lymphomas. IV. Clinicopathologic correlation in 405 cases. *Cancer*, 31: 806-23
—— Salmon, S.E. and Fisher, R. (1979). Adjuvant immunotherapy with BCG in non-Hodgkin's lymphoma: A Southwest Oncology Group controlled clinical trial. In: Salmon, S.E. and Jones, S.E. (eds.), *Adjuvant Therapy of*

Cancer II, Grune and Stratton, New York, p. 163

Kaplan, H.S. (1966a). Evidence for a tumoricidal dose level in the radiotherapy of Hodgkin's disease. *Cancer Research*, 26: 1221-4

——— (1966b). Long-term results of palliative and radical radiotherapy of Hodgkin's disease. *Cancer Research*, 26: 1250-2

——— Dorfman, R.F., Nelsen, T.S. and Rosenberg, S.A. (1973a). Staging laparotomy and splenectomy in Hodgkin's disease: Analysis of indications and patterns of involvement in 285 consecutive unselected patients. *National Cancer Institute Monograph*, 36: 291-301

——— and Stewart, R.J. (1973b). Complications of intensive megavoltage radiotherapy for Hodgkin's disease. *National Cancer Institute Monograph*, 36: 439-44

Kempin, S.J., Cirrincione, C., Straus, D.J., Arlin, Z., Kosiner, B., Pinsky, C. *et al.* (1981). Improved remission rate and duration in nodular non-Hodgkin's lymphoma (NNHL) with the use of mixed bacterial vaccine (MBV). *Proceedings of the American Society of Clinical Oncology*, 22: 514 (abstract)

Kirchhoff, L.V., Evans, A.S., McClelland, K.E., Carvalho, R.P.S. and Pannuti, C.S. (1980). A case-control study of Hodgkin's disease in Brazil. *American Journal of Epidemiology*, 112: 595-608

Koziner, B., Mertelsmann, R., Filippa, D.A., Good, R.A. and Clarkson, B.D. (1978). Adult lymphoid neoplasias of T- and null-cell types. In: Clarkson, B.D., Marks, P.A. and Till, J.E. (eds.), *Differentiation of Normal and Neoplastic Hematopoietic Cells*, Cold Spring Harbor Laboratory, vol. 5, Book B, ch. 8, pp. 843-57

——— Braun, D., Myers, J., Nisce, L., Poussin-Rosillo, H., Straus, D. *et al.* (1981). Combined modality of MOPP chemotherapy and radiotherapy for the treatment of stages I and II Hodgkin's disease. In: Jones, S.E. and Salmon, S.E. (eds.), *Adjuvant Therapy of Cancer III*, Grune and Stratton, New York, p. 77

——— Little, C., Passe, S., Thaler, H.P., Sklaroff, R., Straus, D.J. *et al.* (1982a). Treatment of advanced histiocytic lymphoma: An analysis of prognostic variables. *Cancer*, 49: 1571-9

——— (1982b). Hodgkin's disease: An updated review. In: Molander, D. (ed.), *Diseases of the Lymphatic System*, Springer Verlag, New York (in press)

Lancet (1981). Editorial. Immunocompromised homosexuals. 2: 1325-6

Laurent, G., Pris, J., Delsol, G., Familiades, J. and Fabre, J. (1980). Immunoblastic lymphoma and osteomyelitis. *Lancet*, 1: 258

Lee, B.J., Nelson, J.H. and Schwarz, G. (1964). Evaluation of lymphangiography, inferior venacavography and intravenous pyelography in the clinical staging and management of Hodgkin's disease and lymphosarcoma. *New England Journal of Medicine*, 271: 327-37

Levine, P.H., Kamaraju, L.S., Connelly, R.R., Berard, C.W., Dorfman, R.F., Magrath, I. *et al.* (1982). The American Burkitt's lymphoma registry: eight years' experience. *Cancer*, 49: 1016-22

Li, F.P., Fraumeni, J.F., Mantel, N. and Miller, R.W. (1969). Cancer mortality among chemists. *Journal of National Cancer Institute*, 43: 1159-64

Lilly, F. (1968). The effect of histocompatibility 2 type on response to the Friend leukemia virus in mice. *Journal of Experimental Medicine*, 127: 465-73

Lipton, A. and Lee, B.J. (1971). Prognosis of stage I lymphosarcoma and reticulum cell sarcoma. *New England Journal of Medicine*, 284: 230-3

Loose, L.D., Pittman, K.A., Benitz, K.F. and Silkworth, J.B. (1977). Polychlorinated biphenyl and hexachlorobenzene induced humoral immunosuppression. *Journal of Reticuloendothelial Society*, 22: 253-71

——— Silkworth, J.B., Pittman, K.A., Benitz, K.F. and Mueller, W. (1978). Impaired host resistance to endotoxin and malaria in polychlorinated biphenyl and hexachlorobenzene-treated mice. *Infection and Immunity*, 20: 30-5

Lothe, F. (1963). Kaposi's sarcoma in Ugandan Africans. *Acta Pathologica et Microbiologica Scandinavica*, 161: 1-71

Lukes, R.J. and Butler, J.J. (1966). The pathology and nomenclature of Hodgkin's disease. *Cancer Research*, 26: 1063-81

────── Craver, L.F., Hall, T.C., Rappaport, H. and Rubin, P. (1966a). Report of the nomenclature committee. *Cancer Research*, 26: 1311

────── Butler, J.J. and Hicks, E.B. (1966b). Natural history of Hodgkin's disease as related to its pathologic picture. *Cancer*, 19: 317-44

────── and Collins, R.D. (1974). Functional approach to the classification of malignant lymphoma. *Recent Results in Cancer Research*, 46: 18-25

MacMahon, B. (1966). Epidemiology of Hodgkin's disease. *Cancer Research*, 26: 1189-200

Mangi, R.J., Niederman, J.C., Kelleher, J.E., Jr., Dwyer, J.M., Evans, A.S. and Kantor, F.S. (1974). Depression of cell-mediated immunity during acute infectious mononucleosis. *New England Journal of Medicine*, 291: 1149-53

Mauch, P., Goodman, R. and Hellman, S. (1978). The significance of mediastinal involvement in early stage Hodgkin's disease. *Cancer*, 42: 1039-45

McCaw, B.K., Hecht, F., Harnden, D.G., and Teplitz, R.L. (1975). Somatic rearrangement of chromosome 14 in human lymphocytes. *Proceedings of the National Academy of Sciences*, 72: 2071-5

McKelvey, E.M., Gottlieb, J.A., Wilson, H.E., Haut, A., Talley, R.W., Stephens, R. *et al.* (1976). Hydroxyldaunomycin (adriamycin) combination chemotherapy in malignant lymphoma. *Cancer*, 38: 1484-93

Mellors, R. (1966). Autoimmune disease in NZB/Bl mice. II. Autoimmunity and malignant lymphoma. *Blood*, 27: 435-48

Milder, M.S., Larson, S.M., Bagley, C.M., DeVita, V.T., Johnson, R.E. and Johnston, G.S. (1973). Liver–spleen scan in Hodgkin's disease. *Cancer*, 31: 826-34

Milham, S., Jr. and Hesser, J. (1967). Hodgkin's disease in woodworkers. *Lancet*, 2: 136-7

────── (1979). Mortality in aluminum reduction plant workers. *Journal of Occupational Medicine*, 21: 475-80

Miller, T.P. and Jones, S.E. (1979). Chemotherapy of localized histiocytic lymphoma. *Lancet*, 1: 358-60

Moertel, C.G. and Hagedorn, A.B. (1957). Leukemia or lymphoma and coexistent primary malignant lesions − a review of the literature and study of 120 cases. *Blood*, 12: 788-803

Morrow, R.H., Kisuule, A., Pike, C. and Smith, P.G. (1976). *Journal of National Cancer Institute*, 56: 479-83

Musshoff, K. and Schmidt-Vellmer, H. (1975). Prognostic significance of primary site after radiotherapy in non-Hodgkin's lymphomata. *British Journal of Cancer*, 3 (suppl. II): 425-33

Madler, L.M., Reinherz, E.L., Weinstein, H.J., D'Orsi, C.J. and Schlossman, S.F. (1980). Heterogeneity of T-cell lymphoblastic malignancies. *Blood*, 55: 806-10

Nelson, D.F., Cooper, S., Weston, M.G. and Rubin, P. (1981). Second malignant neoplasms in patients treated for Hodgkin's disease with radiotherapy or radiotherapy and chemotherapy. *Cancer*, 48: 2386-93

Nicholson, W.J. and Selikoff, I.J. (1978). Mortality experience of styrene-polystyrene polymerization workers: initial findings. *Proceedings of the International Symposium on Styrene*, p. 56

Niederman, J.C. (1956). Infectious mononucleosis at Yale-New Haven Medical Center, 1946-1955. *Yale Journal of Biology and Medicine*, 28: 629

O'Conor, G.T. (1970). Persistent immunologic stimulation as a factor in oncogenesis, with special reference to Burkitt's tumor. *American Journal of*

Medicine, 48: 279-85

Öettle, A.G. (1962). Geographical and racial differences in the frequency of Kaposi's sarcoma as evidence of environmental or genetic causes. *Acta Unio Internationalis Cancrum*, 18: 330-63

——— (1963). Geographical and racial differences in frequency of Kaposi's sarcoma as evidence of environmental or genetic causes. In: Ackerman, L.V. and Murray, J.F. (eds.), *Symposium on Kaposi's Sarcoma*, Hafner Publishing Co., New York, p. 17

Ogra, P. (1971). Effect of tonsillectomy and adenoidectomy on nasopharyngeal antibody response to poliovirus. *New England Journal of Medicine*, 284: 59-64

Olin, G.R. (1978). The hazards of a chemical laboratory environment – a study of the mortality in two cohorts of Swedish chemists. *American Industrial Hygiene Association Journal*, 39: 557-62

Olsson, H. and Brandt, L. (1981). Non-Hodgkin's lymphoma of the skin and occupational exposure to herbicides. *Lancet*, 2: 579

Osborne, C.K., Norton, L., Young, R.C., Garvin, A.J., Simon, R.M., Berard, C.W. *et al.* (1980). Nodular histiocytic lymphoma with potential for prolonged disease-free survival. *Blood*, 56: 98-103

Paffenbarger, R.S., Jr., Wing, A.L. and Hyde, R.T. (1977). Characteristics in youth indicative of adult-onset Hodgkin's disease. *Journal of the National Cancer Institute*, 58: 1489-91

Panke, T.W., Langlinais, P.C. and Goyette, R.E. (1978). An 'abnormal' lymphoid proliferation simulating Hodgkin's disease in a burn patient. *Human Pathology*, 9: 716-23

Parker, J.W. (1981). A new look at malignant lymphomas. *Diagnostic Medicine*, June: 77-113

Pattengale, P.K., Smith, R.W. and Gerber, P. (1973). Selective transformation of B lymphocytes by EB virus. *Lancet*, 2: 93-4

Penn, I. (1981). Malignant lymphomas in organ transplant recipients. *Transplantation Proceedings*, 13: 736-8

Peters, M.V. (1950). A study of survivals in Hodgkin's disease treated radiologically. *American Journal of Roentgenology*, 131: 69-73

Portlock, C.S., Rosenberg, S.A., Glatstein, E. and Kaplan, H. (1978). Impact of salvage treatment on initial relapse in patients with Hodgkin's disease, stages I-III. *Blood*, 51: 825-33

——— and Rosenberg, S.A. (1979). No initial therapy for stages III and IV non-Hodgkin's lymphomas of favorable histologic type. *Annals of Internal Medicine*, 90: 10-13

Posnett, D.N., Collins, R.D. and Krantz, S.B. (1979). Osteomyelitis and lymphoma. *Lancet*, 2: 1085

Provisor, A.J., Iacuone, J.J., Chilcote, R.R., Neiburger, R.G., Crussi, F.G. and Baehner, R.L. (1975). Acquired agammaglobulinemia after a life-threatening illness with clinical and laboratory features of infectious mononucleosis in three related male children. *New England Journal of Medicine*, 293: 62-5

Purtilo, D.T., Paquin, L., DeFlorio, D., Virzi, F. and Sakhuja, R. (1979). Immunodiagnosis and immunopathogenesis of the x-linked recessive lymphoproliferative syndrome. *Seminars in Hematology*, 16: 309-43

Ramot, B. and Many, A. (1972). Primary intestinal lymphoma. In: Grundman, H. and Tulinius, H. (eds.), *Current Problems in the Epidemiology of Cancer and Lymphomas*, Springer Verlag, Berlin, Heidelberg, New York, Vol. 39, pp. 194-9

Rappaport, H., Winter, W.J. and Hicks, E.B. (1956). Follicular lymphoma. A re-evaluation of its position in the scheme of malignant lymphomas, based on a survey of 253 cases. *Cancer*, 9: 792-821

Razis, D.V., Diamond, H.D. and Craver, L.F. (1959). Familial Hodgkin's disease: its significance and implications. *Annals of Internal Medicine*, 51: 933-77

Reeves, B.R. (1973). Cytogenetics of malignant lymphomas. Studies utilizing a Giemsa-banding technique. *Human Genetics*, 20: 231

Rege, V., Patel, R. and Briggs, W.A. (1972). Leukocyte antigens and disease. II. Association of HL-A5 and lymphomas. *American Journal of Clinical Pathology*, 58: 14-16

Rinaldo, C.R., Carney, W.P., Richter, B.S., Black, P.H. and Hirsch, M.S. (1980). Mechanisms of immunosuppression in cytomegaloviral mononucleosis. *Journal of Infectious Diseases*, 141: 488-95

Robinson, J.E., Brown, N., Andiman, W., Halliday, K., Francke, U., Robert, M.F. *et al.* (1980). Diffuse polyclonal B-cell lymphoma during primary infection with Epstein-Barr virus. *New England Journal of Medicine*, 302: 1293-7

Rosenberg, S.A. (1975). Bone marrow involvement in the non-Hodgkin's lymphomata. *British Journal of Cancer*, 31 (suppl. II): 261-4

—— Boiron, M., DeVita, V.T., Johnson, R.E., Lee, B.J., Ultmann, E. *et al.* (1971). Report of the committee on Hodgkin's disease staging procedures. *Cancer Research*, 31: 1862-3

Roth, D.G., Cimino, M., Variakojis, D., Golomb, H. and Rowley, J. (1979). B cell acute lymphoblastic leukemia (ALL) with a 14q+ chromosomal abnormality. *Blood*, 53: 235-43

Rothman, S. (1962). Remarks on sex, age and racial distribution of Kaposi's sarcoma and on possible pathogenetic factors. *Acta Unio Internationalis Cancrum*, 18: 326-9

Safai, B., Mike, V., Giraldo, G., Beth, E. and Good, R. (1980). Association of Kaposi's sarcoma with second primary malignancies: possible etiopathogenic implications. *Cancer*, 45: 1472-9

—— and Good, R.A. (1981). Kaposi's sarcoma: A review and recent developments. *CA-A Cancer Journal for Clinicians*, 31: 2-12

Santoro, A., Bonadonna, G., Bonfante, V. and Valagussa, P. (1982). Alternating drug combinations in the treatment of advanced Hodgkin's disease. *New England Journal of Medicine*, 306: 770-5

Schein, P.S., DeVita, V.T., Hubbard, S., Chabner, B.A., Canellos, G.P., Berard, C. *et al.* (1976). Bleomycin, adriamycin, cyclophosphamide, vincristine and prednisone (BACOP) combination chemotherapy in the treatment of advanced diffuse histiocytic lymphoma. *Annals of Internal Medicine*, 85: 417-22

Schimpff, S.C., Schimpff, C.R., Brager, D.M. and Wiernik, P.H. (1975). Leukemia and lymphoma patients interlinked by prior social contact. *Lancet*, 1: 124-9

Schwartz, R.S. (1980). Epstein-Barr virus – oncogen or mitogen? *New England Journal of Medicine*, 302: 1307-8

Searle, C.E. and Waterhouse, A.H. (1978). Epidemiological study of the mortality of British chemists (meetings abstract). *British Journal of Cancer*, 38: 192-3

Shah-Reddy, I., Mayeda, K., Mirchandani, I. and Koppitch, F.C. (1982). Sezary syndrome with a 14:14 (q 12: q 31) translocation. *Cancer*, 49: 75-9

Slocumb, J.C. and MacMahon, B. (1963). Changes in mortality rates from leukemia in the first five years of life. *New England Journal of Medicine*, 268: 922-5

Spector, B.D., Perry, G.S. III and Kersey, J.H. (1978). Genetically determined immunodeficiency diseases (GDID) and malignancy: Report from the immunodeficiency-cancer registry. *Clinical Immunology and Immunopathology*, 11: 12-29

Stein, R.S., Golomb, H.M., Wiernik, P.H., Mauch, P., Hellman, S., Ultman, J.E. *et al.* (1982). Anatomic substages of stage IIIA Hodgkin's disease: Follow-up of a collaborative study. *Cancer Treatment Reports*, 66: 733-41

Stewart, A., Webb, J. and Hewitt, D. (1958). A survey of childhood malignancies. *British Medical Journal*, 1: 1495-505

Straus, D.J., Lee, B.J., Koziner, B., Nisce, L.Z., Young, C.W. and Clarkson, B.D. (1981). The treatment of advanced Hodgkin's disease. *Blut*, 43: 119-24

—— Filippa, D.A., Lieberman, P.H., Koziner, B., Thaler, H.T. and Clarkson, B.D. (1983). The non-Hodgkin's lymphomas. I. A retrospective clinical and pathologic analysis of 499 cases diagnosed between 1958 and 1969. *Cancer*, 51: 101-9

Sweet, D.L., Golomb, H.M., Ultmann, J.E., Miller, J.B., Stein, R.S., Lester, E.P. *et al.* (1980). Cyclophosphamide, vincristine, methotrexate with leucuvorin rescue and cytarabine (COMLA) combination sequential chemotherapy for advanced diffuse histiocytic lymphoma. *Annals of Internal Medicine*, 92: 785-90

—— Kinzie, J., Gaeke, M.E., Golomb, H.M., Ferguson, D.L. and Ultmann, J.E. (1981). Survival of patients with localized diffuse histiocytic lymphoma. *Blood*, 58: 1218-23

Tajima, K., Tominaga, S., Shimizu, H. and Suchi, T. (1981). A hypothesis on the etiology of adult T-cell leukemia/lymphoma. *Gann*, 72: 684-91

Taqi, A.M., Abdurrahman, M.B., Yakubu, A.M. and Fleming, A.F. (1981). Regression of Hodgkin's disease after measles. *Lancet*, 1: 1112

Thigpen, J.E., Faith, R.E., McConnell, E.E. and Moore, J.A. (1975). Increased susceptibility to bacterial infection as a sequela of exposure to 2, 3, 7, 8-tetrachlorodibenzo-p-dioxin. *Infection and Immunity*, 12: 1319-24

Vianna, N.J. (1975). Epidemiology of Hodgkin's disease: Review and etiologic leads. In: King, J. and Faulkner, W. (eds.), *Critical Reviews in Clinical Laboratory Sciences*, CRC Press, Cleveland, p. 245

—— (1977). The malignant lymphomas: epidemiology and related aspects. In: Ioachim, H.L. (ed.), *Pathobiology Annual*, Appleton-Century-Crofts, New York, p. 231

—— and Essman, L.J. (1971). Suppression of chronic lymphocytic leukemia by polycythemia vera. *Cancer*, 27: 1337-41

—— Greenwald, P. and Davies, J.N.P. (1971). Tonsillectomy and Hodgkin's disease: the lymphoid tissue barrier. *Lancet*, 1: 431-2

—— Greenwald, P., Brady, J., Polan, A.K., Dwork, A. and Davies, J.N.P. (1972). Hodgkin's disease: cases with features of a community outbreak. *Annals of Internal Medicine*, 77: 169-80

—— and Polan, A.K. (1973). Epidemiologic evidence for transmission of Hodgkin's disease. *New England Journal of Medicine*, 289: 499-502

—— Davies, J.N.P., Polan, A.K. and Wolfgang, P.E. (1974). Familial Hodgkin's disease: an environmental and genetic disorder. *Lancet*, 2: 854-7

—— Polan, A.K., Keogh, M.D., Greenwald, P. and Davies, J.N.P. (1974a). Tonsillectomy and Hodgkin's disease. *Lancet*, 2: 168-9

—— and Polan, A. (1976). Childhood lymphatic leukemia: prenatal seasonality and possible association with congenital varicella. *American Journal of Epidemiology*, 103: 321-32

—— Thind, I.S., Louria, D.B., Polan, A., Kirmss, V. and Davies, J.N.P. (1977). Epidemiologic and histologic patterns of Hodgkin's disease in blacks. *Cancer*, 40: 3133-9

—— and Polan, A.K. (1978). Immunity in Hodgkin's disease: Importance of age at exposure. *Annals of Internal Medicine*, 89: 550-6

—— and Polan, A.K. (1979). Lymphomas and occupational benzene exposure. *Lancet*, 1: 1394-5

—— Davies, J., Harris, S., Lawrence, C.E., Arbuckle, J., Marani, W. *et al.* (1980). Tonsillectomy and childhood Hodgkin's disease. *Lancet*, 2: 338-40

Vinciguerra, V. and Silver, R.T. (1973). The importance of bone marrow biopsy in the staging of patients with lymphosarcoma. *Blood*, 41: 913-20

Vos, J.G., Moore, J.A. and Zinkl, J.G. (1973). Effect of 2, 3, 7, 8-tetrachlorodi-benzo-p-dioxin on the immune system of laboratory animals. *Environmental Health Perspectives*, 5: 149-62

Weh, H.J. and Andrieu, J.M. (1979). Axillary forms of Hodgkin's disease. Considerations of etiology and clinical characteristics. *Medizinische Welt* (Stuttgart), 30: 1460-2

Weingard, D.N., DeCosse, D., Sherlock, P., Straus, D., Lieberman, P.H. and Filippa, D.A. (1982). Primary gastrointestinal lymphoma: A 30-year review. *Cancer*, 49: 1258-65

Weiss, P. (1954). Casos de limfosarcoma de la raris. *Actas Dermo-sifiliograficas* (Madrid), 45: 1

Wiernik, P.H. and Slawson, R.G. (1982). Hodgkin's disease with direct extension into pulmonary parenchyma from a mediastinal mass: A presentation requiring special therapeutic considerations. *Cancer Treatment Reports*, 66: 711-16

Wollner, N. (1982). LSA_2L_2 in childhood non-Hodgkin's lymphoma. In: Rosenberg, S.A. and Kaplan, H.S. (eds.), *Malignant Lymphomas*, Academic Press, New York, ch. 36, p. 603

Young, C.W., Straus, D.J., Myers, J., Passe, S., Nisce, L.Z., Lee, B.J. *et al.* (1982). Multidisciplinary treatment of advanced Hodgkin's disease by an alternative chemotherapeutic regimen of MOPP/ABDV and low-dose radiation therapy restricted to originally bulky disease. *Cancer Treatment Reports*, 66: 907-14

Zack, M.M., Heath, C.W., Andares, M.D., Girivas, A.S. and Christine, B.W. (1977). High school contact among persons with leukemia and lymphoma. *Journal of the National Cancer Institute*, 59: 1343-49

Zech, L., Haglund, U., Nilsson, K., and Klein, G. (1976). Characteristic chromosomal abnormalities in biopsies and lymphoid-cell lines from patients with Burkitt and non-Burkitt lymphomas. *International Journal of Cancer*, 17: 47-56

Ziegler, J.L., (1981). Burkitt's lymphoma. *New England Journal of Medicine*, 305: 735-45

Zygiert, Z. (1971). Hodgkin's disease: remissions after measles. *Lancet*, 1: 593

14 CANCER OF THE PROSTATE AND TESTIS
C. Mettlin

Introduction

Cancers of the prostate gland and of the testicles are, collectively, the most common tumours of the male genitourinary system. Next to lung cancer, in the United States of America (USA), cancer of the prostate is the most frequently occurring cancer among men, regardless of age, and among young men, testicular cancer is the most commonly occurring malignant neoplasm. Despite their shared importance as sources of cancer mortality and morbidity, these two diseases differ markedly in their epidemiological features. Each has a unique pattern of incidence and, although the aetiology of neither of the diseases is well understood, the avenues for research into their causes are divergent.

Incidence and Mortality Rates

Prostate Cancer

The National Cancer Institute Surveillance Epidemiology and End Results (SEER) reports for 1973-7 provide incidence data on cancer in five States and five metropolitan areas in the USA and Puerto Rico (Young et al., 1981). The age-specific incidence rates of prostatic cancer for the combined areas (excluding Puerto Rico) for all races combined and for whites and blacks nearly doubles every five-year age interval between ages 55 and 74 (Table 14.1). Rates for black males exceed those of white males at every age. The difference in incidence is greatest in the age group 55-59 years where the rate among blacks is almost 2.5 times that of whites.

Mortality rates for prostate cancer also increase with age. For all races combined, mortality rates nearly double from one age group to the next up to age 84. Overall, the average annual mortality rate from prostate cancer was 87 per cent higher in blacks than in whites for the 1973-7 period. The largest difference between black and white mortality rates occurred in the younger age groups where the rates for blacks were 3 to 4 times higher than rates for whites. The average age of death from prostate cancer was 77 years for white males and 72.4 for black males.

Table 14.1: United States Annual Age-specific Incidence Rates of Prostatic Cancer by Race, 1973-1977

Age group	Rate per 100,000 population		
	All races	White males	Black males
<40	0.04	0.04	0.08
40-44	1.0	0.7	3.5
45-49	4.8	4.1	12.4
50-54	20.8	19.3	42.7
55-59	67.8	61.6	146.8
60-64	165.7	154.4	326.5
65-69	318.5	303.0	538.4
70-74	514.1	487.6	851.7
75-79	735.1	705.6	1020.9
80-84	961.2	949.5	1293.4
85+	1060.7	1043.9	1258.5

Source: Young *et al.*, 1981.

Complete mortality statistics have been collected on a nationwide basis in the USA since 1930. As shown in Figure 14.1, prostatic cancer mortality rates for both white and non-white males in the USA have increased since 1930 (Devesa and Silverman, 1978). For all races combined, an overall increase in mortality from prostate cancer of about 150 per cent has occurred between 1930 and 1974. The increase in mortality for non-whites has been much greater than for whites. In white males, there was a 44 per cent increase in prostate cancer mortality between 1930 and 1940. Since 1940, the mortality rates for white males have been more stable. Among non-white males, a different pattern of rising mortality occurred with steadily increasing rates apparent from 1930 to the present. Until 1945, whites had a higher mortality rate from prostate cancer than non-whites but since then mortality has been greater among black men.

Higher mortality rates from prostate cancer are observed in northern European countries, New Zealand, Australia, the USA and Canada (Segi, 1978). The lowest mortality rates are found among South and Southeast Asian countries. Comparable data on cancer incidence are available from 28 countries (Waterhouse *et al.*, 1976). The incidence rates for prostate cancer follow the same pattern as mortality rates with the

Figure 14.1: Trends in Mortality from Prostatic Cancer in the USA, 1930-1974

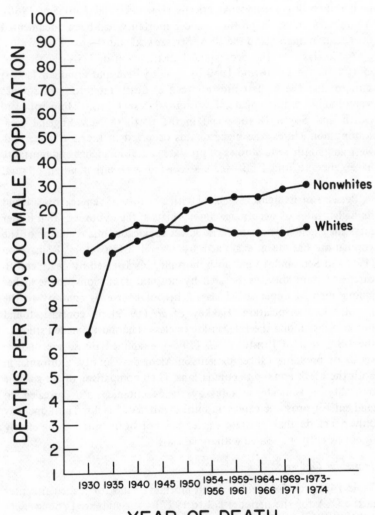

Source: adapted from Devesa and Silverman, 1978.

highest rates occurring in northern European countries, New Zealand, the USA and Canada. Intermediate rates are observed in eastern European and Latin America regions and the lowest rates occur in Asian countries.

Comparison of prostate cancer mortality rates of Japanese immigrants to the USA with those of Japanese in Japan shows substantially higher rates for Japanese-Americans (Haenszel and Kurihara, 1968). A similar increase in prostate cancer mortality had been documented for Polish immigrants to the USA (Straszewski and Haenszel, 1965).

An analysis of the geographical distribution of USA cancer mortality rates for the period 1950 to 1969 by Blair and Fraumeni (1978) showed that the highest prostatic cancer death rates for white males were found in the upper midwestern states of Iowa, Minnesota and North and South Dakota, and in the northern New England area. Among non-whites, the highest rates occurred in the northeast, midwest and southwest. Studies of prostate cancer incidence and mortality have generally found no excess associated with either urban or rural residence.

Because of its being associated with a history of venereal disease and its higher rates of occurrence among blacks, the hypothesis that higher rates may generally characterise lower socioeconomic segments of the population has been examined by several investigators. Richardson (1965) in Scotland, found both mortality, as assessed by death certificate, and morbidity, as assessed by hospital admissions, to be higher among men of upper social class. This, of course, is contrary to the hypothesised association. Hakkey *et al.* (1979), in contrast, found higher rates among the English lower class. The most detailed study in the USA, that of Ernster *et al.* (1977), examined the socioeconomic status of prostatic cancer patients in Alemedea County, California, in both the black and white populations. Their comparison of age-specific mortality and incidence rates by socioeconomic status revealed no gradient for prostatic cancer in either whites or blacks. Thus, one may only conclude that prostate cancer has not been found to be clearly or consistently associated with social class.

Testicular Cancer

Table 14.2 provides incidence and mortality rates for testicular cancer in the USA for the period 1973 to 1977 by age and race (Young *et al.*, 1981). Incidence and mortality rates tend to be bimodal, with a prominent peak in the age group 25-34 years and a lesser peak beginning after age 75. The incidence of testicular cancer is four times greater in whites than in blacks in the USA and mortality from this cancer is 2.5 times higher in whites.

The overall mortality rate from testicular cancer in the USA has changed little during the past 40 years (Devesa and Silverman, 1978).

Table 14.2: United States Average Annual Incidence and Mortality Rates for Testicular Cancer by Race, 1973-1977

| Age (years) | Rate per 100,000 population | | | |
| | White males | | Black males | |
	Incidence	Mortality	Incidence	Mortality
0-14	0.22	0.06	0.31	—
15-24	4.74	1.40	0.41	0.20
25-34	9.32	1.50	2.16	0.43
35-44	6.60	1.33	1.31	0.65
45-54	4.17	0.95	0.65	0.43
55-64	2.32	0.54	0.63	0.63
65-74	1.12	0.76	—	—
75+	1.78	1.29	2.66	—
Overall[a]	3.60	0.80	0.80	0.30

Note: a. Age-adjusted to 1970 USA population.
Source: Young *et al.*, 1981.

Incidence, however, has increased among white males. In 1937-9, the incidence of testicular cancer was 2.0 per 100,000 and in 1973-7 it was 3.6 per 100,000. Increases in incidence were greatest for the age group 15 to 29 years.

Among countries reporting cancer incidence statistics, the highest rates of testicular cancer are reported for Denmark, North American whites, the United Kingdom and northern European countries (Waterhouse *et al.*, 1976). The lowest rates are reported for North American blacks and African blacks.

As with prostate cancer, the black–white differential in risk suggests the possible importance of socioeconomic status. In contrast to the lack of such an association for prostate cancer, testicular cancer more clearly and consistently is linked to social class. Graham *et al.* (1977) reported that in New York State, the risk of testicular cancer was greatest among professionals, a finding similar to that of Mustacchi and Millmore (1976) in California. Ross *et al.* (1978) found greater incidence among upper social class persons but this only was true for cancers occurring among younger men. The major exception to this research is the finding of Grumet and MacMahon (1958) that no gradient of risk was associated with social class.

Aetiology

Prostate Cancer

The aetiology of prostate cancer is not understood. Some of the leading hypotheses suggest the importance of a genetic predisposition, as well as hormonal, viral, sexual and dietary factors. The higher rate of prostatic cancer among American blacks compared to whites and the relatively lower rates among Hispanics and Asians suggest a possible genetic aetiology. Also, some studies show a higher rate of prostatic cancer among the male relatives of prostate cancer patients (Woolf, 1960).

Because many prostate cancers respond to hormone treatment it has been suspected that hormonal factors are involved in its cause. Evidence in support of this hypothesis included the fact that androgen is needed for normal prostatic development and the observation that prostate cancer does not frequently, if ever, develop in males who have been castrated. Studies have reported hormonal differences in patients with prostatic cancer, compared to disease-free subjects, but it is not clear if the hormonal change preceded or occurred as a result of the cancer.

Evidence in favour of a viral aetiology for prostatic cancer comes from studies which have identified certain viruses occurring more frequently in prostate cancer patients compared with patients with non-urogenital diseases. Heshmat *et al.* (1975) found an association between previous gonorrhoeal infection and prostate cancer but this association may reflect the effects of therapeutic procedures to control the gonorrhoea infection rather than the effect of some underlying common venereal cause.

The involvement of sexual factors in the aetiology of prostate cancer has been suggested by the findings that the risk varies with marital status, sexual experience and history of venereal disease. Prostate cancer patients have been found more likely to have been married (Armenian *et al.*, 1975), to have had more marital partners, to have had more premarital and extramarital sexual partners, and to report greater coital frequency in the ten years preceding hospitalisation than patients with no genitourinary or cancerous condition (Steele *et al.*, 1971; Krain, 1973). Michalek *et al.* (1981) found a lower mortality rate for prostatic cancer in Catholic priests in New York State compared with a general population of white males of comparable ages. Kaplan (1980) reported similar results from a national survey of deaths among priests, but the study of Ross *et al.* (1981) of priests' deaths in the Los Angeles area did not find standardised mortality ratios for prostate cancer to be significantly low or high.

Research has just begun on associations between dietary consumption patterns and cancers at a number of sites. A correlation was found between prostatic cancer mortality and *per capita* consumption of dietary fat from 40 countries (Howell, 1974). An analysis of prostatic cancer mortality rates for USA counties between 1950 and 1969 revealed that the highest rates occurred in those areas with the highest consumption of beef, milk products, fats and eggs (Blair and Fraumeni, 1978). Other impetus to search for dietary factors comes from the findings of lower rates of prostatic cancer among certain ethnic and religious groups. The low rate of prostatic cancer in Japanese men relative to USA males may be related to dietary differences (Hirayama, 1979). Mettlin (1980) suggested that the lower rates of consumption of fruits and vegetables of USA blacks may be linked to their greater rates of prostate cancer. In spite of these interesting associations, the available evidence associating dietary factors to prostatic cancer is weak and no biological mechanism by which diet might produce prostate cancer has been identified.

Occupational exposure to rubber (Goldsmith *et al.*, 1980) and cadmium (Lemen *et al.*, 1976) have been associated with prostatic cancer and Winkelstein and Kantor (1969) found an association between air pollution and prostatic cancer mortality. In general, cigarette smoking and alcohol consumption have not been found to be related to prostate cancer. Some studies have reported a lower rate of prostate cancer in patients with cirrhosis of the liver (Glantz, 1964; Robson, 1966). These findings may be explained by the effects of limited oestrogen metabolism capability in the cirrhotic liver.

Benign prostatic hypertrophy (BPH), because of its high prevalence in older men, has been suggested as a possible precursor to carcinoma of the prostate. Fifty per cent of men over 50 years of age and 80 per cent of prostatic cancer cases have some degree of prostatic hypertrophy. Armenian *et al.* (1974) in a retrospective case-control study found men with a history of BPH significantly more likely to be cases than controls. However, detection bias is likely to confound this observation and Greenwald *et al.* (1974) studied men with BPH and controls prospectively to avoid this effect. They found that the populations when followed an average of over ten years experienced no significant differences in prostate cancer mortality.

Testicular Cancer

No single causal factor has been identified in cancer of the testis. A major known risk factor for testis cancer is cryptorchidism (Mostofi, 1973; Morrison, 1976; Henderson *et al.*, 1979). The risk of developing a malignant tumour is estimated to be five times greater in a patient with an undescended testis than in a patient with normally descended testes and the frequency of undescended testes in USA white males is thought to be increasing. The concomitant patterns of increasing incidence of testicular cancer in young adults, and increasing incidence of undescended testes, could result from a common underlying cause. *In utero* exposure to diethylstilboestrol is a possible underlying factor but this has not yet been conclusively demonstrated in epidemiological studies.

Various authors have studied the question of prenatal exposure to hormones. Henderson *et al.* (1979) found six mothers of patients who reported use of 'hormones' during pregnancy compared to only one among the control series, but this difference was not significant. Schottenfeld (1980) observed exposure to diethylstilboestrol or other hormones in 5.8 per cent of mothers of cases compared to 2.5 per cent of hospital controls and 2.1 per cent of neighbourhood controls. Again, although suggestive, the result was not statistically significant.

Prognosis

Prostate Cancer

Data from a recent survey on patterns of care of prostate cancer patients in the USA conducted by the American College of Surgeons show that patient survival is largely dependent on the clinical stage of disease at diagnosis. The overall five-year survival rate for the patients whose disease was confined to the prostate gland was 78 per cent; for patients with localised to distant spread of the disease the overall five-year survival rates ranged from 68 per cent to 23 per cent (Mettlin *et al.*, 1982). Data from the National Cancer Institute's End Results Program on men with prostatic cancer diagnosed between 1950 and 1973 indicate substantial improvements in patient survival since 1950 (Asire *et al.*, 1978). Between 1950 and 1973 survival rates increased substantially for both white and black men, with blacks experiencing the biggest gain. Accompanying the increase in survival rates between 1950 and 1973 was an increase in the percentage of prostate cancer patients diagnosed in the most curable, localised stage. One explanation for the poorer survival rate among black males may be that they tend to be diagnosed at later stages of disease.

Testicular Cancer

The treatment and prognosis of testicular cancers vary according to the cell type of the tumour as well as by the stage of the disease at diagnosis. Seminomas of the germ cell are the type most often diagnosed among middle-aged and younger men accounting for 30 to 40 per cent of all testicular cancers. It is this type of tumour that is associated with the most favourable prognosis. USA SEER data indicate that overall, 88 per cent of seminoma patients diagnosed between 1973 and 1976 survived five years and that this rate appears to be changing little in recent years (Li *et al.*, 1982).

The nonseminoma tumours bear a markedly poorer prognosis. Less than 60 per cent of patients diagnosed between 1973 and 1976 with tumours other than seminomas survived five years. However, recent data (Li *et al.*, 1982) suggest that improved therapy for these tumour types is significantly improving their prognosis. The 30-month survival rates for patients diagnosed in 1973-6 was 65 per cent, but for patients diagnosed between 1977 and 1979 the comparable rate was 77 per cent. Increased survival rates are observed for both localised and advanced nonseminomas.

Detection

Prostate Cancer

The first symptoms of prostate cancer usually include urinary difficulties such as weak or interrupted flow of urine, inability to urinate or difficulty in starting urination. Unfortunately, the presence of symptoms usually is associated with disease that is advanced beyond its earliest stages. Most localised prostate cancer is found among asymptomatic persons and often only at autopsy where it is known as occult disease. Digital rectal examination is a common method for screening for prostate cancer and according to Guinan (1980) it is the most cost-effective. By palpation of the prostate, a physician can feel for a nodule or unusually firm areas that may indicate a tumour. About 50 per cent of prostatic nodules detected by digital rectal examination ultimately are found to be cancerous. The American Cancer Society recommends that all men over the age of 40 years have an annual digital rectal examination (American Cancer Society, 1980). If cancer is suspected, a biopsy should be performed.

A survey by the American College of Surgeons of patients diagnosed with prostate cancer in 1974 and 1979 found that the proportion of patients diagnosed with localised disease increased during that five-year interval (Mettlin *et al.*, 1982). These findings are consistent with trends observed earlier. The percentage of clinically localised tumours detected in whites increased from 48 per cent in 1950-1 to 61 per cent in 1970-3 (Asire *et al.*, 1978). For black patients the number of clincally localised tumours detected increased from 41 per cent in 1950 to 54 per cent in 1970.

Testicular Cancer

The usual symptoms of testicular cancer include a lump in the testicle, painless swelling or altered consistency of the testis. In many patients the tumour is discovered incidentally during the course of a routine medical examination. The mildness of the typical early symptoms combined with ignorance or fear of cancer may often lead patients to delay seeking medical attention until the disease has spread to other parts of the body. It is believed that persons may facilitate early detection of testicular cancer by a self-examination procedure to check for any small lumps or changes in size of the testis. An emphasis on self-detection of early disease would require greater health education directed toward the population at greatest risk. However, those at greatest risk are younger men who less frequently interact with health care providers and health education in schools may prove to be the best route of intervention to promote early detection.

Special Considerations

Prostate Cancer

Epidemiologically, prostate cancer presents problems of research that are not characteristic of other cancers. First, and most troublesome, is the fact that the prevalence of undiagnosed prostate cancer in older men is believed to be quite high, much higher than that clinically evident. Evidence for this comes from the fact that a large number of prostate cancers are diagnosed from pathological examination of trans-urethral resection specimens obtained in the course of treating what had been presumed to be benign obstruction. Furthermore, detailed studies of the prostate at autopsy very often reveal carcinoma that had been previously unsuspected. These so-called latent carcinomas have been observed in large autopsy series in the USA in 26.1 per cent of men over 80 and in 53.4 per cent of men over 70 (Halpert *et al.*, 1963; Berg *et al.*, 1971). Such observations support the common notion that men are more likely to die *with* prostate cancer than *because* of it.

Although there is a question as to whether or not all of these latent tumours are biologically the same as clinical cancer, their widespread prevalence does present a dilemma for aetiological researchers. Because the disease is so age-related, any controlled comparisons such as in a case-control study would require that subjects be matched by age. If the disease is widely prevalent subclinically among the control population, the power of inference of the study is markedly reduced. Since the prevalence of latent disease is likely to be greatest in populations where the risk of manifest disease is greatest, the usual approach of conducting case-control studies among high-risk groups may not be particularly advantageous. Thus, prostate cancer may be a disease in which the most powerful research is that conducted in populations where the disease is rarest and the likelihood that the presumed healthy control bears latent prostate cancer is least. Another approach to the problem of latent disease in the control population is to select, as comparison subjects, men who have recently undergone examination for signs of the disease including, at least, a digital rectal examination. Such control populations are obviously more difficult to obtain.

The question of latent disease is also an important consideration in comparison of rates in populations receiving different levels of medical care. The degree of diagnostic effort may determine, in part, the frequency of diagnosis of prostate cancer. Rising rates in American blacks may be partly attributable to improvements in the distribution of medical care. Similarly, international variations may be explained by such medical care variables rather than by the true underlying frequency of the disease. As Templeton (1981) has observed in underdeveloped areas of Africa, cancers of internal organs, compared to superficial tumours, are far less likely to be correctly recorded as incident cancer.

Another special consideration arises from the fact that the disease occurs so predominently among the oldest segment of the population. In a sense, men who manifest prostate cancer are among the longest survivors in the overall population. If aspects of life style are important aetiological determinants it is conceivable that what would otherwise be considered as 'healthy' practices of daily living may be factors in this disease. In other words, it may be that it is men who take such good care of themselves to survive to old age who are at greatest risk of disease. Thus, the risk factors for prostate cancer can be distinctly different from those known or suspected to play a role in the aetiology of diseases which are likely to cause death at an earlier age. This may explain why Mormons who are at a reduced risk for so many types of cancer appear to have rates comparable to, or slightly above, the remainder of the USA white male population (Enstrom, 1978).

Testicular Cancer

In addition to the special problems presented by its relative rarity, research on testicular cancer is complicated by its tendency towards a bimodal age-specific incidence distribution and its predominant occurrence in young men. The bimodal nature of the incidence curve and recent evidence that incidence is increasing in younger men (Davies, 1981) may indicate that although the same diagnosis applies, the two populations are at risk for different forms of the disease. For this reason it may be particularly important to consider the detailed histological classification of the tumour and to not make general epidemiological characterisations of tumours of different types. Alternatively, the bimodal incidence curve may suggest that distinct aetiologies affect the occurrence of disease among young men as opposed to the older group.

Finally, testicular cancer shares with Hodgkin's disease, leukaemia and other cancers affecting young people, the likelihood that its aetiology extends to early childhood or to foetal development. Thus, the person with testicular cancer may not be the appropriate source of information on exposures of aetiological significance. Prenatal or early childhood experiences may be addressed by information from a parent, and the inclusion of multiple sources of data complicates the conduct of research of this disease.

Summary

In terms of the common epidemiological considerations of time, person and place it is apparent that both of the cancer sites considered here are extremely interesting. While they are diseases of the same anatomic system, their epidemiologies are, in may respects, opposite. Prostatic cancer occurs most often in older men and, in the USA, most often among black men. Testicular cancer, on the other hand, is most frequent among younger, white men. Prostatic cancer is very common in the population at risk, in either a clinically evident or occult form, while cancer of the testis is relatively uncommon. Although it is difficult to know the impact of increasing diagnostic efforts, both of these diseases appear to share trends of rising incidence among high-risk segments of the population. They also share a pattern of increasing survival after diagnosis owing to either earlier diagnosis and more effective therapy, or both.

Many interesting associations have been observed for these diseases and some may be of aetiological significance. However, the range of types of exogenous exposures that have been identified and the fact that no single exposure has been found to greatly enhance risk suggest that prevention of prostatic or testicular cancer is not feasible on the basis of current knowledge. Future inquiry regarding the roles of diet, hormonal phenomena, chemical carcinogenesis and life style is important and may shed further light on the poorly understood aetiologies of these cancers.

References

American Cancer Society (1980). ACS report on the cancer-related health checkup. *Ca – A Cancer Journal for Clinicians*, 30: 195-231

Armenian, H.K., Lilienfeld, A.M., Diamond, E.L. and Bross, I.D.J. (1974). Relation between benign prostatic hyperplasia and cancer of the prostate. *Lancet*, 2: 115-17

——— Lilienfeld, A.M., Diamond, E.L. and Bross, I.D.J. (1975). Epidemiologic characteristics of patients with prostatic neoplasms. *American Journal of Epidemiology*, 102: 47-54

Asire, A.J., Shambaugh, E.M. and Heise, H.W. (1978). *Survival for Cancers of the Genital Organs*. DHEW Publication No. (NIH), 78-1543

Berg, J.W., Hajdu, S.I. and Foote, F.W. (1971). The prevalence of latent cancers in cancer patients. *Archives of Pathology*, 91: 183-6

Blair, A. and Fraumeni, J.F. (1978). Geographic patterns of prostate cancer in the United States. *Journal of the National Cancer Institute*, 61: 1379-84

Davies, J.M. (1981). Testicular cancer in England and Wales: some epidemiological aspects. *Lancet*, 1: 928-32

Devesa, S.S. and Silverman, D.T. (1978). Cancer incidence and morbidity trends in the United States: 1935-1974. *Journal of the National Cancer Institute*, 60: 545-71

Enstrom, J.E. (1978). Cancer and total mortality among active Mormons. *Cancer*, 42: 1943-71

Ernster, V.L., Winkelstein, W., Selvin, S., Brown, S.M., Sacks, S.T., Austin, D.F. *et al.* (1977). Race, socioeconomic status, and prostate cancer. *Cancer Treatment Reports*, 61: 187-91

Glantz, G.M. (1964). Cirrhosis and carcinoma of the prostate gland. *Journal of Urology*, 91: 291-3

Goldsmith, D.F., Smith, A.H. and McMichael, A.J. (1980). A case-control study of prostate cancer within a cohort of rubber and tire workers. *Journal of Occupational Medicine*, 22: 533-41

Graham, S., Gibson, R., West, D., Swanson, M., Burnett, H. and Dayal, H. (1977). Epidemiology of prostate cancer in upstate New York. *Journal of the National Cancer Institute*, 58: 1255-61

Greenwald, P., Kirmss, V., Polan, A.K. and Dick, V.S. (1974). Cancer of the prostate among men with benign prostate hyperplasia. *Journal of the National Cancer Institute*, 53(2): 335-40

Grumet, R. and MacMahon, B. (1958). Trends in mortality from neoplasms of the testis. *Cancer*, 11: 790-7

Guinan, P., Gilham, N., Nagubadi, S.R., Bush, I., Rhee, H. and McKiel, C. (1981). What is the best test to detect prostate cancer? *Ca – A Cancer Journal for Clinicians*, 31: 141-5

Haenszel, W. and Kurihara, M. (1968). Studies of Japanese migrants. 1. Mortality from cancer and other diseases. *Journal of the National Cancer Institute*, 40: 43-68

Hakky, S.I., Chisholm, G.D. and Skeet, R.G. (1979). Social class and carcinoma of the prostate. *British Journal of Urology*, 51: 393-6

Halpert, B., Sheehan, E.E., Schmathorst, W.R. and Scott, R. (1963). Carcinoma of the prostate. A survey of 5,000 autopsies. *Cancer*, 16: 737-42

Henderson, B.E., Benton, B., Jing, J., Yu, M.C. and Pike, M.C. (1979). Risk factors for cancer of the testis in young men. *International Journal of Cancer*, 23: 589-602

Heshmat, M.Y., Herson, J., Kovi, J. and Niles, R. (1973). An epidemiologic study of gonorrhea and cancer of the prostate gland. *Medical Annals of the District of Columbia*, 42: 378-83

Hirayama, T. (1979). Epidemiology of prostate cancer with special reference to the role of diet. *National Cancer Institute Monograph*, 53, United States Printing Office, pp. 149-54

Howell, M.A. (1974). Factor analysis of international cancer mortality data and per capita food consumption. *British Journal of Cancer*, 29: 328-36

Kaplan, S. (1980). Personal communication

Krain, L.S. (1973). Epidemiologic variables in prostatic cancer. *Geriatrics*, 28: 93-8

Lemen, R.A., Lee, J.S., Wagoner, J.K. and Blejer, H.P. (1976). Cancer mortality among cadmium production workers. *Annals of the New York Academy of Sciences*, 271: 273-9

Li, F.P., Connelly, R.R. and Myers, M. (1982). Improved survival rates among testis cancer patients in the United States. *Journal of the American Medical Association*, 247: 825-6

Mettlin, C. (1980). Nutritional habits of blacks and whites. *Preventive Medicine*, 9: 601-6

—— Natarajan, N. and Murphy, G.P. (1982). Recent patterns of care of prostate cancer patients in the United States. *International Advances in Surgical Oncology*, 5(2): 277-321

Michalek, A.M., Mettlin, C. and Priore, R.L. (1981). Prostate cancer among Catholic priests. *Journal of Surgical Oncology*, 17: 129-33

Morrison, A.S. (1976). Cryptorchidism, hernia and cancer of the testis. *Journal of the National Cancer Institute*, 56: 731-3

Mostofi, F.K. (1973). Testicular tumors: epidemiologic, etiologic and pathologic features. *Cancer*, 32: 1186-201

Mustacchi, P. and Millmore, D. (1976). Racial and occupational variations in cancer of the testis: San Francisco, 1956-65. *Journal of the National Cancer Institute*, 56: 717-20

Richardson, I.M. (1965). Prostatic cancer and social class. *British Journal of Preventive and Social Medicine*, 19: 140-2

Robson, M.C. (1966). Cirrhosis and prostatic neoplasms. *Geriatrics*, 21: 150-4

Ross, R.K., Deapen, D.M., Casagrande, J.T., Paganini-Hill, A. and Henderson, B.E. (1981). A cohort study of mortality from cancer of the prostate in Catholic priests. *British Journal of Cancer*, 43: 233-5

Schottenfeld, D., Warshauer, M.E., Sherlock, S., Zauber, A.G., Leder, M. and Payne, R. (1980). The epidemiology of testicular cancer in young adults. *American Journal of Epidemiology*, 112: 232-46

Segi, M. (1978). *Age-adjusted Death Rates for Selected Sites in 52 Countries in 1973*. 'World Population' Cancer Incidence in Five Continents, Segi Institute of Cancer Epidemiology, Japan, vol. III, p. 456

Steele, R., Lees, R.E.M., Kraus, A.S. and Rao, C. (1971). Sexual factors in the epidemiology of cancer of the prostate. *Journal of Chronic Diseases*, 24: 29-37

Straszewski, J. and Haenszel, W. (1965). Cancer mortality among the Polish born in the United States. *Journal of the National Cancer Institute*, 35: 291-7

Templeton, A.C. (1981). Cancer patterns in Africa. The influence of registration bias. In: Mettlin, C. and Murphy, G.P. (eds.), *Cancer Among Black Populations*, Alan R. Liss, New York, 53: 99-110

Waterhouse, J., Muir, C., Correa, P. and Powell, J. (1976). *Cancer Incidence in Five Continents*, vol. III, International Agency for Research on Cancer, Publication No. 15, Lyon

Winkelstein, W. and Kantor, S. (1969). Prostatic cancer: relationship to suspended particulate air pollution. *American Journal of Public Health*, 59: 1134-8

Woolf, G.M. (1960). An investigation of familial aspects of cancer of the prostate. *Cancer*, 13: 739-43

Young, J.L., Percey, C.L. and Asire, A.J. (1981). Surveillance, epidemiology, and end results: Incidence and mortality data, 1973-1977. *National Cancer Institute Monograph*, 57: DHHS Publication No. (NIH) 81-2330, pp. 1-9

15 OCCUPATIONAL CANCER

P. Cole and F. Merletti

Introduction

Interest in occupationally-induced cancer has increased greatly during the last 10 to 15 years. There seem to be four major reasons for this. The first is the growing concern about the quality of the environment. It would appear self-evident that, while industrial effluents and products may produce illness in the general population, exposed workers are likely to be the first and most severely affected persons. Thus workers warrant special attention both for their own protection and so that hazards to the public may be identified as early as possible. A second reason for the interest in occupational carcinogenesis is more subtle; it relates to an expanding social consciousness in many countries. This gives rise to the viewpoint that workers are entitled to know the likely long-term health effects of their exposures in so far as such information exists. A third reason is the perception that when specific carcinogenic agents are identified in the occupational environment they can be readily controlled. This is in contrast to aspects of life style, such as smoking or dietary habits, whose control requires modification of cultural and personal behaviour patterns. A fourth major reason is the current disenchantment with the idea that viruses are a major cause of human cancer. Despite decades of intensive study, the role of viruses in human cancer remains unknown. Yet it was established long ago that some chemicals are human carcinogens. In fact occupational exposures to complex chemical mixtures were among the first causes of cancer to be identified. And in many instances this led to the identification of specific causative agents. Much of the information now available on human carcinogenesis, including a large amount with direct implications for prevention, derives from observations in the occupational setting.

The Magnitude of the Problem

Caution must be used in attempting to interpret estimates of the magnitude of the occupational cancer problem. Recent estimates for the United States of America (USA) have ranged from 1 per cent to as much as 20-40 per cent of all cancers (Bridbord *et al.*, 1978; Doll and Peto, 1981; Higginson and Muir, 1979; Wynder and Gori, 1977). The wide range of these estimates makes it evident that this is an area of uncertainty. However, if a reasonably valid estimate of the proportion of cancer attributable to occupation could be developed, it might serve at least two purposes. Firstly, such an estimate could be useful in health education, and secondly, the estimate might contribute to the establishment of cancer research priorities by permitting major categories of carcinogenic exposures, such as smoking, drugs and occupation, to be ranked according to public health impact.

Yet it must be recognised that all such estimates are very difficult to develop because they depend on the proportion of the population experiencing the exposure of interest and the magnitude of the excess risk among such persons. Further, each of these figures is itself difficult to estimate. In addition, it is widely believed that any single, summary estimate of the proportion of cancer attributable to occupational exposures will be difficult to defend and interpret. No single measure can accord two facts. These are, first, that 'cancer' is a group of diseases probably as diverse in its aetiology as are diseases in general. Second, and similarly, the heterogeneity of occupational exposures is so great, and these exposures vary so much from region to region and over time, that an estimate of the proportion of all cancer due to all occupational exposures defies interpretation in any particular context.

An alternative preferable to any overall estimate is to view occupationally-induced cancer as a series of more-or-less independent problems. This focuses attention on specific occupational experiences that warrant evaluation and on others where control is indicated. This view should prove useful both for understanding occupational carcinogenesis and for preventing it. For example, it was suggested that in Boston in 1967 and 1968 about 18 per cent of bladder cancer in men was due to occupational exposures. Such an estimate is specific for place, time, gender and cancer site; and its validity and precision can be assessed by evaluating the study that developed it (Cole *et al.*, 1972).

The various estimates of occupational cancer have been used by legislators, policy-makers and others to exaggerate (or, alternatively, to minimise) the importance of the problem. But occupational cancer should have a high priority in aetiological research and in programmes of cancer prevention, regardless of its proportional importance. There are three pragmatic reasons for this:

(1) Occupational cancer is concentrated among relatively small groups of people. For these people the risk of developing a particular form of cancer may be very large.

(2) Among the known causes of cancer, occupational hazards are among the few that are susceptible to regulatory control and thus especially suitable for prevention.

(3) Even if only 1 or 2 per cent of the cancer burden is due to occupational exposures, this would mean 8,000 to 16,000 'preventable' cases and 4,000 to 8,000 preventable deaths each year in the USA alone.

There are also several more 'abstract' or 'academic' reasons for assigning a high priority to the study of occupational cancer. For one, the occupational setting has sometimes served as the framework for a 'natural experiment' in which human beings are exposed to multiple agents. Even if evidence of carcinogenicity in animals is used for preventive purposes, there are work environments involving exposure to complex mixtures of substances that cannot be studied in the laboratory, or can be studied only with great difficulty. For another, monitoring the cancer experience of groups of exposed workers by means of epidemiological studies may lead to the detection of previously unknown carcinogenic agents or to the re-evaluation of 'safe' levels of known hazards.

Finally, as a practical matter, most studies of occupational 'carcinogens' are of the follow-up design. Such studies provide estimates of the frequency of all causes of death, not just of cancer. Thus, the study of persons occupationally exposed to suspect carcinogens may provide knowledge regarding health hazards of all types.

Occupation as an Epidemiological Variable

In the USA, among persons of working age, about 77 per cent of men and 67 per cent of women are gainfully employed (US Bureau of the Census, 1980). For most men and many women, employment is a major part of life's experience. Yet, despite their obvious significance, occupational exposures have not been of much concern to the general public. This indifference, and the great diversity of occupational exposures, make them less susceptible to epidemiological study.

There are also several more specific problems that make occupation difficult to study. Many workers are unaware of the conditions surrounding them or the substances they handle. The latter difficulty often results because a particular agent is known by a trivial chemical or trade name. Many persons change occupations from time to time, and may forget or lose interest in the experiences of former occupations. Further difficulties arise because many occupational titles have no specific exposure connotation — a single title may refer to occupations involving exposure to very different substances. Equally problematical, a particular exposure may be sustained in occupations with dissimilar titles or duties. The value of occupational titles as an index of exposure is further reduced by their 'upward social drift', particularly on death certificates. These difficulties are vexing in case-control studies, which are dependent on memory for the recall of exposures, and in any study that uses titles rather than description of duties or exposures to characterise occupations. Such studies, especially when negative, are not persuasive.

Two more difficulties affect virtually all studies of occupational carcinogenesis. Most cancers probably have an 'induction' period of 20 years or more. In industrialised countries, technological advances and changing needs are such that many industries evolve rapidly. As they do, new jobs and exposures come into being and others cease to exist. Thus, a given study might uncover a carcinogenic exposure that no longer occurs. At the same time, the more recent replacement exposure cannot be evaluated because the requisite induction period has not elapsed. Finally a problem results because occupation is so closely related to social class. Indeed, in many studies occupational 'title' — not exposure — is used to designate an individual's social class. Social class, in turn, is a correlate of risk for many cancers, including some for which the association is quite strong. The possible confounding by social class and other characteristics (e.g. race) of an employed group should be evaluated before it is inferred that a causal association exists between the occupational exposure and a cancer. For example, soft-coal miners were reported to be at increased risk of cancer of the stomach (Matolo *et al.*, 1972) but when the effects of social class were evaluated (Creagan *et al.*, 1974), the association was virtually eliminated.

To balance the discussion of occupation as an epidemiological variable, we should mention some characteristics that make it suitable for study. For certain types of occupations, such as skilled trades and professions, exposures are reasonably easy to delineate and are experienced for a working lifetime. Less often, unskilled workers in some industries hold a single position for decades. In such cases, if investigations are conducted in collaboration with management or a trade union, highly valid long-term exposure information may be available.

Objectives of Occupational Studies

Studies of occupational carcinogenesis usually report only if an apparent association between an occupation suspected of being hazardous and a particular malignancy is statistically significant. When possible, the identity of the responsible agent is also given. Often, considerably more valuable information is available. For example, many studies give no idea of the magnitude (relative risk) of the increased cancer risk. And when they do the standardised mortality ratio (SMR) is usually employed. However, the SMR is an 'indirectly' standardised summary measure of effect and, as such, is not guaranteed to be truly standardised. As a result SMRs for two or more groups are not necessarily comparable. This is a particular problem when the SMR is used to describe 'dose-response' relationships. Typically, the more exposed group of subjects will be older than the less exposed. If so, and if in addition the carcinogenic effect of the occupational exposure varies over age, the SMRs should not be compared among these groups. Instead, directly-standardised relative risks should be employed. Usually the attributable risk per cent (ARP) is also missing from occupational studies. The ARP among the exposed is the proportion of cases of the cancer in question among the workers that results from the exposure under study. Instead of estimating the proportion of cancers among the exposed, the proportion of cancers attributable to exposure can be calculated among the population of all workers. This population ARP (PARP) should prove a useful measure for comparing results between studies. The magnitude of the relative risk will differ between similar studies depending on the criteria used to characterise an 'exposed worker'. However, the PARP is much less susceptible to this difficulty because as the criteria for exposure are relaxed, with concomitant reduction in relative risk, the proportion of the referent population that is exposed increases and the PARP remains relatively constant.

Another potentially interesting item, since it could have profound implications for prevention, is the relationship of excess risk to age at first exposure. In one study all the excess risk of bladder cancer among men with occupational exposures was confined to those whose exposure began prior to age 25 (Cole *et al.*, 1972). If this finding were confirmed, it would have considerable significance. Studies of occupational carcinogenesis are needed to determine the relationship of excess risk to age at first exposure. At least two issues appear involved: Firstly, younger persons might be more susceptible to cancer induction; and secondly, only persons who are first exposed while young may work long enough to sustain exposures sufficient to be carcinogenic. (The latter explanation did not apply in the bladder cancer study cited.) In either case, the implication is that only older persons should be placed in potentially carcinogenic work environments. Yet on the basis of existing knowledge this recommendation cannot be made. Several studies (Hoover and Cole, 1973; Doll, 1962) suggested that elderly persons are actually more susceptible than the young to cancer induction. The relationship should be worked out in detail so that their preventive implications can be exploited. It may be that both the young and the old are susceptible, but that the middle aged are relatively resistant to carcinogenesis.

Closely tied to the age at first exposure issue is duration of exposure. Several studies (Cole *et al.*, 1972; Case *et al.*, 1954) suggested that relatively short occupational exposures (e.g. six months to a year) appreciably increase cancer risk. However, it seems there is also a relationship of increased excess risk with increasing duration of exposure. Again, preventive strategies might follow from an understanding of these temporal factors.

An additional temporal factor is the duration of the interval between beginning exposure and the manifestation of disease, the induction period. Concepts of carcinogenesis and cancer growth are not very helpful here, nor are the lessons learned from infectious disease epidemiology. Detailed knowledge of this interval, its components (induction and incubation periods), length, variability and determinants would contribute to the understanding of human carcinogenesis. Such knowledge might also have important implications for screening schedules.

Largely ignored have been the determinants of cancer among workers in addition to the occupational exposure. One exception is the important finding (Selikoff *et al.*, 1968) that cigarette smoking potentiates the carcinogenic effects of asbestos on the lung. Other such agent–agent and host–agent interactions should be sought. The implications would seem to be both of a general scientific and preventive nature.

Table 15.1: Substances and Industrial Processes for which there is Sufficient or Limited Evidence of Carcinogenicity for Man, as Derived from Occupational Settings

Substance[1]	Category of evidence and site[2]			Evaluation by IARC[3]				References[4]
	Sufficient	Limited	Inadequate	Evidence of carcinogenicity in humans	Evidence of carcinogenicity in animals	Evidence of activity in short-term tests	Summary of carcinogenic risk to humans	
Acrylonitrile		lung; colon	lymphatic tissues; stomach; brain; kidney; urinary bladder	limited	sufficient	sufficient	2A	NIOSH[a], 1977; Monson, 1978; O'Berg, 1980; Thies et al., 1980; Werner & Carter, 1981
4-Amino-biphenyl	urinary bladder			sufficient	sufficient	sufficient	1	Clayson, 1976
Arsenic[5]	skin; lung; liver; (angio-sarcoma)		haemato-poietic tissues (leukaemia)	sufficient	inadequate	limited	1	Kyle & Pease, 1965; Kjeldsberg & Ward, 1972; Ott et al., 1974; Lander et al., 1975; Sunderman, 1976; Doll et al., 1977; Tokudome & Karatsune, 1976; Brady et al., 1977; Hernberg, 1977; Mabuchi, 1979; Wall, 1980

Note: a. National Institute of Occupational Safety and Health.

Chemical	Site(s)						Degree	References
Asbestos	lung; pleura, peritoneum (mesothelioma)	larynx	large bowel; prostate; stomach	sufficient	sufficient	inadequate	1	Stell & McGill, 1973; Stell & McGill, 1975; Newhouse & Berry, 1976; Morgan & Shettigara, 1976; Graham et al., 1977; Elmes & Simpson, 1977; Peto et al., 1977; Acheson et al., 1981a; Clemmesen & Hjalgrim-Jensen, 1981
Auramine[5]	urinary bladder			sufficient	sufficient	inadequate	1	Case & Pearson, 1954
Benzene	hemato-poietic tissues (leukaemia)			sufficient	limited	limited	1	Vigliani, 1976; Infante & Epstein, 1977; Zenz, 1978; Aksoy & Erdem, 1978; Ott et al., 1978; Aksoy, 1980
Benzidine	urinary bladder			sufficient	sufficient	sufficient	1	Case et al., 1954; Ferber et al., 1976
Beryllium[5]		lung		limited	sufficient	inadequate	2A	Mancuso, 1980; Infante et al., 1980; Wagoner et al., 1980b; Smith, 1981

Table 15.1: (continued)

| Substance[1] | Category of evidence and site[2] | | | Evaluation by IARC[3] | | | | References[4] |
	Sufficient	Limited	Inadequate	Evidence of carcinogenicity in humans	Evidence of carcinogenicity in animals	Evidence of activity in short-term tests	Summary of carcinogenic risk to humans	
Bis (Chloromethyl) Ether (BCME); Chloromethyl[6] methyl ether (CMME)	lung			sufficient	sufficient	limited	1	Albert et al., 1975; DeFonso & Kelton, 1976; Pasternack et al., 1977; Figueroa et al., 1973
Cadmium[5]		prostate; kidney; lung	nasopharynx	limited	sufficient	inadequate	2B	Hernberg, 1977; Potts, 1965; Kipling & Waterhouse, 1967; Buell, 1975; Kolonel, 1976; Lemen et al., 1976; Kjellström et al., 1979
Chromium[5]	lung	nasal cavity and sinuses; larynx		sufficient	sufficient	sufficient	1	Hernberg, 1977; Sunderman, 1976; Royle, 1975; Langard & Norseth, 1975; Davies, 1978; Hayes et al., 1979; Davies, 1979; Langard et al., 1980

Diethyl[5] sulfate	larynx		limited	sufficient	sufficient	2A	Lynch et al., 1979
Hematite[5]	lung	larynx	sufficient			1	Hernberg, 1977
Isopropyl[5] oils	nasal sinuses	larynx; mouth; pharynx	sufficient			1	IARC, 1982; Alderson & Rattan, 1980
Magenta[5]	urinary bladder		limited	limited		2A	Case & Pearson, 1954; Clayson, 1976
Leather[5] dusts	nasal cavity and sinuses; urinary bladder		inadequate			3	IARC, 1982
Mustard gas	lung	larynx; pharynx	trachea; nasal sinuses	sufficient	limited	sufficient	1	Norman, 1975
β-Naphthyla-mine	urinary bladder		sufficient	sufficient	sufficient	1	Case et al., 1954; Clayson, 1976
Nickel[5]	lung; nasal sinuses		sufficient			1	Hernberg, 1977; Sunderman, 1976; Roush et al., 1980; Acheson et al., 1981b; Cox et al., 1981; Doll et al., 1977
Wood dust[5]	nasal cavity; sinuses		inadequate		inadequate	3	IARC, 1982

Table 15.1: (continued)

| Substance[1] | Category of evidence and site[2] | | | Evaluation by IARC[3] | | | | References[4] |
	Sufficient	Limited	Inadequate	Evidence of carcinogenicity in humans	Evidence of carcinogenicity in animals	Evidence of activity in short-term tests	Summary of carcinogenic risk to humans	
Soots, tars and certain mineral oils	lung; skin; scrotum	larynx; kidney; nasal cavity; urinary bladder		sufficient	sufficient	sufficient	1	Kipling & Waldron, 1976; Redmond et al., 1976; Decoufle, 1976
Trichloro-phenoxyacetic acid[7]	soft tissues			limited			2B	Cook, 1981
Vinyl chloride	liver (angio-sarcoma)	lung; brain	lymphoid and haemato-poietic tissues	sufficient	sufficient	sufficient	1	Brady et al., 1977; Fox & Collier, 1977; Spirtas & Kaminski, 1978; Buffler et al., 1979; Wagoner et al., 1980a

1. This table is restricted to chemical substances for which there is evidence of carcinogenicity to man derived from occupational settings.
2. The explanation of the categories of evidence is as follows: 'Sufficient' — human data are considered persuasive of carcinogenicity for humans; 'limited' — evidence exists for humans but is too limited to be persuasive; 'inadequate' — human data have been considered qualitatively or quantitatively insufficient to allow any conclusion regarding carcinogenicity of the substance to humans.

Table 15.1: continued

3. This column refers to an evaluation of the evidence of the carcinogenic risk to humans of chemicals (industries and industrial processes) made by a working group of the International Agency for Research on Cancer (IARC, 1982). The evaluation was based on consideration of human and animal data and activity in short-term tests. For a complete explanation of the categories of evidence in humans, animals, short-term tests and the summary evaluation, the reader should consult the IARC's report. Briefly the explanation of the summary evaluation is as follows: '1' — carcinogenic for humans; '2A' — probably carcinogenic for humans; '2B' — probably carcinogenic for humans, high degree of evidence; '2B' — probably carcinogenic for humans, lower degree of evidence; '3' — inadequate data to evaluate.

4. Two previous reports (Cole & Goldman, 1975; Cole & Merletti, 1980) include approximately 150 citations not included here.

5. For auramine, diethyl sulphate, hematite, isopropyl oils, magenta, nickel, leather dusts, wood dusts, the evidence of carcinogenicity pertains to processes involving the substance. For minerals and metals it may be that only some compounds or industrial processes are carcinogenic. Note on evaluation of IARC for the substances: auramine, 2B; hematite, 3; isopropyl oils, 3; magenta, 3; leather dusts, 3; nickel, 2A; wood dusts, 3.

6. Carcinogenic activity may reflect contamination with the previously listed substance.

7. Carcinogenic activity probably reflects contamination by 2, 3, 7, 8-tetrachlorodibenzodioxin ('dioxin').

Table 15.2: Substances for which the Evidence of Carcinogenicity to Man Derived from Occupational Settings is Inadequate for Specific Sites

Substance	Site	Evaluation by IARC				References
		Evidence of carcinogenicity in humans	Evidence of carcinogenicity in animals	Evidence of activity in short-term tests	Summary of carcinogenic risk to humans	
Amitrole	lung	inadequate	sufficient	inadequate	2B	Axelson & Sundell, 1974; Axelson et al., 1980
Aniline	urinary bladder	inadequate	limited	inadequate	3	Case & Pearson, 1954; Case et al., 1954
Benzal Chloride	lung	inadequate	limited	limited	3	Sakabe et al., 1976; Sakabe & Fukuda, 1977
Benzotrichloride	lung	inadequate	sufficient	limited	2B	Sakabe et al., 1976; Sakabe & Fukuda, 1977
Benzoylchloride	lung	inadequate	inadequate	inadequate	3	Sakabe et al., 1976; Sakabe & Fukuda, 1977
Benzyl chloride	lung	inadequate	limited	sufficient	3	Sakabe et al., 1976; Sakabe & Fukuda, 1977
Carbon tetrachloride	liver	inadequate	sufficient	inadequate	2B	Simler et al., 1964; Tracey & Sherlock, 1968
Chlordane/heptachlor	central nervous system; haematopoietic tissues (leukaemia); skin; bladder; lung	inadequate	limited	inadequate	3	Infante & Newton, 1975; Wang & MacMahon, 1979a; Wang & MacMahon, 1979b

Table 15.2: continued

					Group	
Chloroprene	liver (angiosarcoma); lung	inadequate	inadequate	sufficient	3	Khachatryan, 1972; Pell, 1978
Ortho and para dichlorobenzene	haematopoietic tissues (leukaemia)	inadequate	inadequate	inadequate	3	Girard et al., 1969
Dimethyl sulphate	lung; eye (choroidal melanoma)	inadequate	sufficient	sufficient	2A	Druckrey et al., 1966; Albert & Puliafito, 1977
Epichlorohydrin	haematopoietic tissues (leukaemia); lung	inadequate	sufficient	sufficient	2B	Enterline, 1980
Ethylene oxide	stomach; lymphoid and haematopoietic tissues (leukaemia, Hodgkin's disease); central nervous system	inadequate	limited	sufficient	2B	Hogstedt et al., 1979; Morgan et al., 1981
Formaldehyde	skin; prostate	inadequate	sufficient	sufficient	2B	Marsh, 1980; Walrath & Fraumeni, 1980; Wong, 1980
Hexachloro-cyclohexane (BHC/lindane)	haematopoietic tissues (leukaemia); lung	inadequate	limited	inadequate	3	Jedlicka et al., 1958; Barthel, 1976; EPA, 1978
Lead	lung	inadequate	sufficient (for some salts)	inadequate	3	Kang et al., 1980; Cooper, 1981; Baker et al., 1980
Polychlorinated biphenyls	skin; rectum; liver; lymphoid and haematopoietic tissues	inadequate	sufficient	inadequate	2B	Bahn et al., 1976; Bahn et al., 1977; Brown & Jones, 1981; Bertazzi et al., 1981

Table 15.2: continued

Substance	Site	Evaluation by IARC				References
		Evidence of carcinogenicity in humans	Evidence of carcinogenicity in animals	Evidence of activity in short-term tests	Summary of carcinogenic risk to humans	
Styrene	lymphoid and haemapoeitic tissues (leukaemia, lymphoma)	inadequate	limited	sufficient	3	Proceedings of NIOSH, 1976; McMichael et al., 1976; Ott et al., 1980
Tetra chloroethylene	haematopoietic tissues (leukaemia)	inadequate	limited	inadequate	3	Blair et al., 1979
Trichloroethylene	oesophagus; liver	inadequate	limited	inadequate	3	Blair, 1980
Orthotoluidine	urinary bladder	inadequate	sufficient	sufficient	2A	IARC, 1982

Carcinogens in Occupational Settings

Tables 15.1 and 15.2 summarise the information available on occupational carcinogenesis. The information is a modified and updated version of prior compilations in which evidence relating to carcinogenicity for animals was not used (Cole and Goldman, 1975; Cole and Merletti, 1980). Table 15.1 relates to substances for which information derives from occupational settings and for which the evidence of carcinogenicity in man is either 'sufficient' or 'limited'. The likelihood that the substance poses a carcinogenic risk to humans has been assessed by a working group assembled for that purpose by the International Agency for Research on Cancer (IARC, 1982). The working group used evidence both from human beings and from animals as well as information from short-term (mutagenicity) tests to make its judgements. For an explanation of the categories used, the reader may consult the group's report. The references listed (Table 15.1) are not necessarily the primary sources which substantiate the Table; rather they are a selection of the few most informative or recent papers, including negative reports and reviews. Table 15.2 is similar to Table 15.1, but is restricted to substances for which all of the available evidence for man in occupational settings permits only the judgement of 'inadequate' evidence of carcinogenicity. Table 15.3 lists occupations with sufficient evidence of increased cancer risk, as derived from epidemiological studies (Simonato and Saracci, 1982).

Some points are important when considering occupations with sufficient or suspected evidence of increased cancer risk. Firstly, although it can be relatively simple to identify an occupational setting as carcinogenic, the identification of the carcinogenic compound is problematical and, because of ignorance about the industrial environment, may have little direct implication. Secondly, the carcinogenic hazard to man posed by most industrial processes has never been investigated and is unknown. Thirdly, even within a particular industrial process exposure may differ from plant to plant or, within a plant, from one time period to another. Thus, generalisations must be made with caution. Nonetheless Tables 15.1 and 15.3 suggest that:

1. The known carcinogenic effects of occupationally encountered chemicals have involved rather strong associations or have pertained to relatively uncommon tumours. Examples are vinyl chloride which was identified mainly because it causes a very rare tumour (angiosarcoma)

Table 15.3: Occupations with Sufficient Evidence of Increased Cancer Risk as Derived from Epidemiological Studies

Industry	Occupation	Site	Substance known or suspected to be the causative agent
Agriculture, forestry and fishing	vineyard workers using arsenical insecticides	lung; skin	arsenic
Pesticides, herbicides production	arsenical insecticides production & packaging	lung	arsenic
Petroleum	wax pressmen	scrotum	polycyclic hydrocarbons
Gas	coke plant workers	lung	benzo(a)pyrene
	gas workers	lung; bladder; scrotum	coal carbonisation products; α-naphthylamine
	gas retort house workers	bladder	α/β-naphthylamine
Metal	copper smelting	lung	arsenic
	chromate producing	lung	chromium
	chromium plating	lung	chromium
	ferrochromium producing	lung	chromium
	steel production	lung	benzo(a)pyrene
	nickel refining	nasal sinuses; lung	nickel[1]
Extractive	arsenic mining	lung; skin	arsenic
	iron ore mining	lung	not identified

Table 15.3: continued

	asbestos mining	lung; pleural & peritoneal mesothelioma	asbestos
	uranium mining	lung	radon
Rubber	rubber manufacture	lymphoid & haematopoietic tissues (leukaemia); bladder	benzene aromatic amines
	calendering; tyre curing; tyre building	lymphoid & haematopoietic tissues (leukaemia)	benzene
	millers; mixers	bladder	aromatic amines
	synthetic latex producers; tyre curing; calender operatives; reclaim workers; cable makers	bladder	aromatic amines
Leather	boot & shoe manufacturers, repairers	nose; haematopoietic tissues (leukaemia); urinary bladder	leather dust; benzene
Furniture	furniture & cabinet workers	nose (adenocarcinoma)	wood dust
Asbestos production	insulated material production (pipes, sheeting, textile, cloths, masks); asbestos cement manufacturers	lung; pleural & peritoneal mesothelioma	asbestos
Construction	insulators & pipe coverers	lung; pleural & peritoneal mesothelioma	asbestos
Shipbuilding, motor vehicles & transport	shipyard & dockyard workers	lung; pleural & peritoneal mesothelioma	asbestos
Chemical	BCME & CMME products & users	lung (oat cell carcinoma)	BCME; CMME (see Table 15.1)

Table 15.3: continued

Industry	Occupation	Site	Substance known or suspected to be the causative agent
Chemical	vinyl chloride producers	liver (angiosarcoma)	vinyl chloride monomer
	isopropyl alcohol manufacturing (strong acid process) workers	paranasal sinuses	causative agent not identified
	pigment chromate producing	lung	chromium
	dye manufacturers & users	bladder	benzidine; 2-naphthylamine; 4-aminodiphenyl
	auramine manufacture	bladder	auramine[2]
Other	roofers, asphalt workers	lung	benzo(a)pyrene

1. The specific compound(s) responsible for a carcinogenic effect cannot be specified precisely.
2. Together with the other aromatic amines used in the process.

Source: Simonato and Saracci (1982); by kind permission of the authors and publisher.

of the liver and beta-naphthylamine, a substance which increases bladder cancer risk 30-fold or more.

2. The most common element leading to the discovery of carcinogenic effects has been a suspicion that arises in the mind of a clinician or pathologist. Typically a concentration of cases is noted by the observer and related to a place of employment. Subsequently, the causative factor may be identified through epidemiological or experimental studies. An excellent example was the first realisation that an occupational exposure was carcinogenic. In 1775, a surgeon linked cancer of the scrotum in chimney sweeps to their exposure to soot (Pott, 1775). It was not until much later that a carcinogen, benzo(a)-pyrene, was identified in soot (Cook *et al.*, 1932).

The same pattern can be seen in two other classical examples. In 1879 Harting and Hesse identified pulmonary cancer as an occupational disease among metal miners in Central Europe but radioactivity was not identified as the causal agent until almost a century later (Hueper, 1966). In 1895 Rehn pointed out that tumours of the urinary bladder had an origin in the German dyestuffs industry (Rehn, 1895), but the identity of the specific causative agents, primarily benzidine and beta-napthylamine, was not established until 60 years later (Case and Pearson, 1954). Other occupational carcinogens were first identified as a result of experimental studies of animals or epidemiological studies of human beings. Table 15.4 gives examples of carcinogens identified by these methods.

3. Special circumstances favourable to the discovery of a carcinogen operated in many of the instances listed in Table 15.4 (Acheson, 1979). In some instances, e.g. hepatic angiosarcoma, nasal cancer, bone sarcoma and mesothelioma, the baseline frequency of the cancer was so low that the occurrence of even a small number of cases in the experience of one observer was sufficient to bring a cause-effect relationship to attention. In others, e.g. nasal sinus cancer, the geographical concentration of the hazardous industry, furniture-making, in a small town caused the association to come to light.

4. The demonstration of a cause-effect relationship in laboratory animals has rarely been the initial factor leading to the discovery of an effect in man. Doll found only four examples of this: carcinoma of the bronchus in gas retort house workers, due to polycyclic hydrocarbons; respiratory cancer in mustard gas manufacturers; angiosarcoma of the liver in manufacturers of polyvinyl chloride; and bladder cancer in chemical workers using 4-amino-diphenyl (Doll, 1976). Similarly, although they are usually necessary for refining risk estimates,

Table 15.4: Occupational Carcinogens by Site, Occupation and Method by which they were First Disclosed

(a) First noted by clinicians or pathologists		
scrotum	polycylcic hydrocarbons	sweeps
pleura	asbestos	miners
skin	ionising radiation; ultra-violet light; arsenic	radiologists; outdoor workers; sheep dip makers
nose	wood dust; isopropyl oil	furniture makers; chemical workers
nose and bronchus	nickel oxide	smelters
leukaemia	benzene	leather workers
bone	radium	luminisers
bladder	2-naphthylamine	dye workers
bronchus	chrome pigments; bichromethyl ether	refiners; ion exchange makers
liver	vinyl chloride	PVC manufacturers
(b) First noted in work in animals		
bronchus, nose, larynx	mustard gas	chemical workers
bladder	4-aminodiphenyl	chemical workers
(c) First noted by epidemiologists		
bladder	2-naphthylamine 2-naphthylamine	coal gas producers; rubber workers
nose	leather dust	boot and shoe operatives

Source: Acheson, E.D. (1979) after Doll, R. (1976).

epidemiological studies have only occasionally brought about the initial identification of the existence of a human carcinogen (Acheson, 1979).

5. As has been pointed out (Acheson, 1979), there is no logical reason why carcinogenic effects should manifest themselves predominantly in unusual situations or in terms of tumours that are otherwise rare. It seems reasonable to assume that many occupational exposures that have induced cancer are as yet undetected. Up to now we seem to have detected only those agents that produce a large increase in the risk of a particular cancer or a small increase in the risk of a rare cancer. There have been relatively few systematic approaches to the discovery

of occupational carcinogens. Thus, it is possible that the systematic approaches now beginning (primarily prospective follow-up studies done in the context of large industrial organisations) will lead to the identification of a number of occupational carcinogens.

On the other hand, it appears that the heyday of the discovery of occupational carcinogens was over long ago. Indeed it was during the 1960s and early 1970s that the majority of established occupational carcinogens was identified. Despite ever more intense scrutiny, the occupational setting appears to be yielding no additional agents that can meet our own or the International Agency for Research on Cancer's criteria for an established human carcinogen. In fact, since 1973 only one agent, 2, 3, 7, 8-tetrachlorodibenzodioxin ('dioxin'), has become so established.

Relationships Between Epidemiology, Occupational Cancer and Experimental Carcinogenesis

An ongoing debate in the scientific community relates to the usefulness of animal data on carcinogenicity for generalising (usually aggrandised by the term extrapolating) to man. There are several points to consider when comparing data on carcinogenesis from animals and human beings.

1. Three categories of substances or occupations associated with human carcinogenesis can be identified:

(a) well-defined chemicals or occupations for which evidence of carcinogenicity in humans is sufficient, such as asbestos or gas retort house workers.

(b) well-defined professions known to pose a carcinogenic risk to humans, but within which the specific causative agents have not been identified. An example is work in the wood industry, which is associated with adenocarcinoma of the nasal sinuses. Nevertheless the causal agent is unknown and it can only be stated that, at least in England, it was present from 1920 to 1940 (Acheson, 1976).

(c) chemicals found to be carcinogenic but for which information on carcinogenic effects in human beings is either limited or inadequate, such as epichlorohydrin or formaldehyde.

There is a fourth category which consists of chemicals considered carcinogenic in animals but for which there are no epidemiological studies. It is notable that of 535 compounds selected by the International

Agency for Research on Cancer for carcinogenicity evaluation (either because human exposure occurs or because there is some suspicion that the chemical may be carcinogenic), 142 have sufficient evidence of carcinogenicity in animals. For only 60 of these is there any published data pertaining to humans.

2. There are more chemicals known to be carcinogenic to animals than are known to be carcinogenic to man. There may be several explanations for this, including interspecies metabolic differences; other factors (such as endogenous viruses) causing laboratory animals to be more sensitive to carcinogens than are human beings; insufficient numbers of epidemiological studies; limitations of the available epidemiological methods especially with respect to cancers of multiple aetiology involving relatively weak carcinogens.

3. Of the 13 chemicals for which there is sufficient evidence of carcinogenicity in human beings only one (arsenic) is not an established animal carcinogen. (For two others, benzene and mustard gas, the evidence for animals is limited.)

4. Human beings experience more complex chemical exposures than do animals. Some of these mixtures have been found to be associated with cancer through *ad hoc* epidemiological studies. However, it has usually been the case that the specific substance involved in the carcinogenic process has not been identified. The design and conduct of an epidemiological study that can identify the specific culpable compound in a mixture is extremely difficult.

5. Negative epidemiological studies cannot be relied upon to establish the absence of causation unless at least a moderately large population has been exposed and 'at risk' for 20 or more years.

Preventing Occupational Cancer

Numerous methods have been proposed to reduce the frequency of occupational cancer. For a new compound, these pertain to every aspect of its 'natural history' from its first synthesis to its manufacture and ultimate use. For compounds already in use, proposals range from testing or re-testing in animals or in 'short-term' assay systems to sophisticated innovations in industrial hygiene. A number of approaches are now presented by the authors which relate to the contributions which epidemiology can make to prevention.

It should prove of value to have at least one organisation responsible for developing and maintaining a list of known and suspect animal and human carcinogens. Naturally, such a list of agents would be of greatest use if explicit, objective criteria were used to define various categories of the certainty of carcinogenicity. An organisation appropriate to this task would be one comprised of scientists; it should not be a regulatory or statutory agency or an organisation closely related to such an agency. Specifically, the authors suggest that the International Agency for Research on Cancer, an arm of the World Health Organization, is well suited to this purpose. The Agency has a long record of evaluating substances for carcinogenicity, primarily using animal evidence. However, it is also concerned with epidemiological data and recently has given special attention to assessing the evidence of the human carcinogenicity of many substances (IARC, 1982).

The second suggestion is that there be developed a classification and coding system for occupations which will relate to the exposures known or suspected to be experienced in occupational settings. Most existing coding schemes relate much more to the social status or pay scale of occupations than to the exposures sustained. The recommended 'exposure-based' code would greatly expedite epidemiological research of several sorts, especially case-control studies and prevalence surveys. Our efforts to develop such a code, as well as the efforts of others, suggest that it would have to be computerised. This is so because of the great amount of information involved and because many interacting and hierarchical variables are necessary to give the code flexibility.

A third suggestion, for a National Death Index, has recently been realised, though it is still too soon for it to be operative or evaluated. All deaths of United States citizens occurring as of 1 January 1979 will be identifiable via a single record system. This Index can serve many useful purposes. The major purpose relevant to our concern is that the Index should greatly facilitate and improve retrospective follow-up studies. However, it will be several years before the Index begins to approach maximum value. It is therefore suggested by the authors that consideration be given to extending the Index back in time to include deaths from 1 January 1974. Such an Index would have great immediate value even if limited by economic considerations to deaths of adult males.

The fourth suggestion is made to complement the National Death Index. It is that there be established registries of workers who sustain exposure to known or suspect hazardous substances. These registries would serve to maintain updated information on the degree of exposure and might record information on some potentially confounding variables such as cigarette smoking.

A fifth suggestion is simply the repetition of a request for a record-linkage system. The authors propose that linkage be limited to medical and occupational information. There are numerous advantages of such a limited system over a grandiose proposal that would include items pertinent to, for example, credit risk and law violations. The advantages relate to feasibility and popular support.

The final suggestion is that it would be appropriate to encourage research into ways by which the methodology of certain types of epidemiological studies could be improved. The study types we have in mind are the proportional mortality survey and the case-control-within-a-cohort study. Proportional mortality studies are frequently done in occupational settings and their methodology could be improved substantially. The case-control-within-a-cohort study has been little used in general. However, it appears uniquely well suited to the occupational setting (Liddel *et al.*, 1977). The development of its methodology might permit it to replace the less efficient retrospective follow-up studies that now typify epidemiological approaches to occupational hazards.

It is important to warn again that screening is not to be relied upon as a cancer control activity. For one thing screening is obviously not a primary preventive measure. More important, there is no real evidence that screening for occupationally-induced cancer brings about any benefit. There is some, albeit meagre, evidence to the contrary. This is not to say that screening should not be done, but it should supplement, and not substitute for, any other approach to cancer control. If screening is conducted it should probably only be done under circumstances where its effects can be evaluated. This recommendation is made because screening has the potential to do more harm than good (Cole and Morrison, 1978).

A review of six suggestions by the authors reveals that only one of them, that relating to a 'clearing house' for information on carcinogens, is uniquely addressed to the cancer problem. All of the others, just as those made previously (Cole and Goldman, 1975), have a much broader reference to all diseases of long induction period which may arise in the occupational setting. The broad applicability of these approaches to disease prevention should help bring about their implementation.

Acknowledgements

We are indebted to Dr John Waterbor for assistance in technical editing. The work of Dr Cole was supported by a grant (5 P30 CA13148) from the National Cancer Institute, Department of Health and Human Services, USA; and that of Dr Merletti by a Fellowship from the International Agency for Research on Cancer, Lyon, France.

References

Acheson, E.D. (1976). Nasal cancer in the furniture and boot and shoe manufacturing industries. *Preventive Medicine*, 5: 295-315
—— (1979). Record linkage and the identification of long-term environmental hazards. *Proc. Roy. Soc. London*, *205*, 165-78
—— Bennett, C., Gardner, M.J., and Winter, P.D. (1981a). Mesothelioma in a factory using amosite and chrysotile asbestos. *Lancet*, 2: 1403-6
—— Cowdell, R.H. and Rang, E.H. (1981b). Nasal cancer in England and Wales: An occupational survey. *British Journal of Industrial Medicine*, 38: 218-24
Aksoy, M. (1980). Different types of malignancies due to occupational exposure to benzene: A review of recent observations in Turkey. *Environmental Research*, 23: 181-90
—— and Erdem, S. (1978). Follow-up study on the mortality and the development of leukemia in 44 pancytopenic patients with chronic exposure to benzene. *Blood*, 52: 285-92
Albert, D.M. and Puliafito, C.A. (1977). Choroidal melanoma possible exposure to industrial toxins. *New England Journal of Medicine*, 296: 634-5
Albert, R.E., Pasternack, B.S., Shore, R.E., Lippman, M., Nelson, N. and Ferris, B. (1975). Mortality patterns among workers exposed to chloromethyl ethers – A preliminary report. *Environmental Health Perspectives*, 11: 209-14
Alderson, M.R. and Rattan, N.S. (1980). Mortality of workers on an isopropyl alcohol plant and two MEK dewaxing plants. *British Journal of Industrial Medicine*, 37: 85-9
Axelson, O. and Sundell, L. (1974). Herbicide exposure, mortality and tumour incidence. An epidemiological investigation on Swedish railroad workers. *Scandinavian Journal of Work-Environment-Health*, 11: 21-8
—— Sundell, L., Andersson, K., Edling, C., Hogstedt, C. and Kling, H. (1980). Herbicide exposure and tumour mortality. *Scandinavian Journal of Work-Environment-Health*, 6: 73-9
Bahn, A.K., Rosenwaike, I., Herrmann, N., Grover, P., Stellman, J. and O'Leary, K. (1976). Melanoma after exposure to PCB's. *New England Journal of Medicine*, 295: 450
—— Grover, P., Rosenwaike, I., O'Leary, K. and Stellman, J. (1977). PCB? and melanoma. *New England Journal of Medicine*, 296: 108
Baker, E.L., Goyer, R.A., Fowler, B.A., Khettry, V., Bernard, D.B., Adler, S. *et al.* (1980). Occupational lead exposure, nephropathy, and renal cancer. *American Journal of Industrial Medicine*, 1: 139-48
Barthel, E. (1976). High incidence of any lung cancer in persons with chronic professional exposure to pesticides in agriculture. *Zeitschrift fur Erkrankungen*

der Atmungsorgane mit Folia Bronchologica, 146: 266-74

Bertazzi, P.A., Zocchetti, C., Guercilena, S., Foglia, M.D., Pesatori, A. and Riboldi, L. (1981). Mortality study of male and female workers exposed to PCB's. *International Symposium on Prevention of Occupational Cancer*, International Labour Office, Geneva, Switzerland, pp. 242-8

Blair, A. (1980). Mortality among workers in the metal polishing and plating industry, 1951-1969. *Journal of Occupational Medicine*, 22: 158-62

—— Decoufle, P., and Grauman, D. (1979). Causes of death among laundry and dry cleaning workers. *American Journal of Public Health*, 69: 508-11

Brady, J., Liberatore, F., Harper, P., Greenwald, P., Burnett, W., Davies, J.N.P. *et al.* (1977). Angiosarcoma of the liver: An epidemiologic survey. *Journal of the National Cancer Institute*, 59: 1383-5

Bridbord, K., Decoufle, P., Fraumeni, J.F., Hoel, D.G., Hoover, R.N., Rall, D.P. *et al.* (1978). Estimates of the fraction of cancer in the United States related to occupational factors. *National Cancer Institute, National Institute of Environmental Health Sciences, and National Institute for Occupational Safety and Health*, Bethesda, Maryland, USA

Brown, D.P. and Jones, M. (1981). Mortality and industrial hygiene study of workers exposed to polychlorinated biphenyls. *Archives of Environmental Health*, 36: 120-9

Buell, G. (1975). Some biochemical aspects of cadmium toxicology. *Journal of Occupational Medicine*, 17: 189-95

Buffler, P.S., Wood, S., Eifler, C., Suarez, L. and Kilian, D.J. (1979). Mortality experience of workers in a vinyl chloride monomer production plant. *Journal of Occupational Medicine*, 21: 195-203

Case, R.A.M. and Pearson, J.T. (1954). Tumours of the urinary bladder in workmen engaged in the manufacture and use of certain dyestuff intermediates in the British chemical industry. II. Further considerations on the role of aniline and of the manufacture of auramine and magenta (Fuchsine) as possible causative agents. *British Journal of Industrial Medicine*, 11: 213-16

—— Hosker, M.E., McDonald, D.B. and Pearson, J.T. (1954). Tumours of the urinary bladder in workmen engaged in the manufacture and use of certain dyestuff intermediates in the British chemical industry. Part I. *British Journal of Industrial Medicine*, 11: 75-104

Clayson, D.W. (1976). Occupational bladder cancer. *Preventive Medicine*, 5: 228-44

Clemmesen, J. and Hjalgrim-Jensen, S. (1981). Cancer incidence among 5686 asbestos-cement workers followed from 1943 through 1976. *Ecotoxicology and Environmental Safety*, 5: 15-23

Cole, P., Hoover, R. and Friedell, G.H. (1972). Occupation and cancer of the lower urinary tract. *Cancer*, 29: 1250-60

—— and Goldman, M.B. (1975). Occupation. In: Fraumeni, J.F., Jr. (ed.), *Persons at High Risk of Cancer: An Approach to Cancer Etiology and Control*, Academic Press, New York, p. 167

—— and Morrison, A.S. (1978). Basic issues in cancer screening. In: Miller, A.B. (ed.), *Screening in Cancer*, UICC Technical Report Series 40, Geneva, pp. 7-39

—— and Merletti, F. (1980). Chemical agents and occupational cancer. *Journal of Environmental Pathology and Toxicology*, 3: 399-417

Cook, J.W., Hieger, I., Kennaway, E.L. and Mayneord, W.V. (1932). The production of cancer by pure hydrocarbons − Part 1. *Proceedings of the Royal Society*, Series B, 111, 455

Cook, R.R. (1981). Dioxin, chloracne and soft tissue sarcoma (letter). *Lancet*, 1: 618-19

Cooper, W.C. (1981). Mortality in employees of lead production facilities and lead battery plants, 1971-1975. In: *Environmental Lead*, Academic Press, New York, p. 111

Cox, J.E., Doll, R., Scott, W.A. and Smith, S. (1981). Mortality of nickel workers: Experience of men working with metallic nickel. *British Journal of Industrial Medicine*, 38: 235-9

Creagan, E.T., Hoover, R.N. and Fraumeni, J.F., Jr. (1974). Mortality from stomach cancer in coal mining regions. *Archives of Environmental Health*, 28: 28-30

Davies, J.M. (1978). Lung-cancer mortality of workers making chrome pigments. *Lancet*, 1: 384

Davies, J.M. (1979). Lung cancer mortality of workers in chromate pigment manufacture: an epidemiological survey. *Journal of the Oil and Colour Chemists' Association*, 62: 157-63

Decoufle, P. (1976). Cancer mortality among workers exposed to cutting-oil mist. *Annals of the New York Academy of Science*, 271: 94-101

DeFonso, R. and Kelton, S.C., Jr. (1976). Lung cancer following exposure to chloromethyl methyl ether. *Archives of Environmental Health*, 31: 125-30

Doll, R. (1962). Susceptibility to carcinogenesis at different ages. *Gerontologia Clinica*, 4: 211-21

—— (1976). The contribution of epidemiology to knowledge of cancer. *Revue d'Epidemiologie Médecine Sociale et Santé Publique*, 24(2): 107-21

—— Matthews, J.D. and Morgan, L.G. (1977). Cancers of the lung and nasal sinuses in nickel workers: A reassessment of the period of risk. *British Journal of Industrial Medicine*, 34: 102-5

—— and Peto, R. (1981). The causes of cancer: Quantitative estimates of avoidable risks of cancer in the United States today. *Journal of the National Cancer Institute*, 66: 1193-308

Druckrey, H., Preussmann, R., Nashed, N. and Ivankovic, S. (1966). Carcinogenic alkylicrende substanzen. 1. Dimethylsulfat, carcinogene wirkung an ratten und wahrscheinliche ursache von berufskrebs. *Zeitschrift für Krebsforschung und Klinische Onkologie*, 68: 103-11

Elmes, P.C. and Simpson, M.J.C. (1977). Insulation workers in Belfast. A further study of mortality due to asbestos exposure (1940-1975). *British Journal of Industrial Medicine*, 34: 174-80

Enterline, P.E. (1980). Importance of sequential exposure in the production of epichlorohydrin and isopropanol. Presented at the workshop on brain tumors in the chemical industry, New York, NY, Oct. 27-29

Environmental Protection Agency. (1978). Summary for reported incidents involving toxaphene. In: Human Effects Monitoring Branch, Benefits and Field Studies Division, Office of Pesticides Program, *Pesticide Incident Monitoring System – Report No. 113*

Ferber, K.H., Hill, W.J. and Cobb, D.A. (1976). An assessment of the effect of improved working conditions on bladder tumor incidence in a benzidine manufacturing facility. *American Industrial Hygiene Association Journal*, 37: 61-8

Figueroa, W.G., Raszkowski, R. and Weiss, W. (1973). Lung cancer in chloromethyl methyl ether workers. *New England Journal of Medicine*, 288: 1096-7

Fox, A.J. and Collier, P.F. (1977). Mortality experience of workers exposed to vinyl chloride monomer in the manufacture of polyvinyl chloride in Great Britain. *British Journal of Industrial Medicine*, 34: 1-10

Girard, R., Tolot, F., Martin, P. and Bourret, J. (1969). Hémopathies graves et exposition à des dérivés chlorés du benzène (à propos de 7 cas). *Journal de Médecine de Lyon*, 50: 771-3

Graham, S., Blanchet, M. and Rohrer, T. (1977). Cancer in asbestos-mining and other areas of Quebec. *Journal of the National Cancer Institute*, 59: 1139-45

Hayes, R.B., Lilienfeld, A.M. and Snell, L.M. (1979). Mortality in chromium chemical production workers: A prospective study. *International Journal of Epidemiology*, 8: 365-74

Hernberg, S. (1977). Incidence of cancer in population with exceptional exposure to metals. In: Hiatt, H.H., Watson, J.D. and Winsten, J.A. (eds.), *Origins of Human Cancer*, Book A, vol. 4, Cold Spring Harbor, Cold Spring Harbor Laboratory, pp. 147-57

Higginson, J. and Muir, C.S. (1979). Environmental carcinogenesis. Misconceptions and limitations to cancer control. *Journal of the National Cancer Institute*, 63: 1291-8

Hogstedt, C., Rohlén, O., Berndstsson, B.S., Axelson, O. and Ehrenberg, L. (1979). A cohort study of mortality and cancer incidence in ethylene oxide production workers. *British Journal of Industrial Medicine*, 36: 276-80

Hoover, R. and Cole, P. (1973). Temporal aspects of occupational bladder carcinogenesis. *New England Journal of Medicine*, 288: 1040-3

Hueper, W.C. (1966). *Occupational and Environmental Cancers of the Respiratory system*, Springer Verlag, New York

IARC Working Group on the Evaluation of the Carcinogenic Risk of Chemicals to Humans (1982). *Chemicals, Industrial Processes and Industries associated with Cancer in Humans*, IARC Monographs, vol. 1-29, Suppl. 4

Infante, P.F. and Epstein, S.S. (1977). Blood dyscrasias and childhood tumor and exposure to chlorinated hydrocarbon pesticides. In: Bingham, E. (ed.), *Proceedings, Conference on Women and the Workplace, June 17-19, 1976, Washington, DC*, Washington, DC, Society for Occupational and Environmental Health, pp. 51-73

——— and Newton, W.A., Jr. (1975). Prenatal chlordane exposure and neuroblastoma. *New England Journal of Medicine*, 293: 308

——— Wagoner, J.K. and Sprince, N.L. (1980). Mortality patterns from lung cancer and nonneoplastic respiratory disease among white males in the beryllium case registry. *Environmental Research*, 21: 35-43

Jedlicka, V.L., Hermanska, Z., Smida, I. and Kouba, A. (1958). Paramyeloblastic leukemia appearing simultaneously in two blood cousins after simultaneous contact with gammexane (Hexachlorcyclohexane). *Acta Medica Scandinavica*, 161: 447-51

Kang, H.K., Infante, P.F. and Carr, J.S. (1980). Occupational lead exposure and cancer. *Science*, 207: 935-6

Khachatryan, E.A. (1972). The occurrence of lung cancer among people working with chloroprene. *Problems in Oncology*, 18: 85

Kipling, M.D. and Waterhouse, J.A.H. (1967). Cadmium and prostatic carcinoma. *Lancet*, 1: 730-1

——— and Waldron, H.A. (1976). Polycyclic aromatic hydrocarbons in mineral oil, tar, and pitch, excluding petroleum pitch. *Preventive Medicine*, 5: 262-78

Kjeldsberg, C.R. and Ward, H.P. (1972). Leukemia in arsenic poisoning. *Annals of Internal Medicine*, 77: 935-7

Kjellström, T., Friberg, L. and Rahnster, B. (1979). Mortality and cancer morbidity among cadmium-exposed workers. *Environmental Health Perspectives*, 28: 199-204

Kolonel, L.N. (1976). Association of cadmium with renal cancer. *Cancer*, 37: 1782-7

Kyle, R.A. and Pease, G.L. (1965). Hematologic aspects of arsenic intoxication. *New England Journal of Medicine*, 273: 18-23

Lander, J.J., Stanley, R.J., Sumner, H.W., Boswell, D.C. and Aach, R.D. (1975). Angiosarcoma of the liver associated with Fowler's solution (potassium arsenite). *Gastroenterology*, 68: 1582-6

Langard, S. and Norseth, T. (1975). A cohort study of bronchial carcinomas in workers producing chromate pigments. *British Journal of Industrial Medicine*, 32: 62-5

—— Andersen, A. and Gylseth, B. (1980). Incidence of cancer among ferrochromium and ferrosilicon workers. *British Journal of Industrial Medicine*, 37: 114-20

Lemen, R.A., Lee, J.S., Wagoner, J.K. and Blejer, H.P. (1976). Cancer mortality among cadmium production workers. *Annals of the New York Academy of Sciences*, 271: 273-9

Liddel, F.D.K., McDonald, J.C. and Thomas, D.C. (1977). Methods of cohort analysis: Appraisal by application to asbestos mining. *Journal of the Royal Statistical Society*, Series A 140: 469-91

Lynch, J., Hanis, N.M., Bird, M.G., Murray, K.J. and Walsh, J.P. (1979). An association of upper respiratory cancer with exposure to diethyl sulfate. *Journal of Occupational Medicine*, 21: 333-41

Mabuchi, K., Lilienfeld, A.M. and Snell, L.M. (1979). Lung cancer among pesticide workers exposed to inorganic arsenicals. *Archives of Environmental Health*, 34: 312-20

Mancuso, T.F. (1980). Mortality study of beryllium industry workers' occupational lung cancer. *Environmental Research*, 21: 48-55

Marsh, G.M. (1980). Proportional mortality among chemical workers exposed to formaldehyde. Presented at the Third Chemical Industry Institute of Toxicology Conference on Toxicology: Formaldehyde Toxicity. Raleigh, North Carolina, USA

Matolo, N.M., Klauber, M.R., Gorishek, W.M. and Dixon, J.A. (1972). High incidence of gastric carcinoma in a coal mining region. *Cancer*, 29: 733-7

McMichael, A.J., Spirtas, R., Gamble, J.F. and Tousey, P.M. (1976). Mortality among rubber workers: Relationship to specific jobs. *Journal of Occupational Medicine*, 18: 178-85

Monson, R.R. (1978). Mortality and cancer morbidity among chemical workers with potential exposure to acrylonitrile. *Report to the B.F. Goodrich Company and to the United Rubber Workers*. Prepared for submission in the posthearing comment period to the OSHA Acrylonitrile Hearing, 22 April 1978

Morgan, R.W. and Shettigara, P.T. (1976). Occupational asbestos exposure, smoking, and laryngeal carcinoma. *Annals of the New York Academy of Science*, 271: 308-10

—— Claxton, K.W., Divine, B.J., Kaplan, S.D. and Harris, V.B. (1981). Mortality among ethylene oxide workers. *Journal of Occupational Medicine*, 23: 767-70

Newhouse, M.L. and Berry, G. (1976). Predictions of mortality from mesothelial tumours in asbestos factory workers. *British Journal of Industrial Medicine*, 33: 147-51

NIOSH (National Institute of Occupational Safety and Health) Current Intelligence Bulletin 18: Acrylonitrile (1977). Rockville, Maryland, DHEW (NIOSH) Publication

Norman, J.E. (1975). Lung cancer mortality in World War I veterans with mustard-gas injury: 1919-1965. *Journal of the National Cancer Institute*, 54: 311-17

O'Berg, M.T. (1980). Epidemiologic study of workers exposed to acrylonitrile. *Journal of Occupational Medicine*, 22: 245-52

Ott, M.G., Holder, B.B. and Gordon, H.L. (1974). Respiratory cancer and occupation exposure to arsenicals. *Archives of Environmental Health*, 29: 250-5

—— Townsend, J.C., Fishbeck, W.A. and Langner, R.A. (1978). Mortality among individuals occupationally exposed to benzene. *Archives of Environ-*

mental Health, 33: 3-10
—— Kolesar, R.C., Scharnweber, H.C., Schneider, E.J. and Venable, J.R. (1980). A mortality survey of employees engaged in the development or manufacture of styrene-based products. *Journal of Occupational Medicine*, 22: 445-60

Pasternack, B.S., Shore, R.E. and Albert, R.E. (1977). Occupational exposure to chloromethyl ethers. A retrospective cohort mortality study (1948-1972). *Journal of Occupational Medicine*, 19: 741-6

Pell, S. (1978). Mortality of workers exposed to chloroprene. *Journal of Occupational Medicine*, 20: 21-9

Peto, J., Doll, R., Howard, S.V., Kinlen, L.J. and Lewinsohn, H.C. (1977). A mortality study among workers in an English asbestos factory. *British Journal of Industrial Medicine*, 34: 169-73

Pott, P. (1775). *Chirurgical Observations*. Hawes, Clarke and Collings, London

Potts, C.L. (1965). Cadmium proteinuria – The health of battery workers exposed to cadmium oxide dust. *Annals of Occupational Hygiene*, 8: 55-61

Proceedings of the NIOSH Styrene-Butadiene Briefing (1976). Covington, Kentucky, Cincinnati, Ohio, Government Printing Office, DHEW

Redmond, C.K., Strobino, B.R. and Cypess, R.H. (1976). Cancer experience among coke by-product workers. *Annals of the New York Academy of Science*, 271: 102-15

Rehn, L. (1895). Blasengeschwulste bei Fuchsm-Arbeitern. *Archiv fur Klinische Chirurgie*, 50: 588-600

Roush, G.C., Meigs, J.W., Kelley, J., Flannery, J.T. and Burdo, H. (1980). Sino-nasal cancer and occupation: a case-control study. *American Journal of Epidemiology*, 111: 183

Royle, M. (1975). Toxicity of chromic acid in the chromium plating industry. *Environmental Research*, 10: 39-53

Sakabe, H., Matsushita, H. and Koshi, S. (1976). Cancer among benzoyl chloride manufacturing workers. *Annals of the New York Academy of Sciences*, 271: 67-70

—— and Fukuda, K. (1977). An updating report on cancer among benzoyl chloride manufacturing workers. *Industrial Health*, 15: 173-4

Selikoff, I.J., Hammond, E.C. and Churg, J. (1968). Asbestos exposure, smoking and neoplasia. *Journal of the American Medical Association*, 204: 106-12

Simler, M., Maurer, M. and Mandard, J.C. (1964). Cancer du foie sur cirrhose au tetrachlorure de carbone. *Strasbourg Médical*, 15: 910-18

Simonato, L. and Saracci, R. (1982). Occupational cancer. In: *ILO Encyclopaedia on Occupational Health*, Geneva

Smith, R.J. (1981). Beryllium report disputed by listed author. *Science*, 211: 556-7

Spirtas, R. and Kaminski, R. (1978). Angiosarcoma of the liver in vinyl chloride/polyvinyl chloride workers. 1977 update of the NIOSH register. *Journal of Occupational Medicine*, 20: 427-9

Stell, P.M. and McGill, T. (1973). Asbestos and laryngeal carcinoma. *Lancet*, 2: 416-7

—— and McGill, T. (1975). Exposure to asbestos and laryngeal carcinoma. *Journal of Laryngology and Otology*, 89: 513-17

Sunderman, F.W., Jr. (1976). A review of the carcinogenicities of nickel, chromium and arsenic compounds in man and animals. *Preventive Medicine*, 5: 279-4

Thiess, A.M., Frentzel-Beyme, R., Link, R. and Wild, H. (1980). Mortalitätsstudie bei chemiefacharbeitern verschiedener produktionsbetriebe mit exposition auch gegenuber acrylnitril. *Zentralblatt fur Arbeitsmedizin und Arbeits-*

schutz, 30: 259-67

Tokudome, S. and Kuratsune, M. (1976). A cohort study of mortality from cancer and other causes among workers at a metal refinery. *International Journal of Cancer*, 17: 310-17

Tracey, J.P. and Sherlock, P. (1968). Hepatoma following carbon tetrachloride poisoning. *New York State Journal of Medicine*, 68: 2202-4

US Bureau of the Census (1982). *Census of Population 1980*, US Government Printing Office, Washington, DC

Vigliani, E.C. (1976). Leukemia associated with benzene exposure. *Annals of the New York Academy of Sciences*, 271: 143-51

Wagoner, J.K., Infante, P.F. and Apfeldorf, R.B. (1980a). Toxicity of vinyl chloride and polyvinyl chloride as seen through epidemiologic observations. In: Vainio, H., Sorsa, M. and Hemminki, K. (eds.), *Occupational Cancer and Carcinogenesis*, Hemisphere Publishing Corporation, Part Four, p. 181

—— Infante, P.F. and Bayliss, D.L. (1980b). Beryllium: an etiologic agent in the induction of lung cancer, nonneoplastic respiratory disease, and heart disease among industrially exposed workers. *Environmental Research*, 21: 15-34

Wall, S. (1980). Survival and mortality pattern among Swedish smelter workers. *International Journal of Epidemiology*, 9: 73-87

Walrath, J. and Fraumeni, J.F., Jr. (1980). Proportionate mortality among New York embalmers. Presented at the Third Chemical Industry Institute of Toxicology Conference on Toxicology: Formaldehyde Toxicity. Raleigh, North Carolina, USA

Wang, H.H. and MacMahon, B. (1979a). Mortality of pesticide applicators. *Journal of Occupational Medicine*, 21: 741-4

—— and MacMahon, B. (1979b). Mortality of workers employed in the manufacture of chlordane and heptachlor. *Journal of Occupational Medicine*, 21: 745-8

Werner, J.B. and Carter, J.T. (1981). Mortality of United Kingdom acrylonitrile polymerisation workers. *British Journal of Industrial Medicine*, 38: 247-53

Wong, O. (1980). An epidemiologic mortality study of a cohort of chemical workers potentially exposed to formaldehyde, with a discussion on SMR and PMR. Presented at the Third Chemical Industry Institute of Toxicology Conference on Toxicology: Formaldehyde Toxicity, Raleigh, North Carolina, USA

Wynder, E.L. and Gori, G.B. (1977). Contribution of the environment to cancer incidence. An epidemiologic exercise. *Journal of the National Cancer Institute*, 58: 825-32

Zenz, C. (1978). Benzene — Attempts to establish a lower exposure standard in the United States. A review. *Scandinavian Journal of Work-Environment-Health*, 4: 103-13

16 INFECTIONS, INFESTATIONS AND CANCER

G.G. Caldwell

Introduction

Presumably human beings have been afflicted with cancer since ancient times because Hippocrates recorded symptoms (haemoptysis, cachexia) thought to be observed in cases of cancer (Clendening, 1960). However, infectious agents have been thought to cause cancer since Peyrille in 1773 coined the term 'virus' (Bainbridge, 1918), and Nepveu considered some then unknown microbe to be responsible (Triolo, 1974). Pasteur in 1881 also thought submicroscopic infectious agents could cause cancer (Roux, 1903). Moreover, most of the textbooks of the late nineteenth and early twentieth centuries outlined theories and described bacteria, protozoa, metazoa and yeasts, but few reported a possible relationship to the then recently identified filterable viruses (Bainbridge, 1918). Today microbial agents are still considered to have carcinogenic potential through either direct action (viruses) or some intermediate (bacteria, fungi and parasites), but convincing data are sparse.

Bacteria

Infection without mention of a specific organism was invoked as an aetiological mechanism or contributing factor towards cancer development, but few studies provide satisfactory evidence that this relationship is valid (Doll and Hill, 1952). Specific groups of bacteria have been weakly associated with cancer (Heath *et al.*, 1975) and although bacteria *per se* do not have clear-cut carcinogenic capability, they may occasionally be involved in the malignant transformation process as metabolic mediators or cofactors.

Fungi

The fungi are more complicated morphologically and metabolically than the bacteria and their relationship to cancer is also indirect. Cancer can result from potent carcinogenic compounds, the mycotoxins, which are produced by many fungal genuses (Aleksandrowicz and Smyk, 1973; Wogan, 1975). Mycotoxins (more than 46 are known) have been suggested to cause leukaemia, some sarcomas, and cancer of many organs (Wogan, 1975, 1976; Dvorachova, 1976; Nicolev *et al.*, 1978; Wray and O'Steen, 1975).

Mycotoxins were proposed as a cause of human liver cancer because the geographical distribution of primary liver cancer was similar to that of mycotoxin contaminated food (Bulatao-Jayme *et al.*, 1982). Various countries, particularly those in Africa, are known to have mycotoxins in foods, and the amounts correlate well with liver cancer incidence rates (Kew *et al.*, 1977; Linsell and Peers, 1977; Wogan, 1976). Although some reports link particular contaminated foods to liver cancer or to fungal exposure in the home (Aleksandrowicz and Smyk, 1973) or occupation (Dvorachova, 1976), not everyone agrees that mycotoxins *alone* are the responsible agent (Chandra, 1976).

Mycoplasma

Most researchers have abandoned the idea that mycoplasma are carcinogenic and consider them merely commensals and tissue culture contaminants (McAllister, 1973).

Protozoa

A parasitic aetiology for cancer was postulated almost a century ago and a protozoan purportedly was isolated in 1901 (Gaylord, 1901). Four protozoan genera have tentatively been associated with malignant disease: *Entamoeba* (Camacho, 1971), *Plasmodium*, *Toxoplasma* (Schuman *et al.*, 1967) and *Trichomonas* (Patten *et al.*, 1963). However, except for *Plasmodium*, which will be discussed with Epstein-Barr virus and Burkitt's lymphoma, the data are relatively sparse (Burton, 1982).

Trematodes

Infestation with *Schistosoma haematobium* (bilharzia) is common in many parts of the world and, concomitantly, so is bladder cancer, particularly in Egypt (Hashem, 1961; Schwartz, 1981). One study of

3,183 Egyptian autopsies found 83 per cent of 65 bladder cancer patients also with evidence of *S. haematobium* infestation (Hashem *et al.*, 1961).

Carcinomas resulting from bilharzia may be differentiated from nonbilharzial tumours because the patients are younger, more often male, and have a greater likelihood of having a squamous cell rather than a transitional cell carcinoma (Schwartz, 1981). Although the malignancies seem to be directly related to the schistosomes, it is also possible that the eggs, which can induce epithelial proliferation, cause the malignant change because cancer occurrence seems to be increased in patients with a heavy egg load (Kuntz *et al.*, 1972). Other investigators have emphasised chronic tissue irritation, an unknown toxin or a carcinogen such as nitrosamine (El-Merzabani *et al.*, 1979). Although some workers doubt any causal association, there is a considerable body of evidence which cannot be completely denied (Kakizoe *et al.*, 1979).

The data relating schistosomes to other malignancies are less clear. Hepatocellular carcinoma has been associated with *S. japonicum* and *S. mansoni* because of the geographical distribution of both diseases, but less often with *S. haematobium* (Edington, 1979). These organisms cannot be clearly incriminated as the cause of liver cancer because the data also suggest the possibility that aflatoxin or hepatitis B virus infection is involved. Furthermore, the scarce epidemiological data and few animal models have not clarified the situation and additional careful analytical studies are needed (Burton, 1982). Colorectal carcinoma associated with schistosomes was considered uncommon and when found, likely coincidental. However, 17 Chinese and Japanese reports indicated that *S. japonicum* may have promoted the development of colon cancer. The dysplastic changes found with schistosomal colitis is a reasonable basis for the potential malignant transformation (Chen *et al.*, 1981). One report indicated that 63.7 per cent of colorectal carcinoma patients were found to be infested with schistosomes (Chuang *et al.*, 1979). Even with such data one must remember that schistosome infestation (except for Puerto Rican immigrants) is relatively uncommon in the population of the United States of America (USA), in which colon cancer is common; however, other aetiologies may be involved (Young *et al.*, 1981; Gelfand, 1967).

The liver flukes *Clonorchis sinensis*, *Opisthorchis felineus* (*O. tenuicollis*) and *Opisthorchis viverrini* have been associated with primary liver and bile duct cancer for nearly a century. Hou (1956) reported 200 primary liver cancer cases from Hong Kong with 46 associated with clonorchiasis without cirrhosis, 67 per cent of these 46 were considered unimpeachable. Even so, in areas of greatest infestation, the Far East, only about 15 per cent of the cases are clearly associated with the parasite (Hou, 1956). The tumour seems to arise primarily from the epithelial cells of the bile ducts, causing cholangiocarcinoma, with ever increasing hyperplasia a likely precursor (Hou, 1956; Flavell, 1981). The parasites are occasionally seen elsewhere in the world, but infestation with *Clonorchis* and *Opisthorchis* species leading to cholangiocarcinoma is rare except in the Orient (Flavell, 1981). Although infestation with these parasites clearly increases the risk of cholangiocarcinoma in the Far East, other factors, such as a protein deficient diet, eating raw or undercooked fish, hepatitis B virus, other chemical carcinogens and the host's immunological status, may play a role (Hou, 1956; Flavell, 1981).

A number of other parasites have on occasion been suggested as playing some role in the development of cancer, but the data are simply too sparse and uncertain to be considered seriously (Sordillo *et al.*, 1981; Burton, 1982).

Viruses

Although viruses were considered as a cause of cancer in the late eighteenth century (Bainbridge, 1918; Triolo, 1974), most of the major discoveries were not made until the twentieth century. The likely reason for this snail's pace was the lack of effective laboratory tools and methods to deal with submicroscopic intracellular parasites (Gross, 1970). Ciuffo (Bayon, 1927) demonstrated the first human tumour virus (albeit benign) by transmission with cell-free filtrates of human wart tissue. Multiple studies on both deoxyribonucleic acid (DNA) and ribonucleic acid (RNA) viruses in animals followed and many of the viruses were shown to produce tumours in animals. Koch's postulates have been satisfied for many virus–host systems, showing that cancer may be produced directly by the action of viruses in animals (Gross, 1970). The effect of such viruses in humans is more controversial and good, well-studied examples are sparse (Heath *et al.*, 1975); however, some statistical and laboratory data, although not conclusive, are highly suggestive (Doll, 1978).

This animal virus research led to the development of better and ever more sophisticated cell culture and laboratory methods and equipment (Grace *et al.*, 1960; Hsiung, 1977). Concomitantly, scientists searching for a human tumour virus used these same techniques, but the search has been difficult because some of the more useful techniques available to the virologist, such as transplantation, or inoculation of cell-free filtrates into young of the same species, were not possible in humans. Of course, studies could be done by using cell culture and inoculation into other animals, especially primates. The development of elegant molecular biology techniques, along with the demonstration of reverse transcriptase (Baltimore, 1970), culminated in the identification of unique viral-like sequences in human leukaemias, lymphomas and sarcomas (Hehlmann *et al.*, 1973).

Finally, there are the rather crude and imprecise epidemiological and seroepidemiological studies undertaken in human populations, which provide the only *in vivo* evidence of tumour viruses in man (Lilienfeld *et al.*, 1967). Epidemiological studies of potentially infected human populations may be done by review of cancer clusters (Caldwell and Heath, 1976), follow-up of individuals who may inadvertently, through the use of poliomyelitis or yellow fever vaccines, have received viable animal tumour viruses (Heath *et al.*, 1975), and simple case-control serological studies when there is known contact with a potential oncogenic virus (Caldwell *et al.*, 1975).

All of these methods have been used and have resulted in the isolation, description and characterisation of viruses considered to have at least some oncogenic potential.

Deoxyribonucleic Acid Viruses

Viruses are divided into two groups based on the type of nucleic acid within the virion. Studies thus far favour the deoxyribonucleic acid (DNA) viruses, particularly the herpes viruses, as the more likely human tumour viruses. On the other hand ribonucleic acid (RNA) viruses seem more active in animals.

Epstein-Barr Virus (EBV). Burkitt (1958) published his paper about the recognition and observation of a sarcoma (Burkitt's Lymphoma, BL) he thought unique to African children. The considerable variation in the occurrence of this disease cut across tribal and geographical lines, seemed more related to topography and climate than to any other factor and suggested an environmental component in the cause of this tumour (Burkitt 1962, 1964; Burkitt and Wright, 1966). Furthermore, because the disease occurred primarily in children with only rare cases in adult immigrants, Burkitt espoused the idea that this environmental factor was an infectious agent.

Haddow (1964) pointed out that the age distribution of cases was consistent with the hypothesis of an immunity conferring infection and that the geographical distribution coincided quite readily with arthropod-borne virus diseases such as O'nyong-nyong or yellow fever. Suggestions that the virus might tend to cluster within these geographical and climatic boundaries provided further support to the idea of an infectious origin (Williams *et al.*, 1969), but clustering has been recently disputed (Brubaker *et al.*, 1973). Certainly, there is little evidence of clustering except for a specific time period (Williams *et al.*, 1978) and occasional reports in other countries (Richardson, 1977). Seasonal clustering in the latter half of the year has been mentioned (Williams *et al.*, 1974). These studies led to searches for BL in other countries and cases were reported from around the world (e.g. Cohen *et al.*, 1969; Ahlstrom *et al.*, 1967; Hoogstraten, 1967; Wright, 1966). Although these reports led to many studies, further elucidation of the aetiology depended primarily on the evaluation of the role of infectious agents, isolated from African BL cases (Dalldorf and Bergamini, 1964; Bell *et al.*, 1964; Gross, 1970). Electron-microscopic studies of lymphoid tissues from BL patients and cell cultures derived from patients revealed occasional herpes-like particles (Epstein and Achong, 1967) but not in direct preparations of tumour tissue (Bernard and Lambert, 1964).

Other groups developed cell cultures from BL patients and observed that the cells tended to be free-floating rather than adherent to the culture vessel (Burkitt and Wright, 1970; Rabson *et al.*, 1964). Electron-microscopy demonstrated the presence of virus-like particles in a small proportion of lymphoblasts (Epstein *et al.*, 1964). The virus observed in these cultures was approximately 110 to 115 mu in diameter, with immature particles approximately 75 mu in diameter in both nucleus and cytoplasm which was identified and confirmed as a herpes virus by electron-microscopy of purified virus (Epstein *et al.*, 1964).

Continued research on EBV demonstrated its presence in infected tissues (Henle, 1968) and its ability to transform normal cells, primarily B lymphocytes (Klein, 1975). Similar viruses were visualised or isolated from patients with lymphomas in New Guinea and occasionally elsewhere (Pope *et al.*, 1967).

After the isolation of EBV, serological tests were developed and immunofluorescence demonstrated that membrane fluorescence paralleled the presence of EBV as seen by electron-microscopy (Epstein and Achong, 1967).

A number of viral antigens were found by using these methods with the viral capsid antigen (VCA) being equated with the EBV (Ernberg and Klein, 1979). The VCA antibody present was found to be maternally derived in the first few months of life and then to drop to low levels until reinfection occurred. By three years of age nearly every child had developed antibodies, often without clinical illness (Biggar *et al.*, 1978). The antibody levels were maintained for at least 18 months (Kafuko *et al.*, 1972) in persons without BL but patients with BL had very high antibody titres (Henle *et al.*, 1969). Persons who maintained high VCA titres which showed no tendency to decrease with time seemed to be at higher risk for tumour development (Henle *et al.*, 1969).

The data from climatic and geographical studies, along with virus isolation and seroepidemiological data, suggested an arthropod vector (Burkitt, 1972). However, since EBV is ubiquitous and not all EBV infected persons develop BL, some other factor or factors must also be involved (Burkitt, 1969; 1972). Dalldorf *et al.* (1964) noted that malaria also occurred with this same geographical and climatic distribution. Burkitt (1969) suggested that EBV was interacting with a chronically immunosuppressed reticuloendothelial (R-E) system infected with malaria, and others agreed (Kafuko *et al.*, 1969). A large prospective study was begun, but this question has not been resolved, although malaria antibodies were no different in BL patients compared to controls (Feorino and Mathews, 1974). Serological studies in Ghana have shown no urban–rural differences in VCA titre, although malaria was more prevalent in the countryside (Biggar *et al.*, 1981). This suggests that malaria does not affect the immunological response to EBV and if this combination of infections is aetiologically related to BL, they exert their effects independently. Finally, such discussions may become moot if malaria control campaigns and antimalarial therapy lead to a decrease in malaria infection but current data are not yet clear on this point (Morrow *et al.*, 1976).

With the large amount of data available most persons accept EBV as an important aetiological factor in BL, even though cofactors (e.g. malaria, chromosome aberrations, immune deficiency) may also be required (Purtilo, 1980). In addition, serological studies indicate that neonatal or transplacental infection may also be a major factor (de-Thé, 1977).

Once viruses were isolated from BL and investigators developed serological techniques to detect antigen and antibody, many diseases were checked for possible association. In one such study EBV precipitating antibody was found in patients with nasopharyngeal carcinoma

(NPC) (Old *et al.*, 1966). NPC is common in Orientals, particularly the Chinese, but relatively rare in Europe and North America and of intermediate frequency in some African populations (Muir, 1972). Shortly after this first serological association herpes-type viral particles were found in cultured NPC cells from a Chinese patient (de-Thé *et al.*, 1969). Investigations conducting further serological studies comparing anti-EBV antibody titres in sera from patients with a variety of head and neck tumours found that 84 per cent of NPC patients had titres of at least 1:160 whereas non-ill controls and patients with other head and neck tumours had much lower (<1:36) titres (Henle *et al.*, 1970; Lin *et al.*, 1973). Other studies confirmed the EBV serological findings, but elevated titres to other herpes viruses were also found leading to the idea that such results might be fortuitous or simply due to reactivation of a latent virus infection(s) (Feorino *et al.*, 1972).

Elegant DNA homology studies demonstrated that EBV-DNA was present in cells of NPC (Nonoyama and Pagano, 1973) and specifically in the malignant epithelial cells but not in the lymphoid component of the neoplasm (Klein *et al.*, 1974). Later, EBV was isolated from malignant epithelial cells after passage through nude mice (Trumper *et al.*, 1977).

The EBV genome or high antibody titres have been associated with NPC everywhere the neoplasm has occurred (e.g. Henle *et al.*, 1970; Levine *et al.*, 1977). Although most investigators agree that EBV is causally related to NPC, the geographical distribution, familial occurrence and association with specific human leukocyte antigens (HLA) suggest additional genetic or environmental cofactors are also required (Joncas *et al.*, 1976; Gajwani *et al.*, 1980).

Other malignancies investigated for a possible association with EBV have shown that patients with Hodgkin's disease (HD) have elevated anti-EBV antibody titres (Henle and Henle, 1973; Evans and Comstock, 1981) but this may also be the result of reactivation (Lange *et al.*, 1978). Even though Epstein-Barr nuclear antigen (EBNA) has been found in cells in peripheral blood during acute infection, none was present in 17 patients with HD, although EBNA is usually found in cells bearing the EBV genome (Gergely *et al.*, 1979). Occasionally, isolates of EBV have been made from HD patients and immune complexes demonstrated in tissue (Sutherland *et al.*, 1978). Epidemiological data have shown that HD does occasionally occur in time-space clusters and interpersonal contact has been considered a risk factor but no viral transmission has been demonstrated (Heath *et al.*, 1975). Case-control studies and cohort studies of cancer, especially HD following infectious mononucleosis, have shown small relative risks (Rosdahl *et al.*, 1974; Carter *et al.*, 1977). The number of childhood contacts, sibship size and socioeconomic status have been suggested as major modifiers of EBV-HD risk by changing the age of infection to later years (Gutensohn and Cole, 1981). Finally, although it is possible, but not yet proven, that HD is caused by a virus, even EBV, there is no substantive evidence that the infection is directly transmitted from patient to patient (Gallo and Gelman, 1981).

Data relating EBV to leukaemia and non-Hodgkin's lymphomas only suggest a hypothesis for further research (Fraumeni, 1971). Similarly, the evidence for an oncogenic effect in immunosuppressed patients (Hanto *et al.*, 1982) needs to be expanded (Purtilo, 1980).

A variety of non-malignant diseases, notably infectious mono-nucleosis (IM), has been linked to EBV and thus may serve as a reservoir of virus. Patients with IM have been found to excrete EBV from the oral pharynx, and seroconversion has been shown following the clinical disease (Gerber *et al.*, 1972; Ginsberg *et al.*, 1977).

Considerable space has been devoted to this discussion of EBV because no other agent has been so clearly associated with human cancer. EBV has been shown to cause both productive (virus replication causing cell death) and nonproductive (virus genome present but latent) infections with the latter condition expressed under appropriate circumstances (cofactors) causing malignant transformation (Epstein and Achong, 1973). EBV has been uniquely associated with BL and NPC through presence of the viral genome and induced nuclear antigens and represents the best evidence to date of viral causation of any human cancer (zur Hausen, 1980).

Herpes Simplex Type 2 (HSV-2). Cancer of the cervix has long been associated with early menarche, early sexual relations, promiscuity, marital instability, smoking and possible lower socioeconomic conditions (Christopherson and Parker, 1965; Rotkin, 1967), and women without these attributes are relatively free from the disease (Cross *et al.*, 1968). Furthermore, the precise timing of the sexual activity factors with regard to first pregnancy or early adolescence may be important (Sebastian *et al.*, 1978). These characteristics suggested the possibility of venereal transmission of an infectious agent and a viral aetiology had been postulated, but serology for eleven different viruses, including herpes simplex virus (HSV), was negative (Lewis *et al.*, 1965). Later atypical cells were identified in cervical epithelium with acute HSV infection and the viral association was reconsidered (Naib *et al.*, 1966; Nahmias *et al.*, 1967).

Coincidental research on separation of HSV strains revealed at least two types of HSV (Plummer, 1964). Dowdle and co-workers (1967) tested 91 separate isolates from different anatomical sites and showed that all 42 genital strains were type-2 virus. The ability to distinguish between genital HSV (HSV-2) infections and resulting antibodies from those of other herpes viruses permitted more precise investigation of the HSV-2 cervical cancer relationships (Rawls *et al.*, 1968). Transmission of HSV-2 from active penile lesions was shown (Nahmias *et al.*, 1969) along with infection of the cervix uteri (Willcox, 1968).

Seroepidemiological studies found that women with carcinoma of the cervix had HSV-2 antibodies in their serum more often than control women (Rawls *et al.*, 1970; Nahmias *et al.*, 1970). Similar findings occurred in widely separated countries (Menczer *et al.*, 1975), which appeared to agree well with the epidemiological data about socio-economic status (Rawls *et al.*, 1970), promiscuity (Rawls *et al.*, 1968; 1976; Graham *et al.*, 1982), other venereal diseases (Royston *et al.*, 1970) and younger age at first intercourse (Rawls *et al.*, 1976). However, not every finding agreed, raising some doubt about a causal association (Adam *et al.*, 1971).

Cervical carcinoma has been considered a continuum of cervical epithelial abnormality, beginning with mild atypia progressing to dysplasia of varying severity, then carcinoma *in situ* and, finally, invasive carcinoma (Koss *et al.*, 1963). If this natural history is true, then HSV-2 infection and/or antibody ought to be present in those conditions as well and, in general, such is the case (Rawls *et al.*, 1968; 1970; Royston *et al.*, 1970; Nahmias *et al.*, 1970) but not every study agrees (Ozaki *et al.*, 1978). These studies suggested that the HSV-2 infection preceded the earliest atypia (Catalano and Johnson, 1971). Conversely, when considering patients with other cancers, usually there were not greater numbers of persons with HSV-2 antibodies compared with controls (Rawls *et al.*, 1969).

Another property suggesting a possible causal relationship to cancer of the cervix is the ability of HSV-2 to replicate in human cells (Birch *et al.*, 1976) and transform both mammalian and human cells in culture (Aurelian *et al.*, 1981). However, attempts to isolate HSV-2 from cervical cancer cells in culture have usually been unsuccessful except, rarely, from degenerating cervical carcinoma cells in culture (Aurelian *et al.*, 1971). HSV-2 has been demonstrated in exfoliated cells but not biopsies of carcinomas (Aurelian, 1972). Viral DNA has been found in the squamous cervical carcinoma cells on only one occasion (Frenkel *et al.*, 1972) but HSV-2 coded RNA and the presence of tumour associated antigens (Aurelian *et al.*, 1973) suggests an intimate and possibly causal relationship to squamous cervical carcinoma (McDougall *et al.*, 1980).

Because the male sex partner could logically serve as the transmitting vector in coitus, HSV-2 has also been suspected as a causal factor in male genital tract cancer (Rotkin, 1967; Rawls *et al.*, 1968; Nahmias *et al.*, 1969; Graham *et al.*, 1982). Carcinoma of the penis and cervix have been reported to occur together and incidence appears to be correlated although carcinoma of the penis occurs less frequently (Cartwright and Sinson, 1980). The number of cases of cervical cancer in second wives, following cervical cancer in the first wife, and household pairs of penile and cervical cancer are suggestive but few (Payan, 1979).

Prostatic carcinoma, on the other hand, has not been so clearly linked to cancer of the cervix except by the idea that the reservoir and vector for HSV-2 transmission is the male genitourinary tract (Centifano *et al.*, 1972). HSV-2 has been found in prostatic carcinoma cells (Centifano *et al.*, 1973) and one such strain transforms hamster cells in culture (Centifano *et al.*, 1975). Serological studies with different methods have been contradictory (Herbert *et al.*, 1976; Baker *et al.*, 1981) and no virus has been seen by electron-microscopy or isolated (Baker *et al.*, 1981). In 81 prostatic carcinoma patients tested by serum inhibition haemagglutination, 34 had HSV-2 antibodies, compared with 81 of 224 benign prostatic hypertrophy patients, a statistically significant difference ($P < 0.05$) (Baker *et al.*, 1981).

Even though HSV-2 has a strong association with cancer of the cervix (Graham *et al.*, 1982), and a weaker association with male genitourinary cancer (Baker *et al.*, 1981), the circumstantial nature of the evidence cannot conclusively prove causality and further research is needed.

Herpes Simplex Type-1 (HSV-1). HSV-1 appears to be the nongenital form of herpes simplex (Dowdle *et al.*, 1967) but either strain can occasionally infect the preferred site of the other (Chang, 1977; Young *et al.*, 1978). HSV-1 has been found to persist in a latent form in the host (Joncas, 1979); it can transform cells in culture (Rapp, 1981), but viral DNA has not been identified in lip carcinomas (Cassai *et al.*, 1981). HSV-1 has been associated with precancerous oral leukoplakia lesions and carcinomas of the head and neck, lip, skin and, questionably, carcinomas of the cervix and kidney where clear distinctions from HSV-2 were not made (Lehner *et al.*, 1975; Choi *et al.*, 1977; Gecht,

1980). Serological studies have been equivocal because nearly 100 per cent of most populations become HSV-1 antibody positive (Rawls and Campione-Piccardo, 1981). The association with cancer is still anecdotal (Cohen, 1981) and for vaccine development purposes is considered negative (Skinner *et al.*, 1980), but clearly additional work is needed.

Cytomegalovirus (CMV). CMV is ubiquitous in distribution and causes a variety of acute infections beginning during pregnancy (Kriel *et al.*, 1970) and continuing into adulthood (Stern, 1968). Acute infection, particularly a mononucleosis syndrome, may occur following transfusions (Stevens *et al.*, 1970) or organ transplantation (Chatterjee *et al.*, 1978).

CMV was known to be a latent infection associated with venereal disease (Chretien *et al.*, 1977) and appeared to fit the known epidemiological patterns of carcinoma of the cervix nearly as well as HSV-2. It could transform cells in culture (Geder *et al.*, 1976) and CMV antibodies were found in sera of 61 per cent of women with cervical atypia compared to 42 per cent with other cervical disorders and 33 per cent in healthy women (Pasca *et al.*, 1975). This virus has also been isolated from cervical cancer biopsy specimens in cell culture (Melnick *et al.*, 1978). These findings of course do not prove causality but they do raise the possibility that CMV, as well as HSV-2, may be aetiologically related to cervical cancer either separately or synergistically (Melnick *et al.*, 1978; Pacas *et al.*, 1975).

CMV has been found in semen (Lang *et al.*, 1974) and is also associated with prostatic carcinoma, although the data are few (Mandel and Schuman, 1980). One prostatic cancer isolate transforms cells in culture (Geder *et al.*, 1976; 1977) and serum from the patient reacted to CMV specific membrane and intracellular antigens (Geder *et al.*, 1977). Sanford *et al.* (1977) demonstrated that sera of prostatic cancer patients had detectable antibodies (> 1: 4) to CMV more often (95 per cent) than control sera (61 per cent and 78 per cent). However, considerable research, particularly on seroepidemiology and the long-term culture of normal and neoplastic prostate cells (Ziegel *et al.*, 1977), is needed.

Another cancer associated with CMV is Kaposi's sarcoma (KS), a rare cutaneous cancer found primarily in older African males (Giraldo and Beth, 1980). KS also occurs in a disseminated visceral form that is more common in children (Safai and Good, 1981) and has a poorer prognosis (Bhana *et al.*, 1970). The visceral form also occurs after organ transplantation (Myers *et al.*, 1974) with immunosuppression (Master *et al.*, 1970), or other primary malignancies (Safai *et al.*, 1980). KS cells have been cultured and herpes-like viruses resembling CMV identified (Glaser *et al.*, 1977). Serological studies of European and African KS patients compared with healthy matched controls showed that all European KS sera contained CMV-neutralising antibodies, but the African patient sera did not react to CMV and none of the groups had an association to EBV, HSV-1 or HSV-2 (Giraldo *et al.*, 1975). Sera from American KS patients were all positive for CMV antibody (Giraldo *et al.*, 1978). CMV is a persistent virus (Joncas, 1979) and early antigens and DNA have been found in biopsies from KS (Giraldo *et al.*, 1980), although CMV-RNA has not (zur Hausen *et al.*, 1974).

American KS occurred more often in older males of Italian or Jewish lineage (Digiovanna and Safai, 1981); however, now KS has been reported in increasing numbers in younger but homosexual males (Durack, 1981). The lesions in this group are often generalised and death has occurred more rapidly than usual (Centers for Disease Control, 1981). In addition these men suffered other opportunistic infections (Durack, 1981), and like other active homosexual males, frequent sexually transmitted diseases (Darrow *et al.*, 1981). Similarly CMV is more prevalent among homosexuals than among heterosexual men (Drew *et al.*, 1981) and CMV antibody or virus isolation was positive in all homosexual males with KS tested (Hymes *et al.*, 1981). The circumstances are of concern because the number of known cases continues to increase and because cases reported from Europe may represent transmission to another continent of a more virulent CMV or other agent (Thomsen *et al.*, 1981). However, as intriguing as this idea is, the unusual circumstances may be the result not of CMV but of either multiple drug/chemical abuse, secondary immunosuppression, unusual sexual practices or some combination of these with CMV or another unknown agent (Durack, 1981). Extensive studies are under way and should clarify the situation in the near future.

Neuroblastoma, Wilms' tumour, Hodgkin's disease and adenocarcinoma of the colon have been tentatively linked to CMV, but confirmatory data are needed for the understanding of CMV in these cancers (Wertheim and Voute, 1976; Huang and Roche, 1978).

Other Human Herpes Viruses.   Although most other human herpes viruses are viewed as secondary invaders (Wright and Winer, 1961), children born to mothers who suffered chickenpox during pregnancy appear to be at higher risk for cancer (Adelstein and Donovan, 1972). However, serological studies did not confirm this finding (Gahrton *et al.*, 1971).

Pox Viruses. The pox viruses include a number of DNA viruses which produce benign and malignant tumours in rabbits and squirrels and molluscum contagiosum, a benign human tumour (Andrewes *et al.*, 1977). Yaba, a simian pox virus, causes benign histocytomas in monkeys (Niven *et al.*, 1961) and similar histocytomas occurred after accidental inoculation in humans (Griesemer and Manning, 1973). Although considered oncogenic, these viruses appear to be unimportant to human cancer (Bierwolf, 1980).

Adenoviruses. Adenoviruses, in spite of their wide distribution, do not cause serious disease and are not oncogenic in humans, but they are very useful in experimental molecular virology (Flint, 1980).

Papovaviruses. This group of DNA viruses is divided into two genera: papillomavirus and polyomavirus. The first group includes the mostly benign wart viruses of animals and humans. The second group includes the more clearly oncogenic polyomavirus of the mouse, simian vacuolating agent (SV40) and two potentially oncogenic human viruses – BK and JC (Andrewes *et al.*, 1977; Howley, 1980).

The human wart (papilloma) virus was identified more than 70 years ago, but the full range of infection was not appreciated until recent years (zur Hausen and Gissman, 1980). Papillomaviruses have been found in tissue from human laryngeal papillomas, vulvar condylomata acuminata, skin warts, epidermodysplasia verruciformis (zur Hausen, 1980b; Orth *et al.*, 1978). With proper genetic and/or environmental cofactors some benign papillomas may become malignant but confirmatory work is needed, and particular interest should be given to oesophageal papillomatosis (zur Hausen, 1980b).

The polyomavirus group includes two animal viruses of great importance to molecular biology and to the understanding of viral oncology (Andrewes *et al.*, 1977; Howley, 1980). The original polyomavirus is unrelated to human disease, but SV40 is still suspect.

SV40 is oncogenic in hamsters and can transform human cells in culture (Eddy, 1964; Jones *et al.*, 1976). Transformation occurs most readily in cells from persons with genetic susceptibility and may define a group with unusually high risk for cancer (Miller and Todaro, 1969; Blattner *et al.*, 1978). The primary importance of SV40 is the potential for cancer development in persons who received poliomyelitis vaccine made in monkey kidney cell cultures which were naturally contaminated with SV40 (Fraumeni *et al.*, 1963; Eddy, 1964). Fortunately, no evidence has been reported to date showing an increase in cancer occurrence in recipients of such vaccines (Fraumeni *et al.*, 1963; 1970) even though production of humoral antibodies and isolation of SV40 from stools clearly showed inoculation (Eddy, 1964; Gerber, 1967). Continuous follow-up of these persons has been done until recently (Fraumeni *et al.*, 1970) and the proposed termination of active follow-up is controversial (Mortimer, 1982).

Papova-like viruses were identified in electron-microscope studies of progressive multifocal leukoencephalopathy (PML) (ZuRhein and Chou, 1965) and human brain tumours (Bastian, 1971). Similar viruses were isolated from PML patients (Padgett *et al.*, 1971) and a renal transplant patient (Gardner *et al.*, 1971). One of the viruses from a PML patient was SV40; the other PML virus (JCV) and the renal isolate (BKV) were antigenically distinct but related new viruses (Padgett, 1980; Howley, 1980). The viruses were shown to transform cells in culture and induce virus specific tumour antigens which show strong antigenic relationships (Padgett, 1980). Both JCV and BKV will produce a variety of tumours in animals, including primates, with a predilection for the central nervous system (London *et al.*, 1978; Padgett, 1980).

Seroepidemiological studies and surveys show that both viruses are ubiquitous but independent in their distribution and 70-90 per cent of adults are seropositive; infection most likely occurs in childhood (Mantyjarvi, 1979) with BKV transmitted transplacentally (Taguchi *et al.*, 1975). Serological studies and viral isolation have shown these viruses to be associated with a number of illnesses, including some cancers, especially when the host is immunosuppressed as in renal transplantation (Flower *et al.*, 1977; Mantyjarvi, 1979; Padgett, 1980). Although DNA hybridisation studies have been done with cancerous and normal tissues, the results are equivocal and even though these viruses have oncogenic potential their relationship to human cancer is unproven (Padgett, 1980).

Hepatitis B Virus (HBV). In 1965 an antigen was found, Australian antigen (Au), in the serum of an Australian aborigine with leukaemia (Blumberg *et al.*, 1965). Au was found most often in patients with leukaemia, Down's syndrome or multiple transfusions and was then shown to be identical with Prince's serum hepatitis antigen (Blumberg *et al.*, 1968; 1970; Prince, 1968). The Au antigen appeared to be infectious or was associated closely with the infectious agent which ultimately was accepted as HBV (Blumberg *et al.*, 1968). At first the antigen was thought to be unrelated to chronic liver disease or primary liver cancer (PLC) (Blumberg *et al.*, 1968), but occasional workers reported finding HBV antigen or antibody in PLC patients (Prince *et al.*, 1970). PLC was much more common in Africa and Asia but HBV antigenaemia was shown to occur in association with PLC in Africa (Kew *et al.*, 1974; 1979), Asia (Ohbayashi *et al.*, 1972), Europe (Trichopoulos *et al.*, 1978) and America (Omata *et al.*, 1979).

Family members are also likely to be either HBV antigen or antibody positive, especially mothers (Ohbayashi *et al.*, 1972). In fact, the mothers of HBV positive PLC patients were more likely to be positive to HBV surface antigens than mothers of controls (Larouze *et al.*, 1976). Consequently, PLC may be the result of transplacental infection by HBV or very early in life leading to chronic infection possibly with viraemia, chronic hepatitis, cirrhosis and ultimately PLC (Ohbayashi *et al.*, 1972; Larouze *et al.*, 1976).

In countries where this association has not been confirmed, researchers hypothesised that other required environmental cofactors, e.g. aflatoxin, genetic susceptibility, parasites or chemicals such as alcohol, were missing (Omata *et al.*, 1979; Falk, 1982). HBV appears to be able to cause PLC in normal livers or livers affected with non-alcoholic related disease (Omata *et al.*, 1979). Patients with PLC attributed to other environmental factors have not been tested in any great depth for HBV antigens or antibodies.

Laboratory data, such as isolation of HBV or identification of HBV antigens in PLC cells, have lagged behind the seroepidemiological studies (Gerber and Thung, 1979). However, such research including tissue culture and DNA hybridisation studies are under way (zur Hausen, 1980b). Animal models are also being developed (Lapis, 1978).

Finally, although many questions remain, most researchers feel that HBV is causally related to PLC (Lefkowitch, 1981). Furthermore, the development and planned use of the new HBV vaccine may reduce the incidence of HBV-caused hepatitis and, secondarily, PLC — a prevention strategy of worldwide importance (Blumberg and London, 1981).

Ribonucleic Acid (RNA) Virus

The RNA viruses have been associated with viral oncology from the earliest discoveries and have been detected in nearly all animal species (Andrewes *et al.*, 1977; Gross, 1970). Although investigators have made many important virological and oncological discoveries studying these viruses, the scope of this chapter does not permit a complete review and the early historical work has been admirably collected by Gross (1970).

Although humans are infected from time to time with RNA viruses, the data relating such exposure to carcinogenesis are scant and unconvincing (Heath *et al.*, 1975). In addition, humans also have contact with a large number of domestic and wild animals, potential vectors of RNA tumour viruses indigenous to their species, but again there is little evidence to suggest transmission to humans, although the potential exists (Heath *et al.*, 1975).

Contact with animals bearing endogenous leukaemia viruses has been studied and although tumours are occasionally seen in owner and animal (Viola, 1968), such reports are relatively uncommon. A review of cancer clusters reported to the Cancer Branch, Centers for Disease Control, between 1963 and 1976 showed that 32 of 73 clusters involved some animal contact. However, in only two cases were the tumours the same cell type in patient and pet – a lymphosarcoma and, the other, a Burkitt's-like tumour. Furthermore, of 563 leukaemia patients interviewed in Kansas City between 1966 and 1970, 278 had no animal contact and only 18 reported contact with ill (not necessarily with cancer) animals.

Cattle are closely associated with human endeavours, and considerable attention has been given to the association between cancer in cattle and humans following the premier studies by Bendixen (1963), Olson (1974), and Heath and Caldwell (1981). These studies were reinforced by the isolation of bovine leukosis virus (BLV) (Miller *et al.*, 1969), the finding of virus particles in milk (Ferrer *et al.*, 1981), and replication in, but not transformation of, human cells in culture (Diglio and Ferrer, 1976). Horizontal transmission among cattle and across species barriers to sheep and, questionably, to chimpanzees has been shown experimentally (Olson *et al.*, 1972; McClure *et al.*, 1974).

Epidemiological studies in humans have shown increases in the incidence of leukaemia or lymphoma in some circumstances but often without evidence of transmission of BLV from cattle to humans (Donham *et al.*, 1980). Furthermore, scientists conducting seroepidemiological studies have not found BLV antibodies in human sera (Caldwell, 1979). Although recent studies (Donham *et al.*, 1980; Ferrer *et al.*, 1981) have increased interest in BLV, the equivocal epidemiological data, negative serological data, loss of infectivity from pasteurisation (Baumgartener *et al.*, 1976) and negative molecular hybridisation studies (Kettman *et al.*, 1978) seem to eliminate this organism as a human pathogen.

Cats, unlike cattle, do not provide food for humans, but close personal contact as household pets provides ample opportunity for transmission of the feline oncornaviruses. The feline leukaemia virus (FeLV), first isolated by Jarrett (1964) from a leukaemic cat, has been found to be transmitted horizontally, particularly from mother to kitten (Hardy *et al.*, 1977). The virus has been found in nasal secretions, saliva and urine, as well as in cultured cells from respiratory, gastrointestinal and urinary systems, which may be the outflow pathway for transmission (Jarrett, 1975). Furthermore, FeLV can replicate and transform a variety of cells from different animal species, including man (Azocar and Essex, 1979; Hardy, 1980).

Epidemiological studies — some completed before FeLV was isolated when serological testing could not have been done — have shown an increased risk for leukaemia compared with controls (Bross *et al.*, 1972). Other studies involving various data sets and analytical techniques could not confirm an increased risk for malignancies in humans associated with cats (Hardy, 1980). Studies in veterinarians who are likely to have contact with FeLV positive cats have been reviewed by Hardy (1980). Of the five studies reported two were negative, two found increases in the frequency of haematopoietic malignancies and one an excess number of melanoma cases, but no clear conclusion that FeLV was responsible could be drawn.

Seroepidemiological studies and attempts to detect FeLV antigens, also reviewed by Hardy (1980), produced conflicting results with nearly every available method. Although the evidence at present is equivocal, whether or not FeLV ever plays a role in human carcinogenesis remains unresolved and further research is needed to solve the public health dilemma.

Oncornaviruses or retroviruses have been sought in human disease, and although some isolates were made, most of these viruses have not been established as causes of human malignancies (Kaplan *et al.*, 1979) while others clearly have been disproven (Shigematsu *et al.*, 1971). In addition the problem was further confounded because similar particles were found in normal tissues of many species, including humans (Panem *et al.*, 1975) and human sera lyses oncornaviruses (Welsh *et al.*, 1975). Still, such agents may have cancer-causing roles not yet understood (Levy, 1977).

Recently, a retrovirus was isolated from a patient with cutaneous T-cell lymphoma (Poiesz *et al.*, 1980), another from a patient with

T-cell leukaemia (Sézary syndrome), and though similar, both were distinct from other retroviruses by immunological studies, nucleic acid hybridisation and characterisation of the reverse transcriptase (Poiesz *et al.*, 1981; Kalyanaraman *et al.*, 1981). This new virus, human T-cell leukaemia-lymphoma virus (HTLV), transforms T-cells, is not an endogenous virus and thus far has been found only in cells from patients with T-cell neoplasia (Gallo *et al.*, 1981). Natural antibodies have been demonstrated in patients from which HTLV was isolated and are probably the first demonstration of natural retrovirus antibodies in humans (Kalyanaraman *et al.*, 1981).

During this same period Japanese scientists identified an area of high T-cell leukaemia/lymphoma prevalence on Kyushu (Tajima *et al.*, 1981). Sera from Japanese patients with adult T-cell leukaemia were found to have high anti-HTLV antibody titres, not found in normal donors (Kalyanaraman *et al.*, 1982). More recently, antibody against structural protein of HTLV was found in six West Indies blacks with adult T-cell lymphoma (Catovsky *et al.*, 1982). These later findings suggest that HTLV may be a widely distributed true human retrovirus. Nonetheless, this idea awaits confirmation.

Even if this virus, too, proves to be a disappointment and not a human retrovirus, the effort has not been wasted. Much has been learned about the viral aetiology of cancer in both animals and humans (Hehlman and Erfle, 1980; Karpas, 1982). This work led to the formation of the proto-pro-virus and oncogene theories of carcinogenesis, which, although not totally accepted, do have considerable supporting experimental data (Todaro *et al.*, 1980). Reverse transcriptase was discovered and opened new areas of understanding (Baltimore, 1970; Temin and Mizutani, 1970), including the identification of retroviral genes in human nucleic acid (Favera *et al.*, 1982). Nevertheless, the exact role of the retroviruses in human cancer is still unclear.

Case Clustering in Cancer

Because of the variable geographical distribution of cancer and interest in the infectious aetiology, unusual aggregations were suspected of representing transmission of an infectious agent. Occasional reports had been written, but not until Heath and Hasterlik (1963) reported on the extensive studies of a cluster of childhood leukaemia cases in Niles, Illinois, was much emphasis given to these events. Following this report, studies of such unusual occurrences were begun for many cancers, but emphasis was mainly on leukaemia, lymphoma and Hodgkin's disease (HD) (Caldwell and Heath, 1976; Smith, 1982).

In response to the many anecdotal reports, a number of analytical methods were devised to test for temporal, geographical or time-space clustering (Barton *et al.*, 1965; Larsen *et al.*, 1973; Mantel, 1967; Pike and Smith, 1974). However, nearly all methods required arbitrary specification of time and space parameters which could seriously affect the results (Smith, 1982). Such methods do not account for transmission elsewhere than in the individual's usual area of residence (Smith, 1982), individual susceptibility or a variable latent period (Pike and Smith, 1968).

Another type of clustering has been postulated, particularly with regard to HD, i.e. interpersonal contact through 'acquaintance networks'. Although George *et al.* (1965) reported close contact among unrelated HD cases, Vianna and associates (1971) developed the hypothesis that interpersonal contact as a means of transmission was more important than previously considered. Follow-up studies seemed to confirm their ideas (Vianna *et al.*, 1972; Vianna and Polan, 1973). However, many investigators remain cautious and sceptical, particularly because of the difficulty of defining adequate comparison populations for statistical evaluation (Smith and Pike, 1976; Smith, 1978). Even so, the hypothesis remains intriguing and cannot be dismissed out of hand.

The overall assessment is that clustering does occasionally occur, but chance is often an equally likely reason for any cluster, whether or not an infectious agent is involved (Alderson, 1980). However, this does not mean that infection in some form cannot be involved, and further improvement in epidemiological and virological techniques is needed before the issue of infection as a cause of cancer can be completely settled (Heath, 1982).

References

Adam, E., Levy, A.H., Rawls, W.E. and Melnick, J.L. (1971). Seroepidemiologic studies of herpesvirus type 2 and carcinoma of the cervix I. Case-control matching. *Journal of the National Cancer Institute*, 47: 941-51

Adelstein, A.M. and Donovan, J.W. (1972). Malignant disease in children whose mothers had chickenpox, mumps or rubella in pregnancy. *British Medical Journal*, 4: 629-31

Ahlstrom, C.G., Andersson, T., Klein, G. and Akerman, M. (1967). Malignant lymphoma of 'Burkitt type' in Sweden. *International Journal of Cancer*, 2: 583-5

Alderson, M. (1980). The epidemiology of leukemia. *Advances in Cancer Research*, 31: 1-76

Aleksandrowicz, J. and Smyk, B. (1973). The association of neoplastic diseases and mycotoxins in the environment. *Texas Reports on Biology and Medicine*, 31: 715-26

Andrewes, C., Pereira, H.G. and Wudy, P. (1977). *Viruses of Vertebrates*, Baillière Tindall, London, pp. 274-92, 356-89

Aurelian, L. (1972). Possible role of *Herpesvirus hominis*, type 2, in human cervical cancer. *Federation Proceedings; Federation of American Societies for Experimental Biology*, 31: 1651-2

—— Strandberg, J.D., Melendez, L.V. and Johnson, L.A. (1971). Herpesvirus type 2 isolated from cervical cancer cells grown in tissue culture. *Science*, 174: 704-7

—— Schumann, B. and Marcus, R.R. (1973). Antibody to HSV-2 induced tumor specific antigens in sera from patients with cervical carcinoma. *Science*, 181: 161-4

—— Kessler, I.I., Rosenshein, N.D. and Barbour, G. (1981). Viruses and gynecologic cancers: herpesvirus protein (ICP 10/AG-4), a cervical tumor antigen that fulfills the criteria for a marker of carcinogenicity. *Cancer*, 48: 455-71

Azocar, J. and Essex, M. (1979). Susceptibility of human cell lines to feline leukemia virus and feline sarcoma virus. *Journal of the National Cancer Institute*, 63: 1179-84

Bainbridge, W.S. (1918). *The Cancer Problem*, Macmillan, New York, Introduction, p. 106

Baker, L.H., Mebust, W.K., Chin, T.D.Y., Chapman, A.L., Hinthorn, D. and Towle, D. (1981). The relationship of herpesvirus to carcinoma of the prostate. *Journal of Urology*, 125: 370-4

Baltimore, D. (1970). RNA-dependent DNA polymerase in virions of RNA tumour viruses. *Nature*, 226: 1209-11

Barton, D.E., David, F.N. and Merrington, M. (1965). A criterion for testing contagion in time and space. *Annals of Human Genetics*, 29: 97-102

Bastian, F.O. (1971). Papova-like virus particles in human brain tumor. *Laboratory Investigation*, 33: 169-75

Baumgartener, L., Olson, C. and Onuma, M. (1976). Effect of pasteurization and heat treatment on bovine leukemia virus. *Journal of the American Veterinary Medical Association*, 169: 1189-91

Bayon, H.P. (1927). Parasites and malignant proliferations. *Journal of Tropical Medicine and Hygiene*, 39: 73-80

Bell, T.M., Massie, A., Ross, M.G.R. and Williams, M.C. (1964). Isolation of a reovirus from a case of Burkitt's lymphoma. *British Medical Journal*, 1: 1212-13

Bendixen, H.J. (1963). Preventive measures in cattle leukemia leukosis enzootica bovis. *Annals of the New York Academy of Sciences*, 108: 1241-67

Bernard, W. and Lambert, D. (1964). Ultrastructure des tumeurs de Burkitt de l'enfant africain. In: *Symposium on Lymphatic Tumours in Africa (Paris, 1963)*, Karger, Basel and New York, pp. 270-84

Bhana, D., Templeton, A.C., Master S.P. and Kyalwazi, S.K. (1970). Kaposi sarcoma of lymph nodes. *British Journal of Cancer*, 24: 464-70

Bierwolf, D. (1980). Viruses and cancer risk in man. *Archiv fur Geschwulstforschung*, 50: 506-14

Biggar, R.J., Henle, G., Bocker, J., Lennett, E.T., Fleisher, G., Henle, W. (1978). Primary Epstein-Barr virus infections in African infants, II. Clinical and serological observations during seroconversion. *International Journal of Cancer*,

22: 244-50
—— Gardiner, C., Lennett, E.T., Collins, W.E., Nkrumah, F.K. and Henle, W. (1981). Malaria, sex and place of residence as factors in antibody response to Epstein-Barr virus in Ghana, West Africa. *Lancet*, 2: 115-18
Birch, J., Fink, C.G., Skinner, G.R.B., Thomas, G.H. and Jordan, J.A. (1976). Replication of type 2 herpes simplex viruses in human endocervical tissue in organ culture. *British Journal of Experimental Pathology*, 57: 460-71
Blattner, W.A., Lubiniecki, A.S., Mulvihill, J.J., Lalley, P. and Fraumeni, J.F., Jr. (1978). Genetics of SV40 T-antigen expression: studies of twins, heritable syndromes and cancer families. *International Journal of Cancer*, 22: 231-8
Blumberg, B.S., Alter, H.J. and Visnich, S.A. (1965). A 'new' antigen in leukemia sera. *Journal of the American Medical Association*, 191: 541-6
—— Sutnich, A.I. and London, W.T. (1968). Hepatitis and leukemia: their relation to Australian antigen. *Bulletin of the New York Academy of Medicine*, 44: 1566-86
—— Sutnich, A.I., London, W.T. and Millman, I. (1970). Australia antigen and hepatitis. *New England Journal of Medicine*, 283: 349-54
—— and London, W.T. (1981). Hepatitis B virus and the prevention of primary hepatocellular carcinoma. *New England Journal of Medicine*, 304: 782-4
Bross, I.D.J., Bertell, R. and Gibson, R. (1972). Pets and adult leukemia. *American Journal of Public Health*, 62: 1520-32
Brubaker, G., Geser, A. and Pike, M.C. (1973). Burkitt's lymphoma in the North Mara district of Tanzania, 1964-1970 − failure to find evidence of space-time clustering in a high risk isolated area. *British Journal of Cancer*, 28: 469-72
Bulatao-Jayme, J., Almero, E.M., Castro, C.A., Jardeleza, T.R. and Salamat, L.A. (1982). A case-control dietary study of primary liver cancer risk from aflatoxin exposure. *International Journal of Epidemiology*, 11: 112-19
Burkitt, D. (1958). A sarcoma involving the jaws in African children. *British Journal of Surgery*, 46: 218-23
—— (1962). A 'tumour safari' in East and Central Africa. *British Journal of Cancer*, 16: 379-86
—— (1964). A children's cancer dependent on climatic factors. *Nature*, 194: 232-4
—— (1969). Etiology of Burkitt's lymphoma − an alternative hypothesis to a vectored virus. *Journal of the National Cancer Institute*, 42: 19-28
—— (1972). The trail to a virus − a review. In: Biggs, P.M., de-Thé, G. and Payne, L.H. (eds.), *Oncogenesis and Herpesviruses*, International Agency for Research on Cancer, Lyon, pp. 345-8
—— and Wright, D. (1966). Geographic and tribal distribution of the African lymphoma in Uganda. *British Medical Journal*, 1: 569-73
—— and Wright, D.H. (1970). *Burkitt's Lymphoma*. Churchill Livingstone, Edinburgh, London
Burton, G.J. (1982). Parasites. In: Schottenfeld, D. and Fraumeni, J.F., Jr. (eds.), *Cancer, Epidemiology and Prevention*, Saunders Company, Philadelphia, pp. 408-18
Caldwell, G.G. (1979). Bovine leukemia virus. Public Health Serologic Studies. In: *Proceedings of Bovine Leukosis Symposium*, US Department of Agriculture, Washington, pp. 143-59
—— Baumgartener, L., Carter, C., Cotter, S., Currier, R., Essex, M. *et al.* (1975). Serologic testing in man for evidence of antibodies to feline leukemia virus and bovine leukemia virus. *Bibliotheca Haematologica*, 43: 238-41
—— and Heath, C.W., Jr. (1976). Case clustering in cancer. *Southern Medical Journal*, 69: 1598-602
Camacho, E. (1971). Amebic granuloma and its relationship to cancer of the

cecum. *Diseases of the Colon and Rectum*, 14: 12-16

Carter, C.D., Brown, T.M., Jr., Herbert, J.T. and Heath, C.W., Jr. (1977). Cancer incidence following infectious mononucleosis. *American Journal of Epidemiology*, 105: 30-6

Cartwright, R.A. and Sinson, J.D. (1980). Carcinoma of penis and cervix. *Lancet*, 1: 97

Cassai, E., Rotola, A., Meneguzzi, G., Milanesi, G., Garsia, S., Remotti, G. *et al.* (1981a). Herpes simplex virus and human cancer. I. Relationship between human cervical tumours and herpes simplex type 2. *European Journal of Cancer*, 17: 685-93

——— Rotola, A., DiLuca, D., Manservigi, R., Meneguzzi, G., Milanesi, G. (1981b). Herpes simplex virus and human cancer. II. Search for relationship between labial tumours and herpes simplex type 1. *European Journal of Cancer*, 17: 695-702

Catalano, L.W., Jr. and Johnson, L.D. (1971). Herpesvirus antibody and carcinoma in situ of the cervix. *Journal of the American Medical Association*, 217: 447-50

Catovsky, D., Greaves, M.F., Rose, M., Galton, D.A.G., Goolden, A.W.G., McCluskey, D.R. *et al.* (1982). Adult T-cell lymphoma-leukaemia in blacks from the West Indies. *Lancet*, 1: 639-43

Centers for Disease Control (1981). Kaposi's sarcoma and pneumocystis pneumonia among homosexual men − New York City and California. *Morbidity and Mortality Weekly Report*, 30: 305-8

Centifano, Y.M., Drylie, D.M., Deardourff, S.L. and Kaufman, H.E. (1972). Herpesvirus type 2 in the male genitourinary tract. *Science*, 178: 318-9

——— Kaufman, H.E., Zam, Z.S., Drylie, D.M. and Deardourff, S.L. (1973). Herpesvirus particles in prostatic carcinoma cells. *Journal of Virology*, 2: 1608-11

——— Zam, Z.S., Kaufman, H.E. and Drylie, D.M. (1975). *In vitro* transformation of hamster cells by herpes simplex virus type 2 from human prostatic cancer cells. *Cancer Research*, 35: 1880-6

Chandra, R.K. (1976). Nutrition as a critical determinant in susceptibility to infection. *World Review of Nutrition and Dietetics*, 25: 166-88

Chang, T.W. (1977). Genital herpes and type 1 *Herpesvirus hominis*. *Journal of the American Medical Association*, 238: 155

Chatterjee, S.N., Fiala, M., Weiner, J., Stewart, J.A., Stacey, B. and Warner, N. (1978). Primary cytomegalovirus and opportunistic infections. Incidence in renal transplant recipients. *Journal of the American Medical Association*, 240: 2446-9

Chen, M.C., Chang, P.Y., Chuang, C.Y., Chen, Y.J., Wang, F.P., Tang, Y.C. and Chou, S.C. (1981). Colorectal cancer and schistosomiasis. *Lancet*, 1: 971-3

Choi, N.W., Cheltigara, P.T., Abu-Zeid, H.A.H. and Nelson, N.A. (1977). Herpesvirus infection and cervical anaplasia − a seroepidemiological study. *International Journal of Cancer*, 19: 167-71

Chretien, J.H., McGinniss, C.G. and Muller, A. (1977). Venereal causes of cytomegalovirus mononucleosis. *Journal of the American Medical Association*, 238: 1644-5

Christopherson, W.M. and Parker, J.E. (1965). Relation of cervical cancer to early marriage and childbearing. *New England Journal of Medicine*, 273: 235-9

Chuang, C.Y., Chang, P.Y., Hu, J.C. and Chen, M.C. (1979). Pathomorphologic observations on the relation between late schistosomiasis colitis and colorectal cancer. *Chinese Medical Journal*, 92: 113-18

Clendening, L. (1960). *Source Book of Medical History*. Dover Publications, New York, Introduction, pp. 17, 39

Cohen, M.H., Bennett, J.M., Berard, C.W., Ziegler, J.L., Vogel, C.L., Sheagren, J.N. *et al.* (1969). Burkitt's tumor in the United States. *Cancer*, 23: 1259-72

Cohen, W.L. (1981). Herpes simplex virus and oral cancer. *Dental Hygiene*, 55: 31-9

Cross, H.E., Kennell, E.E. and Lilienfeld, A.M. (1968). Cancer of the cervix in an Amish population. *Cancer*, 21: 102-8

Dalldorf, G. and Bergamini, F. (1964). Unidentified, filterable agents isolated from African children with malignant lymphomas. *Proceedings of the National Academy of Sciences of the United States of America*, 51: 263-5

―――― Linsell, C.A., Barnhart, F.E. and Martyn, R. (1964). An epidemiological approach to the lymphomas of African children and Burkitt's sarcoma of the jaws. *Perspectives in Biology and Medicine*, 7: 435-49

Darrow, W.W., Barrett, D., Jay, K. and Young, A. (1981). The gay report on sexually transmitted diseases. *American Journal of Public Health*, 71: 1004-11

de-Thé, G. (1977). Is Burkitt's lymphoma related to perinatal infection by Epstein-Barr virus? *Lancet*, 1: 335-7

―――― Ambrosioni, J.C., Ho, H.C. and Kwan, H.C. (1969). Lymphoblastoid transformation and presence of herpes type viral particles in a Chinese naso-pharyngeal tumor cultured *in vitro*. *Nature*, 221: 770-1

Digiovanna, J.J. and Safai, B. (1981). Kaposi's sarcoma. Retrospective study of 90 cases with particular emphasis on the familial occurrence, ethnic back-ground and prevalence of other diseases. *American Journal of Medicine*, 71: 779-83

Diglio, C.A. and Ferrer, J.F. (1976). Induction of syncytia by the bovine C-type leukemia virus. *Cancer Research*, 36: 1056-67

Doll, R. (1978). An epidemiological perspective of the biology of cancer. *Cancer Research*, 38: 3573-83

―――― and Hill, A.B. (1952). A study of the aetiology of carcinoma of the lung. *British Medical Journal*, 2: 1271-86

Donham, K.J., Berg, J.W. and Sawin, R.S. (1980). Epidemiologic relationships of the bovine population and human leukemia in Iowa. *American Journal of Epidemiology*, 112: 80-92

Dowdle, W.R., Nahmias, A.J., Harwell, R.W. and Pauls, F.P. (1967). Association of antigenic type of *Herpesvirus hominis* with site of viral recovery. *Journal of Immunology*, 99: 974-80

Drew, W.L., Mentz, L., Miner, R.C., Sands, M. and Ketterer, B. (1981). Prevalence of cytomegalovirus isolation in homosexual men. *Journal of Infectious Diseases*, 143: 188-92

Durack, T. (1981). Opportunistic infections and Kaposi's sarcoma in homosexual men. *New England Journal of Medicine*, 305: 1465-7

Dvořáčhová, I. (1976). Aflatoxin inhalation and alveolar cell carcinoma. *British Medical Journal*, 1: 691

Eddy, B.E. (1964). Simian virus 40 (SV-40): An oncogenic virus. *Progress in Experimental Tumor Research*, 4: 1-26

Edington, G.M. (1979). Schistosomiasis and primary liver cell carcinoma. *Trans-actions of the Royal Society of Tropical Medicine and Hygiene*, 73: 351

El-Merzabani, M.M., El-Aaser, A.A. and Zakhary, N.I. (1979). A study on the aetiological factors of bilharzial bladder cancer in Egypt. 1-Nitrosamines and their precursors in urine. *European Journal of Cancer*, 15: 287-91

Epstein, M.A., Achong, B.G. and Barr, Y.M. (1964). Virus particles in cultured lymphoblasts from Burkitt's lymphoma. *Lancet*, 1: 702-3

―――― and Achong, B.G. (1967). Formal discussion: immunologic relationships of the herpes-like EB virus of cultured Burkitt lymphoblasts. *Cancer Research*, 27: 2489-93

—— and Achong, B.G. (1973). Various forms of Epstein-Barr virus infection in man: established facts and a general concept. *Lancet*, 2: 836-9

Ernberg, I. and Klein, G. (1979). EB virus-induced antigens. In: Epstein, M.A. and Achong, B.G. (eds.), *The Epstein-Barr Virus*, Springer Verlag, Berlin-Heidelberg-New York, pp. 39-60

Evans, A.S. and Comstock, G.W. (1981). Presence of elevated antibody titres to Epstein-Barr virus before Hodgkin's disease. *Lancet*, 1: 1183-6

Favera, R.D., Gelmann, E.P., Gallo, R.C. and Wong-Staal, F. (1983). A human gene homologous to the transforming gene (*V-Sis*) of simian sarcoma virus. *Nature* (in press)

Feorino, P., Palmer, E.L. and Martin, M.L. (1972). Incidence of herpesvirus antibody among leukemic and nasopharyngeal carcinoma patients. *Proceedings of the Society for Experimental Biology and Medicine*, 139: 913-15

—— and Mathews, H.M. (1974). Malaria antibody levels in patients with Burkitt's lymphoma. *American Journal of Tropical Medicine and Hygiene*, 23: 574-6

Ferrer, J.F., Kenyon, S.J. and Gupta, P. (1981). Milk of dairy cows frequently contains a leukemogenic virus. *Science*, 213: 1014-6

Flavell, D.J. (1981). Liver-fluke infection as an aetiological factor in bile-duct carcinoma of man. *Transactions of the Royal Society of Tropical Medicine and Hygiene*, 75: 814-24

Flint, S.J. (1980). Molecular biology of adenoviruses. In: Klein, G. (ed.), *Viral Oncology*, Raven Press, New York, pp. 603-63

Flower, A.J.E., Banatvala, J.E. and Chrystie, I.L. (1977). BK antibody and virus-specific IgM response in renal transplant recipients, patients with malignant disease, and healthy people. *British Medical Journal*, 2: 202-23

Fraumeni, J.F., Jr. (1971). Infectious mononucleosis and acute leukemia. *Journal of the American Medical Association*, 215: 1159

—— Ederer, F. and Miller, R.W. (1963). An evaluation of the carcinogenicity of simian virus 40 in man. *Journal of the American Medical Association*, 185: 713-8

—— Stark, C.R., Gold, E. and Lepou, M.L. (1970). Simian virus 40 in polio vaccine: Followup of newborn recipients. *Science*, 167: 59-60

Frenkel, N., Roizman, B., Cassai, E. and Nahmias, A.J. (1972). DNA fragment of herpes simplex 2 and its transcription in human cervical cancer tissue. *Proceedings of the National Academy of Sciences of the United States of America*, 69: 3784-9

Gahrton, G., Wahren, B. and Killander, D. (1971). Epstein-Barr and other herpesvirus antibodies in children with acute leukemia. *International Journal of Cancer*, 8: 242-9

Gajwani, B.S., Devereaux, J.M. and Beg, J.A. (1980). Familial clustering of nasopharyngeal carcinoma. *Cancer*, 46: 2325-7

Gallo, R.C. and Gelman, E.P. (1981). In search of a Hodgkin's disease virus. *New England Journal of Medicine*, 304: 169-70

—— Poiesz, B.J. and Ruscetti, F.W. (1981). Regulation of human T-cell proliferation: T-cell growth factor and isolation of a new class of type-C retroviruses from human T-cells. *Haematologie und Bluttransfusion*, 26: 502-14

Gardner, M.B. (1971). Current information on feline and canine cancers and relationship or lack of relationship to human cancer. *Journal of the National Cancer Institute*, 46: 281-90

Gardner, S.D., Field, A.M., Coleman, D.V. and Hulme, B. (1971). New human papovavirus (BK) isolated from urine after renal transplantation. *Lancet*, 1: 1253-7

Gaylord, H.R. (1901). The protozoan of cancer. *American Journal of the Medical*

Sciences, 121: 503-39

Gecht, M.L. (1980). Carcinoma at the site of herpes simplex infection. *Journal of the American Medical Association*, 244: 1675

Geder, L., Lausch, R., O'Neill, F. and Rapp, F. (1976). Oncogenic transformation of human embryo lung cells by human cytomegalovirus. *Science*, 192: 1134-6

——— Sanford, E.J., Rohner, T.J. and Rapp, F. (1977). Cytomegalovirus and cancer of the prostate: *in vitro* transformation of human cells. *Cancer Treatment Reports*, 61: 139-46

Gelfand, M. (1967). *A Clinical Study of Intestinal Bilharziasis (Schistosoma mansoni) in Africa*, Arnold, London

George, W.K., Miller, M. and George, W.D., Jr. (1965). Hodgkin's disease in roommates. *Journal of the American College Health Association*, 13: 399-402

Gerber, M.A. and Thung, S.A. (1979). The localization of hepatitis viruses in tissues. *International Review of Experimental Pathology*, 20: 49-76

Gerber, P. (1967). Patterns of antibodies to SV40 in children following last booster with inactivated poliomyelitis vaccines. *Proceedings of the Society for Experimental Biology and Medicine*, 125: 1284-7

——— Nonoyama, M., Lucas, S., Perlin, E. and Goldstein, L.I. (1972). Oral excretion of Epstein-Barr virus by healthy subjects with infectious mononucleosis. *Lancet*, 2: 988-9

Gergely, L., Czeglidy, J., Vaczi, L., Scalka, A. and Berenyi, E. (1979). Cells containing Epstein-Barr nuclear antigen (EBNA) in peripheral blood. *Acta Microbiologica Academiae Scientiarum Hungaricae*, 26: 41-5

Ginsberg, C.M., Henle, W., Henle, G. and Horwitz, C.A. (1977). Infectious mononucleosis in children. Evaluation of Epstein-Barr virus-specific serological data. *Journal of the American Medical Association*, 237: 781-5

Giraldo, G., Beth, E., Kourilsky, F.M., Henle, W., Henle, G., Miké, V. *et al.* (1975). Antibody patterns to herpesviruses in Kaposi's sarcoma: serological association of European Kaposi's sarcoma with cytomegalovirus. *International Journal of Cancer*, 15: 839-48

——— Beth, E., Henle, W., Henle, G., Miké, V., Safai, B. *et al.* (1978). Antibody patterns to herpesviruses in Kaposi's sarcoma. II. Serological association of American Kaposi's sarcoma with cytomegalovirus. *International Journal of Cancer*, 22: 126-31

——— and Beth, E. (1980). The relationship of cytomegalovirus to certain human cancers, particularly to Kaposi's sarcoma. In: Giraldo, G. and Beth, E. (eds.), *The Role of Viruses in Human Cancer VI*, Elsevier, New York, pp. 57-73

——— Beth, E. and Huang, E.S. (1980). Kaposi's sarcoma and its relationship to cytomegalovirus (CMV). III. CMV DNA and CMV early antigens in Kaposi's sarcoma. *International Journal of Cancer*, 26: 23-9

Glaser, R., Geder, L., St. Jeor, S., Michelson-Fiske, S. and Haguenau, F. (1977). Partial characterization of a herpes-type virus (K9V) derived from Kaposi's sarcoma. *Journal of the National Cancer Institute*, 59: 55-60

Grace, J.T., Mirand, E.A. and Mount, D.T. (1960). Relationship of viruses to malignant disease. Part II. Oncogenic properties of cell-free filtrates of human tumors. *Archives of Internal Medicine*, 105: 482-91

Graham, S., Rawls, W., Swanson, M. and McCurtis, J. (1982). Sex partners and herpes simplex virus type 2 in the epidemiology of cancer of the cervix. *American Journal of Epidemiology*, 115: 729-35

Griesemer, R.A. and Manning, J.S. (1973). Simian tumor viruses. In: Hellman, A., Oxmon, M.N. and Pallach, R. (eds.), *Biohazards in Biological Research*, Cold Spring Harbor Laboratory, New York, pp. 179-90

Gross, L. (1970). *Oncogenic Viruses*, 2nd edn., Pergamon Press, New York

Gutensohn, N. and Cole, P. (1981). Childhood social environment and Hodgkin's

disease. *New England Journal of Medicine*, 304: 135-40
Haddow, A.J. (1964). Age incidence in Burkitt's lymphoma syndrome. *East African Medical Journal*, 41: 1-6
Hanto, D.W., Frizzera, G., Gajl-Peczalska, K.J., Sakamoto, K., Purtilo, D.T., Balfour, H.H. *et al.* (1982). Epstein-Barr virus-induced B-cell lymphoma after renal transplantation. *New England Journal of Medicine*, 306: 913-18
Hardy, W.D., Jr. (1980). The virology, immunology and epidemiology of the feline leukemia virus. In: Hardy, W.D., Jr., Essex, M. and McClelland, A.J. (eds.), *Feline Leukemia Virus*, Elsevier, New York, Amsterdam, Oxford, pp. 33-78
—— McClelland, A.J., MacEwen, E.G., Hess, P.W., Hayes, A.A. and Zuckerman, E.E. (1977). The epidemiology of the feline leukemia virus (FeLV). *Cancer*, 39: 1850-5
Hashem, M. (1961). The aetiology and pathogenesis of the bilharzial bladder cancer. *Journal of the Egyptian Medical Association*, 44: 857-966
—— Azki, S.A. and Hussein, M. (1961). The bilharzial bladder cancer and its relation to schistosomiasis. A statistical study. *Journal of the Egyptian Medical Association*, 44: 579-97
Heath, C.W., Jr. (1982). The leukemias. In: Schottenfeld, D. and Fraumeni, J., Jr. (eds.), *Cancer Epidemiology and Prevention*, Saunders Company, Philadelphia, pp. 728-38
—— and Hasterlik, R.J. (1963). Leukemia among children in a suburban community. *American Journal of Medicine*, 34: 796-812
—— Caldwell, G.G. and Feorino, P.C. (1975). Viruses and other microbes in persons at high risk of cancer. An approach to cancer etiology and control. In: Fraumeni, J.R., Jr. (ed.), *Proceedings of a Conference*, Key Biscayne, Florida, December 10-12. Academic Press, New York, pp. 241-64
—— and Caldwell, G.G. (1981). Malignancies of cattle which may relate to public health. In: Steel, J.H. and Beran, G.W. (eds.), *Handbook Series in Zoonoses*, vol. II, CRC Press, Boca Raton, Florida, p. 443
Hehlman, R., Baxt, W., Hyle, D. and Spiegelman, S. (1973). Molecular evidence for a viral etiology of human leukemias, lymphomas, and sarcomas. *American Journal of Clinical Pathology*, 60: 65-79
—— and Erfle, V. (1980). Human leukemia viruses? RNA tumor viruses, human malignancies, and concepts of viral carcinogenesis. *Blut*, 41: 247-56
Henle, G., Henle, W., Clifford, P., Diehl, V., Kafuko, G.W., Kirya, B.G. *et al.* (1969). Antibodies to Epstein-Barr virus in Burkitt's lymphoma and control groups. *Journal of the National Cancer Institute*, 43: 1147-57
Henle, W. (1968). Evidence for viruses in acute leukemia and Burkitt's tumor. *Cancer*, 21: 580-6
—— Henle, G., Ho, H.C., Burtin, P., Cachin, Y., Clifford, P. *et al.* (1970). Antibodies to Epstein-Barr virus in nasopharyngeal carcinoma, other head and neck neoplasms, and control groups. *Journal of the National Cancer Institute*, 44: 225-31
—— and Henle, G. (1973). Epstein-Barr Virus (EBV)-related serology in Hodgkin's disease. *National Cancer Institute Monographs*, 36: 79-84
Herbert, J.T., Birkhoff, J.D., Feorino, P.M. and Caldwell, G.G. (1976). Herpes simplex virus type 2 and cancer of the prostate. *Journal of Urology*, 116: 611-12
Hoogstraten, J. (1967). Observations on Burkitt's tumour in central and northern Canada. *International Journal of Cancer*, 2: 566-75
Hou, P.C. (1956). The relationship between primary carcinoma of the liver and infestation with *Clonorchis sinensis*. *Journal of Pathology and Bacteriology*, 72: 239-46

Howley, P.M. (1980). Molecular biology of SV40 and the human polyomaviruses BK and JC. In: Klein, G. (ed.), *Viral Oncology*, Raven Press, New York, pp. 489-550

Hsiung, G.D. (1977). Laboratory diagnosis of viral infections: general principles and recent developments. *Mount Sinai Journal of Medicine*, New York, 44: 1-26

Huang, E.S. and Roche, J.K. (1978). Cytomegalovirus DNA and adenocarcinoma of the colon. *Lancet*, 1: 957-60

Hymes, K.B., Cheung, T., Greene, J.B., Prose, N.S., Marcus, A., Ballard, H. *et al.* (1981). Kaposi's sarcoma in homosexual men – a report of eight cases. *Lancet*, 2: 598-600

Jarrett, W.F.H. (1975). Cat leukemia and its viruses. *Advances in Veterinary Science and Comparative Medicine*, 19: 165-91

—— Crawford, E.M., Martin, W.B. and Davie, F. (1964). Leukaemia in the cat. A virus-like particle associated with leukaemia (lymphosarcoma). *Nature*, 202: 567-8

Joncas, J.H. (1979). Persistence, reactivation, and cell transformation by human herpesviruses: herpes simplex 1, 2 (HSV-1, HSV-2), cytomegalovirus (CMV), varicella-zoster (VZV), Epstein-Barr virus (EBV). *Canadian Journal of Microbiology*, 25: 254-60

—— Rioux, E., Wastiaue, J.P., Leyritz, M., Robellard, L. and Menezes, J. (1976). Nasopharyngeal carcinoma and Burkitt's lymphoma in a Canadian family. I. HLA typing, EBV antibodies and serum immunoglobulins. *Canadian Medical Association Journal*, 115: 858-68

Jones, R.E., Sanford, E.J., Rohner, T.J., Fr., Rapp, F. (1976). In vitro viral transformation of human prostatic carcinoma. *Journal of Urology*, 115: 82-5

Kafuko, G.W., Baingana, N., Knight, E.M. and Tibemanya, J. (1969). Association of Burkitt's tumour and holoendemic malaria in West Nile District, Uganda: Malaria as a possible aetiologic factor. *East African Medical Journal*, 46: 414-16

—— Henderson, B.E., Kirya, B.G., Manube, G.M.R., Tukei, P.M, Day, N.E. *et al.* (1972). Epstein-Barr virus antibody levels in children from the West Nile District of Uganda. Report of a field study. *Lancet*, 1: 706-9

Kakizoe, T., Wang, T., Eng, V.W.S., Furrer, R., Dion, P., Bruce, W.R. *et al.* (1979). Volatile N-nitrosamines in the urine of normal donor and of bladder cancer patients. *Cancer Research*, 39: 829-32

Kalyanaraman, V.S., Sarngadharan, M.G., Poiesz, B., Ruscetti, F.W. and Gallo, R.C. (1981). Immunological properties of a type C retrovirus isolated from cultured human T-lymphoma cells and comparison to other mammalian retroviruses. *Journal of Virology*, 38: 906-15

—— Sarngadharan, M.G., Nakao, Y., Ito, Y., Aoki, T. and Gallo, R.C. (1982). Natural antibodies to the structural core protein (p 24) of the human T-cell leukemia (lymphoma) retrovirus found in sera of leukemia patients in Japan. *Proceedings of the National Academy of Sciences of the United States of America*, Mar 79(5): 1653-7

Kaplan, H.S., Goodenow, R.S., Gartner, S. and Bieber, M.M. (1979). Biology and virology of the human malignant lymphomas. *Cancer*, 43: 1-24

Karpas, A. (1982). Viruses and leukemia. *American Scientist*, 70: 277-85

Kettman, R., Burny, A., Cleuter, Y., Ghysdael, J. and Mammerickx, M. (1978). Distribution of bovine leukemia virus proviral DNA sequences in tissues of animals with enzootic bovine leucosis. *Leukemia Research*, 2: 23-32

Kew, M.C., Geddes, E.W., Macnab, G.M. and Bersohn, I. (1974). Hepatitis-B antigen and cirrhosis in Bantu patients with primary liver cancer. *Cancer*, 34: 539-41

———— Marcus, R. and Geddes, E.W. (1977). Some characteristics of Mozambican Shangaans with primary hepatocellular cancer. *South African Medical Journal*, 51: 306-9

———— Desmyter, J., Bradburne, A.F. and Macnab, G.M. (1979). Hepatitis B virus infection in Southern African blacks with hepatocellular cancer. *Journal of the National Cancer Institute*, 62: 517-620

Klein, G. (1975). The Epstein-Barr virus and neoplasia. *New England Journal of Medicine*, 293: 1353-7

———— Giovanella, B.C., Lendahl, T., Fialkow, P.J., Singh, S. and Stehlin, J.S. (1974). Direct evidence for the presence of Epstein-Barr virus DNA and nuclear antigen in epithelial cells from patients with poorly differentiated carcinoma of the nasopharynx. *Proceedings of the National Academy of Sciences of the United States of America*, 71: 4737-41

Koss, L.G., Stewart, F.W., Foote, F.W., Jordan, M.J., Bader, G.M. and Day, E. (1963). Some histological aspects of behavior of epidermoid carcinoma *in situ* and related lesions of the uterine cervix. A long-term prospective study. *Cancer*, 16: 1160-211

Kriel, R., Gates, G.A., Wulff, H., Powell, N., Poland, J. and Chin, T.B.Y. (1970). Cytomegalovirus isolations associated with pregnancy wastage. *American Journal of Obstetrics and Gynecology*, 1067: 885-92

Kuntz, R.E., Cheever, A.W. and Myers, B.J. (1972). Proliferative epithelial lesions of the urinary bladder of non-human primates infected with *Schistosoma haematobium. Journal of the National Cancer Institute*, 48: 223-35

Lang, D.J., Kummer, J.F. and Hartley, D.P. (1974). Cytomegalovirus in semen: persistence and demonstration in extracellular fluids. *New England Journal of Medicine*, 291: 121-3

Lange, B., Arbeter, A., Hewetson, J. and Henle, W. (1978). Longitudinal study of Epstein-Barr virus antibody titers and excretion in pediatric patients with Hodgkin's disease. *International Journal of Cancer*, 22: 521-7

Lapis, K. (1978). Pathogenesis and biological features of virus-induced primary liver cancer in chickens and its established transplantable form. In: Remmer, H., Balt, H.M., Bannasch, P. and Popper, H. (eds.), *Primary Liver Tumors*, MTP Press, Lancaster, England, pp. 437-48

Larouze, B., London, W.T., Saimot, G., Werner, B.G., Lustbader, E.D., Payet, M. *et al.* (1976). Host responses to hepatitis-B infection in patients with primary hepatic carcinoma and their families. A case/control study in Senegal, West Africa. *Lancet*, 2: 534-8

Larsen, R.J., Holmes, C.L. and Heath, C.W., Jr. (1973). A statistical test for measuring unimodal clustering: a description of the test and its application to cases of acute leukemia in metropolitan Atlanta, Georgia. *Biometrics*, 29: 301-9

Lefkowitch, J.H. (1981). The epidemiology and morphology of primary malignant liver tumors. *Surgical Clinics of North America*, 61: 169-89

Lehner, T., Wilton, J.M.A. and Shillitoe, E.J. (1975). Immunological basis for latency, recurrences, and putative oncogenicity of herpes simplex virus. *Lancet*, 2: 60-7

Levine, P.H., Wallen, W.C., Ablashi, D.V., Granlund, D.J. and Connelly, R. (1977). Comparative studies on immunity to EBV-associated antigens in NPC patients in North America, Tunisia, France and Hong Kong. *International Journal of Cancer*, 20: 332-8

Levy, J.A. (1977). Endogenous C-type viruses in normal and 'abnormal' cell development. *Cancer Research*, 37: 2957-68

Lewis, G.C., Jr., Rowe, W.P., Dell Angelo, R.J. and Brodsky, I. (1965). Investigation of viral etiology for cervical cancer. *American Journal of Obstetrics and*

Gynecology, 93: 659-66

Lilienfeld, A.M., Pedersen, E. and Dowd, J.E. (1967). *Cancer Epidemiology: Methods of Study*, Johns Hopkins Press, Baltimore

Lin, T.M., Yang, C.S., Chiou, J.F., Tu, S.M., Lin, C.C., Liu, C.H. *et al.* (1973). Seroepidemiological studies on carcinoma of the nasopharynx. *Cancer Research*, 33: 2603-8

Linsell, C.A. and Peers, F.G. (1977). Aflatoxin and liver cell cancer. *Transactions of the Royal Society of Tropical Medicine and Hygiene*, 71: 471-3

London, W.T., Houff, S.A., Madden, D.L., Fuccillo, D.A., Gravell, M., Wallen, W.C. *et al.* (1978). Brain tumors in owl monkeys inoculated with a human polyomavirus (JC virus). *Science*, 201: 1246-9

Mandel, J.S. and Schuman, L.M. (1980). Epidemiology of cancer of the prostate. *Reviews of Cancer Epidemiology*, 1: 1-83

Mantel, N. (1967). The detection of disease clustering and a generalized regression approach. *Cancer Research*, 27: 209-20

Mantyjarvi, R.A. (1979). New oncogenic human papovaviruses. *Medical Biology*, 57: 29-35

Master, S.P., Taylor, J.F., Kyalwazi, S.K. and Ziegler, J.L. (1970). Immunological studies in Kaposi's sarcoma in Uganda. *British Medical Journal*, 1:600-2

McAllister, R.M. (1973). Viruses in human carcinogenesis. *Progress in Medical Virology*, 16: 48-85

McClure, H.M., Keeling, M.E., Custer, R.P., Marshak, R.R., Abt, D.A. and Ferrer, J.F. (1974). Erythroleukemia in two infant chimpanzees fed milk from cows naturally infected with bovine C-type virus. *Cancer Research*, 34: 2745-57

McDougall, J.K., Galloway, D.A. and Fenoglio, C.M. (1980). Cervical carcinoma detection of herpes simplex virus RNA in cells undergoing neoplastic change. *International Journal of Cancer*, 25: 1-8

Melnick, J.L., Lewis, R., Wimberly, I., Kaufman, R.H. and Adam, E. (1978). Association of cytomegalovirus (CMV) infection with cervical cancer: Isolation of CMV from cell cultures derived from cervical biopsy. *Interviology*, 10: 115-9

Menczer, J., Leventon-Kriss, S., Modan, M., Oelsner, G. and Gerichter, C.B. (1975). Antibodies to herpes simplex virus in Jewish women with cervical cancer and in healthy Jewish women of Israel. *Journal of the National Cancer Institute*, 55: 3-6

Miller, J.M., Miller, L.D., Olson, C. and Gillette, K.G. (1969). Virus-like particles in phytohemagglutinin stimulated lymphocyte cultures with reference to bovine lymphosarcoma. *Journal of the National Cancer Institute*, 43: 1297-305

Miller, R.W. and Todaro, G.J. (1969). Viral transformation of cells from persons at high risk of cancer. *Lancet*, 1: 81-2

Morrow, R.H., Gutensohn, N. and Smith, P.G. (1976). Epstein-Barr virus-malaria interaction models for Burkitt's lymphoma: Implications for preventive trials. *Cancer Research*, 36: 667-9

Mortimer, E.A., Jr. (1982). Long-term follow-up after SV40 inoculation. *Lancet*, 306: 1177

Muir, C.S. (1972). Cancer of the head and neck-nasopharyngeal cancer. Epidemiology and etiology. *Journal of the American Medical Association*, 220: 393-4

Myers, B.D., Kessler, E., Levi, J., Pick, A. and Rosenfeld, J.B. (1974). Kaposi's sarcoma in kidney transplant recipients. *Archives of Internal Medicine*, 133: 307-11

Nahmias, A.J., Naib, Z.M., Josey, W.E. and Clepper, A.C. (1967). Genital herpes simplex infection. Virologic and cytologic studies. *Obstetrics and Gynecology*, 29: 395-400

―――― Dowdle, W.R., Naib, Z.M., Josey, W.E., McLane, D. and Domescik, G.

(1969). Genital infection with type 2 *herpes virus hominis*. A commonly occurring venereal disease. *British Journal of Venereal Diseases*, 45: 294-8

—— Josey, W.E., Naib, Z.M., Luce, C.V. and Guest, B.A. (1970). Antibodies to *Herpesvirus hominis* Types 1 and 2 in humans. II. Women with cervical cancer. *American Journal of Epidemiology*, 91: 547-52

Naib, Z.M., Nahmias, A.J. and Josey, W.E. (1966). Cytology and histopathology of cervical herpes simplex infection. *Cancer*, 19: 1026-31

Nicolev, I.G., Chernozemsky, I.N., Petkova-Bocharova, T., Stoyanov, I.S., and Stoichev, I.I. (1978). Epidemiologic characteristics of urinary system tumors and Balkan nephropathy in an endemic region of Bulgaria. *European Journal of Cancer*, 14: 1237-42

Niven, J.S.F., Armstrong, J.A., Andrews, C.H., Pereira, H.G. and Valentine, R.C. (1961). Subcutaneous 'growths' in monkeys produced by a poxvirus. *Journal of Pathology and Bacteriology*, 81: 1-14

Nonoyama, M. and Pagano, J.S. (1973). Homology between Epstein-Barr virus DNA and viral DNA from Burkitt's lymphoma and nasopharyngeal carcinoma determined by DNA-DNA reassociation kinetics. *Nature*, 242: 44-7

Ohbayashi, A., Okochi, K. and Mayumi, M. (1972). Familial clustering of asymptomatic carriers of Australia antigen and patients with chronic liver disease or primary liver cancer. *Gastroenterology*, 62: 618-25

Old, L.J., Bayse, E.A., Oettgen, H.F., de Hardven, E., Geering, G., Williamson, B. *et al.* (1966). Precipitating antibody in human serum to an antigen present in cultured Burkitt's lymphoma cells. *Proceedings of the National Academy of Sciences of the United States of America*, 56: 1699-704

Olson, C. (1974). Bovine lymphosarcoma (leukemia) — A synopsis. *Journal of the American Veterinary Medical Association*, 165: 630-2

—— Miller, L.D., Miller, J.M. and Hoss, H.E. (1972). Transmission of lymphosarcoma from cattle to sheep. *Journal of the National Cancer Institute*, 49: 1463-7

Omata, M., Ashcavai, M., Lieu, C.T. and Peters, R.L. (1979). Hepatocellular carcinoma in the U.S.A. Etiologic considerations. Localization of hepatitis B antigens. *Gastroenterology*, 78: 279-87

Orth, G., Jablonska, S., Breitlurd, F., Favre, M., Croissant, O. (1978). The human papillomaviruses. *Bulletin du Cancer*, 65: 151-64

Ozaki, Y., Ishiguro, T., Ohashi, M., Sawaragi, I. and Ito, Y. (1978). Antibodies to herpesvirus type 1 and type 2 among Japanese cervical cancer patients. *Gann; Japanese Journal of Cancer Research*, 69: 119-22

Pacsa, A.S., Kummerlander, L., Pejtsch, B. and Pali, K. (1975). Herpesvirus antibodies and antigens in patients with cervical anaplasia and in controls. *Journal of the National Cancer Institute*, 55: 775-81

Padgett, B.L. (1980). Investigations into the possible role of the human polyomaviruses in human cancer. In: Giraldo, G. and Beth, E. (eds.), *The Role of Viruses in Human Cancer*, vol. 1, Elsevier, New York, pp. 117-23

—— Walker, D.L., ZuRhein, G.M., Eckroade, R.J. and Dessel, B.H. (1971). Cultivation of a papova-like virus from human brain with progressive multifocal leucoencephalopathy. *Lancet*, 1: 1257-60

Panem, S., Prochownik, E.V., Reale, F.R. and Kirsten, W.H. (1975). Isolation of type C virions from a normal human fibroblast strain. *Science*, 189: 297-9

Patten, S.F., Hughes, C.P. and Reagon, J.W. (1963). An experimental study of the relationship between *Trichomonas vaginalis* and dysplasia in the uterine cervix. *Acta Cytologica*, 7: 187-90

Payan, H.M. (1979). Cancer in married couples. *Southern Medical Journal*, 72: 17-19

Pike, M.C. and Smith, P.G. (1968). Disease clustering: A generalization of Knox's

approach to the detection of space-time interactions. *Biometrics,* 24: 541-56
——— and Smith, P.G. (1974). A case-control approach to examine diseases for evidence of contagion, including diseases with long latent periods. *Biometrics,* 30: 263-79

Plummer, G. (1964). Serological comparison of the herpes viruses. *British Journal of Experimental Pathology,* 45: 135-41

Poiesz, B.J., Ruscetti, F.W., Gazdar, A.F., Bunn, P.A., Minna, J.D. and Gallo, R.C. (1980). Detection and isolation of type C retrovirus particles from fresh and cultured lymphocytes of a patient with cutaneous T-cell lymphoma. *Proceedings of the National Academy of Sciences of the United States of America,* 77: 7415-19

——— Ruscetti, F.W., Reitz, M.S., Kalyanaraman, V.S. and Gallo, R.C. (1981). Isolation of a new type C retrovirus (HTLV) in primary uncultured cells of a patient with Sézary T-cell leukaemia. *Nature,* 294: 268-71

Pope, J.H., Achong, B.G., Epstein, M.A. and Beddulph, J. (1967). Burkitt's lymphoma in New Guinea: Establishment of a line of lymphoblasts *in vitro* and description of their fine structure. *Journal of the National Cancer Institute,* 39: 933-45

Prince, A.M. (1968). An antigen detected in the blood during the incubation period of serum hepatitis. *Proceedings of the National Academy of Sciences of the United States of America,* 60: 814-21

——— Leblanc, L., Krohn, K., Masseyeff, R. and Albert, M.E. (1970). S.H. antigen and chronic liver disease. *Lancet,* 2: 717-18

Purtilo, D.T. (1980). Epstein-Barr-virus-induced oncogenesis in immune-deficient individuals. *Lancet,* 1: 300-3

Rabson, A.S., O'Conor, G.T., Baron, S., Whong, J.J. and Legallais, F.Y. (1964). Morphologic, cytogenetic and virologic studies *in vitro* of a malignant lymphoma from an African child. *International Journal of Cancer,* 1: 228-32

Rapp, F. (1981). Transformation by the herpes simplex viruses. In: Nahmias, A.J., Dowdle, W.R. and Schinazi, R.E. (eds.), *The Human Herpesviruses. An Interdisciplinary Perspective,* Elsevier, New York, Oxford, pp. 221-7

Rawls, W.E., Laurel, D., Melnick, J.L., Glicksmon, J.M. and Kaufman, R.H. (1968). A search for viruses in smegma, premalignant and early malignant cervical tissues. The isolation of herpesviruses with distinct antigenic properties. *American Journal of Epidemiology,* 87: 647-55

——— Tompkens, W.A.F. and Melnick, J.L. (1969). The association of herpesvirus type 2 and carcinoma of the uterine cervix. *American Journal of Epidemiology,* 89: 547-54

——— Gardner, H.L. and Kaufman, R.L. (1970). Antibodies to genital herpesvirus in patients with carcinoma of the cervix. *American Journal of Obstetrics and Gynecology,* 107: 710-16

——— Garfield, C.H., Steh, P. and Adam, E. (1976). Serological and epidemiological considerations of the role of herpes simplex virus type 2 in cervical cancer. *Cancer Research,* 36: 829-35

——— and Campione-Piccardo, J. (1981). Epidemiology of herpes simplex virus type 1 and 2 infections. In: Nahmias, A.J., Dowdle, W.R. and Schinazi, R.F. (eds.), *The Human Herpesviruses. An Interdisciplinary Perspective,* Elsevier, New York, Oxford, pp. 137-52

Richardson, D.H. (1977). Burkitt's lymphoma clusters in a Virginia community. *Virginia Medicine,* 104: 19-21

Rosdahl, N., Larsen, S.O. and Clemmesen, J. (1974). Hodgkin's disease in patients with previous infectious mononucleosis: 30 years experience. *British Medical Journal,* 2: 253-6

Rotkin, I.D. (1967). Sexual characteristics of a cervical cancer population. *Ameri-*

can Journal of Public Health, 57: 815-29

Roux, E. (1903). Sur les microbes dits 'invisibles'. *Revue Bulletin Institute Pasteur*. 1: 7-12, Introduction

Royston, I., Aurelian, L. and Davis, H.J. (1970). Genital herpes virus findings in relation to cervical neoplasia. *Journal of Reproductive Medicine*, 4: 9-13

Safai, B., Miki, V., Giraldo, G., Beth, E. and Good, R.A. (1980). Association of Kaposi's sarcoma with secondary primary malignancies. Possible etiopathogenic implications. *Cancer*, 45: 1472-9

——— and Good, R.A. (1981). Kaposi's sarcoma: A review and recent developments. *Cancer*, 31: 2-12

Sanford, E.J., Geder, L., Laychock, A., Rohner, T.J. and Rapp, F. (1977). Evidence for the association of a cytomegalovirus with carcinoma of the prostate. *Journal of Urology*, 118: 789-92

Schuman, L.M., Choi, N.W. and Gullen, W.H. (1967). Relationship of central nervous system neoplasms to *Toxoplasma gondii* infection. *American Journal of Public Health*, 57: 848-56

Schwartz, D.A. (1981). Helminths in the induction of cancer. II. *Schistosoma haematobium* and bladder cancer. *Tropical and Geographical Medicine*, 33: 1-7

Sebastian, J.A., Leeb, B.O. and See, R. (1978). Cancer of the cervix – a sexually transmitted disease. Cytologic screening in a prostitute population. *American Journal of Obstetrics and Gynecology*, 131: 620-3

Shigematsu, T., Priori, E.S., Dmochowski, L. and Wilburr, J.R. (1971). Immuno-electron microscopic studies of type C virus particles in ESP-1 and HEK-1-HRLV cell lines. *Nature*, 234: 412-14

Skinner, G.R., Buchan, A., Hartley, C.E., Turner, S.P. and Williams, D.R. (1980). The preparation, efficacy and safety of 'antigenoid' vaccine NFV (1)(S–L+) MRC toward prevention of herpes simplex virus infections in human subjects. *Medical Microbiology and Immunology*, 169: 39-51

Smith, P.G. (1978). Current assessment of 'case clustering' of lymphomas and leukemias. *Cancer*, 42: 1026-34

——— (1982). Spatial and temporal clustering. In: Schottenfeld, D. and Fraumeni, J.F., Jr. (eds.), *Cancer Epidemiology and Prevention*, Saunders Company, Philadelphia, pp. 391-407

——— and Pike, M.C. (1976). Current epidemiological evidence for transmission of Hodgkin's disease. *Cancer Research*, 36: 660-2

Sordillo, E.M., Sordillo, P.P., Hajdui, S.I. and Good, R.A. (1981). Lymphangio-sarcoma after filarial infection. *Journal of Dermatologic Surgery and Oncology*, 7: 235-9

Stern, H. (1968). Isolation of cytomegalovirus and clinical manifestations of infection at different ages. *British Medical Journal*, 1: 665-9

Stevens, D.P., Barker, L.F., Ketcham, A.S. and Meyer, H.M., Jr. (1970). Asymptomatic cytomegalovirus infection following blood transfusion in tumor surgery. *Journal of the American Medical Association*, 2311: 1341-4

Sutherland, J.C., Olweny, C.L.M., Levine, P.H., Mardiney, M.R., Jr. (1978). Epstein-Barr virus-immune complexes in postmortem kidneys from African patients with Burkitt's lymphoma and American patients with and without lymphoma. *Journal of the National Cancer Institute*, 60: 941-6

Taguchi, F., Nagaki, D., Saito, M., Haruyama, C., Iwasaki, K. and Suzuki, T. (1975). Transplacental transmission of BK virus in human. *Japanese Journal of Microbiology*, 19: 395-8

Tajima, K., Tominaga, S., Shimizu, H. and Suchi, T. (1981). A hypothesis of the etiology of adult T-cell leukemia/lymphoma. *Gann; Japanese Journal of Cancer Research*, 72: 684-91

Temin, H.M. and Mizutani, S. (1970). RNA-dependent DNA polymerase in virions of Rous sarcoma virus. *Nature*, 226: 1211-3

Thomsen, H.K., Jacobsen, M. and Malchow-Møller, A. (1981). Kaposi sarcoma among homosexual men in Europe. *Lancet*, 2: 688

Todaro, G.J., Callahan, R., Rapp, V.R. and DeLarco, J.E. (1980). Genetic transmission of retroviral genes and cellular oncogenes. *Proceedings of the Royal Society of London, Biological Sciences*, 210: 367-85

Trichopoulos, D., Tabor, E., Gerety, R.J., Xirouchaki, E., Sparros, L., Muñoz, N. et al. (1978). Hepatitis B and primary hepatocellular carcinoma in a European population. *Lancet*, 2: 1217-9

Triolo, V.A. (1974). Nineteenth century foundations of cancer research. *Cancer Research*, 24: 4-27

Trumper, P.A., Epstein, M.A., Giovanella, B.C. and Finerty, S. (1977). Isolation of infectious EB virus from the epithelial tumour cells of nasopharyngeal carcinoma. *International Journal of Cancer*, 20: 655-62

Vianna, N.J., Greenwald, P. and Davies, J.N.P. (1971). Extended epidemic of Hodgkin's disease in high-school students. *Lancet*, 1: 1209-11

—— Greenwald, P., Brady, J., Polan, A.K., Dwork, A., Mauro, J. et al. (1972). Hodgkin's disease: cases with features of a community outbreak. *Annals of Internal Medicine*, 77: 169-80

—— and Polan, A.K. (1973). Epidemiologic evidence for the transmission of Hodgkin's disease. *New England Journal of Medicine*, 289: 499-502

Viola, M.V. (1968). Hematological malignancies in patients and their pets. *Journal of the American Medical Association*, 205: 567-8

Welsh, R.M., Cooper, N.R., Jensen, F.C. and Oldstone, M.B.A. (1975). Human serum lyses RNA tumour viruses. *Nature*, 257: 612-14

Wertheim, P. and Voute, P.A. (1976). Neuroblastoma, Wilms' tumor and cytomegalovirus. *Journal of the National Cancer Institute*, 57: 701-3

Willcox, R.R. (1968). Necrotic cervicitis due to primary infection with the virus of herpes simplex. *British Medical Journal*, 1: 610-11

Williams, E.H., Spit, P. and Pike, M.C. (1969). Further evidence of space-time clustering of Burkitt's lymphoma patients in the West Nile district of Uganda. *British Journal of Cancer*, 23: 235-46

—— Day, N.E. and Geser, A.G. (1974). Seasonal variation in onset of Burkitt's lymphoma in the West Nile district of Uganda. *Lancet*, 2: 19-22

—— Smith, P.G., Day, N.E., Geser, A., Ellice, J. and Tukei, P. (1978). Space-time clustering of Burkitt's lymphoma in the West Nile district of Uganda: 1961-1975. *British Journal of Cancer*, 27: 109-22

Wogan, G.N. (1975). Mycotoxins. *Annual Review of Pharmacology and Toxicology*, 15: 437-51

—— (1976). Aflatoxins and their relation to hepatocellular cancer. In: Okuda, K. and Peters, R.L., (eds.), *Hepatocellular Cancer*, John Wiley and Sons, New York, pp. 25-41

Wray, B.B. and O'Steen, K.C. (1975). Mycotoxin-producing fungi from house associated with leukemia. *Archives of Environmental Health*, 30: 571-3

Wright, D.H. (1966). Burkitt's tumour in England. A comparison with childhood lymphosarcoma. *British Journal of Cancer*, 1: 503-14

Wright, E.T. and Winer, L.H. (1961). Herpes zoster and malignancy. *Archives of Dermatology*, 84: 110-12

Young, E.J., Vainrub, B., Musher, D.M., Kumpuris, A.G., Uribe, G., Gyorkey, P. et al. (1978). Acute pharyngotonsillitis caused by herpesvirus type 2. *Journal of the American Medical Association*, 239: 1885-6

Young, J.L., Percy, C.L., Asire, A.J. (eds.) (1981). Surveillance, epidemiology, and end results: incidence and mortality data, 1973-77. *National Cancer*

Institute Monographs, 57: 14-15

Ziegel, R.F., Arya, S.K., Horoszewicz, J.S. and Carter, W.A. (1977). A status report on human prostatic carcinoma, with emphasis on potential viral etiology. *Oncology; Journal of Clinical and Experimental Cancer Research*, 34: 29-44

zur Hausen, H. (1980a). The role of Epstein-Barr virus in Burkitt's lymphoma and nasopharyngeal carcinoma. In: Rapp, F. (ed.), *Oncogenic Herpesviruses*, vol. II, CRC Press, Boca Raton, Fla., pp. 13-24

—————— (1980b). The role of viruses in human tumours. *Advances in Cancer Research*, 33: 77-107

—————— Schulte-Holthausen, H., Wolf, H., Dorries, K. and Egger, H. (1974). Attempts to detect virus-specific DNA in human tumors. II. Nucleic acid hybridizations with complementary RNA of human herpes group viruses. *International Journal of Cancer*, 13: 657-64

—————— and Gissmann, L. (1980). Papillomaviruses. In: Klein, G. (ed.), *Viral Oncology*, Raven Press, New York, pp. 433-45

ZuRhein, G.M. and Chou, S.M. (1965). Particles resembling papova viruses in human cerebral demyelinating disease. *Science*, 148: 1477-9

17 THE ROLE OF DRUGS IN THE PRODUCTION OF HUMAN CANCER

J.R. Coulter

Introduction

Other than pure placebos all drugs are necessarily biologically active agents. The medical profession must therefore try to predict and balance the benefits and risks to be expected from drug use. Many effects can only be predicted statistically. While knowledge of undesirable acute effects of drugs on humans is often extensive, delayed adverse effects (of which cancer is but one example) are less well understood and documented. This poses a considerable clinical dilemma which it is hoped this chapter will help resolve. Known carcinogenic agents are regularly used in the treatment of advanced malignancies. Some, surviving their original cancer, have developed a second unrelated malignancy very likely as a result of the earlier treatment (Seiber, 1977; Reimer et al., 1977). These consequences notwithstanding, few would question the use of carcinogenic drugs in these situations. The hard problems are posed by non-fatal, sometimes trivial, diseases for which a drug, with limited evidence of carcinogenicity, may be advised. Resort to published lists which classify drugs into apparently firm carcinogen/non-carcinogen categories provides very limited help. Such classifications beg too many questions and lose too much important information. Because the single term 'carcinogen' is used to cover substances acting in quite different ways its application without qualification can be misleading. Help comes from an understanding of carcinogenic mechanisms.

Uncritical reliance on published lists also fails for several practical reasons:

(a) The International Agency for Research on Cancer (IARC), for example, sets up expert panels to review the available literature on carefully selected individual agents. A review panel will not usually be constituted until sufficient evidence has accumulated to stimulate and reward this effort. The absence of a drug from the IARC lists does not establish non-carcinogenicity.

(b) The IARC makes scrupulous assessments and frequently concludes

327

a review with words such as, 'There is limited evidence for the carcinogenicity of clofibrate in experimental animals. The epidemiological data were insufficient. No evaluation of the carcinogenicity of clofibrate to humans could be made' (IARC Monographs 24, 1980a). This 'not proven' verdict is no help to clinicians seeking black and white categories.

(c) Some quantitative estimate of risk is desirable but is not provided in IARC and other lists.

(d) Proof of carcinogenicity is difficult, proof of non-carcinogenicity is impossible. Lack of proof of carcinogenicity is not proof of safety. The history of medical treatments provides many examples of agents, once thought to be safe, which have subsequently been shown to carry a cancer risk (X-ray, oestrogens, cyclophosphamide) and there is every reason to suppose that this progression will continue. For physicians to make their own assessments of carcinogenic risks they will need to consider data from three sources (human epidemiology, animal experiments, and other, strictly laboratory, tests giving endpoints such as cell transformation or mutation) interpreted through an understanding of the processes underlying the transformation of a normal to a malignant cell and ultimately to a clinically detectable cancer.

Carcinogenesis

Initiation

There is a general acceptance that carcinogenesis involves two discrete stages, the first being a single irreversible event called 'initiation' and the second, one, two or more events, possibly spread out in time and called 'promotion' (Miller and Miller, 1981). There is much evidence which points to initiation involving a mutation, a permanent heritable change in the genetic information carried by deoxyribonucleic acid (DNA) in the cell nucleus. Indeed it has been shown that in one human bladder cancer, at least, a single point mutation distinguishes a cancer from a normal cell (Reddy *et al.*, 1982; Tabin *et al.*, 1982). This involves a G-T transversion, precisely the mutation favoured by many bladder carcinogens. This mutation results in a glycine-valine substitution in a single protein of molecular weight 21,000. Mutation proceeds through several steps; DNA damage followed by repair which restores the continuity and hence readability of the DNA chain but in which the base sequence is changed so that the DNA now encodes a different message. Cells containing unrepaired DNA are unlikely to survive and reproduce and are therefore unable to transmit the malignant code to daughter cells. Mutation is not the process of DNA damage, but results from faulty repair following DNA damage; DNA repair is an integral part of mutagenesis. Two observations follow: drugs, such as caffeine (Timson, 1977) and chloroquine (Michael and Williams, 1974), which inhibit DNA repair are more likely to protect against the effect of cancer initiators than to themselves initiate cancer. Secondly, cells which have suffered relatively light DNA damage are more likely to be significant in cancer initiation than those severely damaged and with less chance to survive. This may explain the apparent paradox that chronic lymphatic leukaemia has evidently not been observed after radiation, lymphocytes being particularly prone to cell death after radiation exposure (Boice, 1981). Sigmoid-shaped dose-response curves which describe many physiological and lethal responses provide an inappropriate model to describe a process in which the cells of interest are those which are lightly affected and well able to compete with normal, non-mutated, surrounding cells.

Promutagens and Activation. The chemical structure of the substance (mutagen) which reacts with the DNA and leads to DNA damage is frequently not the same as the drug as administered; the drug is activated by enzymes. Activation converts a 'procarcinogen' to an 'ultimate carcinogen'. Agents, such as phenobarbitone, which enhance the production of activating enzymes may act as enhancers of carcinogenic activity. Microsomal oxidase enzymes are responsible for the activation of many procarcinogens. Drugs and other agents may interfere with these oxidative and other activating reactions. Vitamins C, E and selenium may act as anti-carcinogens by interfering with this step in initiation. Drugs may also interact with other agents, either naturally present in the body on in the diet, to form an ultimate carcinogen. For example, secondary and tertiary amine drugs reacting with nitrite in the acid milieu of the stomach have been shown to form nitrosamines which are potent mutagens and carcinogens.

Two further important consequences stem from the recognition of initiators as mutagens. The DNA alphabet consists of the same four bases in every living cell. Moreover, every cell in a particular individual contains the same sequence of bases (except mature sex cells which contain only half the sequence). A chemical, which can react with a base leading to a mutation, may therefore do so in any cell *provided it can get to the DNA of that cell*. It follows that apparent specificity of a carcinogen (acting as a mutagen) for a particular organ or site depends not on any innate reactivity between the drug and the DNA of particular cells but on other less specific factors such as a higher local concentration of the drug or of activating enzymes. Most cells, possibly all, contain activating enzymes, although often at very low concentration, and physiological barriers vary from time to time depending on age and other conditions. This view provides guidance in interpreting human and animal epidemiological data. How should one ascribe cause when a population exposed to a known or suspect carcinogen exhibits an increase in a number of different cancers, some, or perhaps none, of which individually reach statistical significance? The answer to this question depends critically on one's model of specificity and will profoundly affect regulation of, and attitude to, prescription of suspect drugs. Estimates of cancer risk based exclusively on statistically significantly specific cancers will always, and sometimes very greatly, underestimate the absolute risk.

Secondly, there is no *a priori* reason to suppose that drug-induced mutations will be confined to somatic cells or to mutations leading only to cancer. The same drug will cause other, non-malignant, mutations in somatic cells and mutations in germ line cells, provided again it can reach and penetrate these cells in its reactive form. Germ line mutations, particularly in spermatocytes which, unlike genetically quiescent ova, are continuously producing mature sperm, may lead to the conception of a damaged foetus or transmission into the gene pool of mutant recessive genes. Gene damage may lead to abortion or birth of an affected offspring. Carcinogenicity and birth defect data thus may each help in the interpretation of the other, although teratogenic influences acting directly on the developing foetus are a far more common cause of birth defect than mutation in the gametes. Many teratogens are non-mutagens and have no links to carcinogenesis. However, vinyl chloride monomer, proposed in the 1940s as an anaesthetic (Infante *et al.*, 1976), cigarette smoking (Bridges *et al.*, 1979) and anaesthetic gas exposure (Cohen *et al.*, 1974) have each been associated with all three effects (cancer; abortion; birth defect) and it may be supposed that more comprehensive birth defect registers would point up many other examples of exposure to carcinogens being associated with an increase in the other two indicators. Exposure to each of these substances has also been shown to result in the appearance of mutagens in the urine (McCoy *et al.*, 1977; Yamasaki and Ames, 1977). The exposure of a male parent clearly identifies the mode of transmission as genetic and the primary injury as a mutation. Substances capable of causing this result are therefore potential cancer initiators. Men treated with cyclophosphamide have subsequently sired defective children and this possibility must be considered when prescribing any mutagenic carcinogenic drug. The lack of more evidence in this area gives no assurance of safety but rather reflects the inadequacy of present birth defect statistics. Many mutagens are teratogens. Neubert (1980) gives more detail on these links.

Somatic mutation not leading to cancer is an as yet uncharted sea with some still debatable theoretical work and observations suggesting that this may be the basis of ageing (Burnet, 1974; Bertell, 1977). It is necessary to remain sensitive to new developments in this area.

Promoters

Promoters may be more varied in their action and this action appears to be less well understood. They seem not to interact with DNA but possibly with the cell membrane. Their action, at least initially, appears to be reversible. Some inhibit cell differentiation. Some appear to be organ specific. Promoters, by themselves, will not initiate a cancer but require the prior initiation of a cell by a mutagen. Some agents are capable of generating a clinical cancer without the aid of a second substance; they must therefore be regarded as both initiator and promoter.

Carcinogen: an Ambiguous Term

Factors fulfilling each function in the carcinogenesis cycle are ubiquitous. The administration of a drug or other agent fulfilling only one role may therefore identify that substance as a carcinogen. The description of a substance as 'a carcinogen' is no help in understanding its mode of action. The assumption, implicit in much of the literature, that the term 'carcinogen' describes a single characteristic has led to a great deal of confusion. For example, numerous papers have compared the results of mutagenicity tests in bacteria with carcinogenicity tests in animals and many have commented disparagingly on the former because there is not a 100 per cent correlation. But it is known that many promoters, co-carcinogens and enzyme inducers are not mutagens and *must* therefore be negative in tests for the latter character. Conversely, identifying a drug as a mutagen indicates that it may cause any or all of the genetic consequences mentioned above provided it can reach cellular DNA in a reactive form but does not tell you that it will be able to penetrate a suitable cell.

Sources of Evidence

The most incontrovertible evidence that a substance is a human carcinogen is provided by carefully designed epidemiological studies in humans. Many difficulties attend such studies, a fact well illustrated by the very short list of substances (39) which the IARC regards as providing acceptable evidence as human carcinogens. Of these only ten have been used or suggested for use as human drugs. The long latency with consequent long exposure before a decision as to safety can be made makes exclusive dependence on human data morally indefensible. Chemical carcinogens show a very high correlation between ability to cause cancer in animals and man, although because of the small number of proven human carcinogens this relationship is highly asymmetrical. A standard National Cancer Institute (NCI) test (50 animals per group, two species, both sexes, and two dose levels giving 400 test animals and 200 controls), under good conditions, is capable of revealing a 10-100 per cent increase in the cancer rate. Because of this relative insensitivity and the high cost (approximately $US 300,000 per substance) the high dose chosen is the highest which is tolerated without impairing the general health of the animal, i.e. the sensitivity of the test is maximised by maximising the dose rather than by increasing the number of animals. Most human carcinogens would be rated non-carcinogens if tested in groups of only 50 animals at the doses at which humans are usually exposed. Consider the risk from DES mentioned below. To test reliably animals at these low doses would demand impossibly large and expensive experiments. There is no evidence that non-initiators at low dose will become initiators at high dose or conversely that initiators at high dose will cease to initiate at some suitably low threshold dose. All those substances accepted by the IARC as proven human carcinogens have been shown also to cause cancer in experimental animals, except arsenic and benzene, both of which are acutely toxic at high dose. This probably explains the apparent anomaly. It has been shown that there is about an 85 per cent chance that a substance, carcinogenic in one animal species, will be carcinogenic when tested in a second species (Purchase, 1980). The predictive value of a positive result in two species for a third should theoretically approach $1-(0.15)^2$ or about 98 per cent. These 85 and 98 per cent figures are therefore appropriate when predicting human carcinogenicity from the results of animal tests. Most recognised authorities take positive results in two animals as indicating potential human carcinogenicity. Some anomalous results may be explained by weak carcinogenicity and the failure of real cancer differences to reach statistical significance. However, some strong carcinogens appear not to be carcinogenic in some species; beta naphthylamine is a potent human bladder carcinogen and is carcinogenic in at least three other species but is negative in the rat and rabbit. Certain classes of compound, such as chlorinated hydrocarbons, tend to be positive in one species, the mouse, while negative in the rat, suggesting different metabolism. Phenacetin is carcinogenic in the hamster but not in the rat. Hamster liver S9, but not rat liver S9, will give a positive result with phenacetin in an Ames test (Bartsch *et al.*, 1980).

The third tier of test procedures uses end points other than the production of a cancer. They are cheaper and much quicker to perform than animal tests. From a large number of these tests those with the highest predictive value are transformation of cells in tissue culture and mutation of bacteria, specifically the Ames system which uses several strains of *Salmonella typhimurium*. A substance giving a positive result in either of these tests has a better than 90 per cent chance of being positive in an animal test (Purchase *et al.*, 1978). Extrapolation from a mutagenicity test to cancer production in an animal is therefore as reliable as from one animal species to another. There is thus no logical reason why a positive result in one species together with a positive result in one of these tests should not be accepted as a predictor of potential human carcinogenicity and this was indeed suggested several years ago by the Occupational Safety and Health Administration of the United States of America (USA). However, there has been a general unwillingness to accord a non-cancer end point, such as mutation in a bacterium, the same significance as cancer in an animal model and the simple probabilistic logic of the above statement is not widely accepted. As bacterial mutagenicity tests are statistically far more sensitive than animal tests it is very likely that some agents positive in the former, but negative in the latter, are, in reality, weak carcinogens. The industrial chemical 1, 2 dichloroethane and the food additive AF2 were first thought to be non-carcinogens in animal tests. Positive results in bacterial mutagenicity tests led to retesting in animals and these proved to be positive (Ames, 1979). Tris BP, an agent which came into general use in the USA for fireproofing children's nightwear, vinyl bromide and vinylidene chloride, were shown to be mutagenic in an Ames test before they were shown to be carcinogenic in animals. Like phenacetin, vinylidene chloride is activated by some species but not by others and this property correlates with carcinogenicity (Bartsch *et al.*, 1980). A positive result in a mutagenicity test indicates that the substance, if a carcinogen, is most likely an initiator and warns us that it may cause genetic damage other than that leading to cancer. This aspect of short-term tests has been extensively reviewed by Green (1980).

Quantitation and Acceptibility of Risk

Reasonably accurate estimation of the size of the risk to individual patients can only be based on human epidemiological studies. Large populations, very long and meticulous follow-up and sophisticated statistical analysis are prerequisites and the first two conditions have been met with only a few of the substances of interest. Radiation is the best explored. For many new drugs the exposed populations may always remain too small, too scattered or too confounded with other drugs ever to obtain reliable estimates of risk for any but the most potent carcinogens. To reduce this problem to a minimum much greater attention should be paid to the central storing, collation and analysis of information on drug consumption.

Quantitative molar comparison of different substances has shown that both carcinogenicity in animals and mutagenicity in bacteria range over at least six orders of magnitude (Ames and Hooper, 1978). The species differences mentioned above warn that simple quantitative extrapolation from animals to humans is unwise. Such exercises must be reinforced with a considerable knowledge of species-specific metabolism. However, qualitatively, as explained, there is about a 98 per cent chance that a drug carcinogenic in two species or one species and positive in a bacterial mutagenicity or cell transformation test will be a human carcinogen. Some of the important variables associated with risk are explained by the carcinogenesis model.

Dose Response

If a carcinogenic drug is a mutagen (or converted to a mutagen *in vivo*) it is almost certainly an initiator and linear dose response relationships without threshold should be applied, i.e. any dose above zero carries a risk which is proportional to the size of the dose. This model is applied to radiation and while there is no possibility of directly measuring the risk at very low doses there are several good reasons why this model is appropriate. In bacterial tests, where the results of exposing very large populations can be examined, dose responses at low dose often follow this model. Secondly, the question as to whether or not a very small human exposure to a mutagen carries a risk is often wrongly formulated. It is incorrectly assumed that the population being examined starts at the 'origin', at the x, y intercept, with no other exposure and with otherwise a zero risk. The question is then asked: 'Will exposure to a small dose of a carcinogen move this population, even slightly, along the risk axis? ' But in most Western countries about 25 per cent of the population will get cancer at some time in their lives and about 20 per cent will die of cancer. These cancers result from exposure to thousands of both naturally occurring and man-made agents. Thus, the real human population is already well out in the x, y space and the appropriate question is: 'Will the addition of a small extra amount of carcinogen increase the cancer risk? ' The answer must be 'yes' for the chance of a cancer being initiated is a function of the integrated effective dose of all mutagens combined. For analogous reasons the same model should be applied to germ line genetic effects.

Although this linear model is often applied to all carcinogens without distinction there is no theoretical or experimental evidence which supports its application to carcinogens which work through other parts of the carcinogenesis cycle. The action of promoters seems to be reversible in the early stages suggesting that there is probably a threshold. The response will also depend on the presence of initiated cells; no cells, no cancer no matter how large the dose. Older people should therefore be far more responsive to promoters than younger people. In experiments on bladder cancer the sweeteners saccharin and cyclamate have been shown to be promoters (Hicks *et al.*, 1975). One might therefore predict that smokers or those exposed to other bladder carcinogens may show a carcinogenic response to these sweeteners not shown by non-smokers or those not exposed to such initiators. Similarly, enzyme inducers, sometimes called co-carcinogens, but falling within the broad definition used by the IARC given above (e.g. phenobarbitone), exhibit sigmoid shaped dose responses with effective thresholds. Unfortunately the actual threshold and position of the curve is often unknown and in these cases together with those in which the exact role of the carcinogen is unknown it is safest to assume a linear model.

Age

Most carcinogens are teratogens but many teratogens are not carcinogens. However, teratogenicity does indicate an ability to cross the placenta and therefore a potential to initiate cancer in the unborn. Thirty-eight chemicals have been shown, in animals, to cross the placenta and give rise to cancer in neonatal or later life (Tomatis, 1979). Although the placenta is a rich source of enzyme activity and the mother may activate procarcinogenic drugs, the resulting ultimate carcinogens being chemically highly reactive are unlikely to survive long enough to induce cancers in the foetus. Several factors unique to the foetus bear on this process. Many enzyme systems in the foetus are relatively poorly developed. Procarcinogens may therefore remain inactive. Furthermore, carcinogens may be unable to transform undifferentiated cells (Rice, 1979) and for both these reasons the very young foetus may be relatively resistant to carcinogenic drugs. Initiated cells seem to require normal division for expression of malignancy (Kakunaga, 1975). There is thus a limited period between differentiation and reproductive quiescence during which cells such as nerve cells are susceptible to carcinogens. In many experiments cancers have appeared in the offspring before they have appeared in the mother. Stewart and Kneale (1970) showed that a variety of cancers in children who had been exposed to X-ray *in utero* appeared before the tenth year of postnatal life. Promoters administered postnatally have also been shown to be effective when exposure to low doses of initiators occurred during foetal life. These effects have all been demonstrated in animals. Only DES and arsenic have been clearly linked with human cancers following foetal exposure (Tomatis, 1979). While exposure to initiators during foetal or early childhood life allows the maximum time for the slow transformation into clinical cancers, exposure in old age may be without effect if insufficient lifetime remains for expression. Similarly no germ line damage can be transmitted by those past their reproductive years. For tissues normally under hormonal control emergence and growth of cancers in these tissues continue to be influenced by hormone levels and balances.

Population Size

While most doctors will be concerned with the risk to individual patients, quite a small shift in risk and hence cancer incidence may become a significant public health problem if a carcinogenic drug comes into widespread use. It was estimated in 1978 that 80 million women were taking oral contraceptives (WHO, 1978). A 1 per cent shift in the cancer rate in a population of this size means 200,000 more cancers! Similarly, an increase in the birth defect rate sufficiently small to make unequivocal identification difficult may, nonetheless, cause a problem of considerable magnitude if a large number of foetuses are exposed. A mutagen causing teratogenic effects in a variety of tissues and ways could be difficult to detect; contrast this situation with thalidomide in which a very unusual and highly specific defect was caused.

Hormones and Substances with Hormone Activity

Diethylstilboestrol (DES) is a synthetic chemical with potent oestrogenic properties which came into common use as a treatment for threatened abortion in the 1950s. In 1971 Herbst *et al.* described a number of rare clear cell adenocarcinomas of the vagina in young women who had been exposed to DES *in utero*. Over 350 cases have now been identified and the risk has been estimated as less than 4 per 1,000 (Herbst *et al.*, 1979) and most probably between 0.1 and 1.0 per 1,000 (Hoover and Fraumeni, 1981). The cancers have appeared during puberty, the incidence rising at age 14, peaking at 19 and then falling rapidly.

Menopausal oestrogen treatment has been convincingly associated with increased risk of endometrial and breast cancer and endometrial cancer has also been linked with the oral contraceptive, Oracon, which sequences oestrogen and progestin. There is equivocal evidence linking oral contraceptive use with both an increase and a decrease in breast cancer. Hoover and Fraumeni (1981) give more details on this point. DES is accepted by the IARC as a proven human carcinogen. The mechanisms which underlie the carcinogenicity of oestrogen-like substances and the possibly antagonistic activity of progestins are uncertain. More than one mechanism may be involved. There is some evidence that some oestrogenic substances can be enzymatically activated to initiators (Metzler, 1975). Oestrogen has been shown to enhance mutagenic activity in an Ames test. The sites at which oestrogen-induced cancers appear are all normally under hormonal control which is, as it were, *prima facie* evidence of promotional activity. It has also been suggested that the function of DES in the production of clear cell adenocarcinoma of the vagina is to alter the normal foetal development of the genital tract such that cells which should remain above the cervix become incorporated in the vaginal wall. Cancers arise in some of these aberrant cells when, at puberty, they come under the influence of endogenous oestrogen, rather as cancers arise in teratomas (Herbst *et al.*, 1979; Forsberg, 1979).

Nitrosamines

Nitrite is added to many processed meats but is also present naturally in the saliva. At low pH nitrite reacts with many secondary and tertiary amines to produce nitrosamines which are potent mutagens and carcinogens. Amine drugs may therefore become carcinogens in the acid stomach. Mutagenic and carcinogenic activity in meat and fish (source of amine) incubated with nitrite under simulated gastric conditions has been demonstrated (Weisberger *et al.*, 1980). Different amines react at different rates and the resulting nitrosamines differ in their carcinogenicity. A standard WHO test which simulates gastric conditions produced the following series of percentage nitrosamine yield from various drugs: aminophenozone 50, phenacetin 7, lucanthone 2.4, tolazamide 0.6, chlorpheniramine and oxytetracycline 0.2, quinacrine 0.1, disulphiram and methapyrilene 0.08, chlorpromazine 0.05, methadone 0.04, dextropropoxyphene 0.03. The following additional drugs have been shown to form nitrosamines: piperazine, ephedrine, ethambutol, chlordiazepoxide, chlorpromazine, cyclizine, tripilennamine, nikethamide. A detailed and authoritative discussion of nitrosatable drugs and references to mutagenicity and carcinogenicity is available in IARC Monograph 24 (1980b).

Carcinogenesis Inhibitors

A number of epidemiological studies have pointed to a high incidence of gastrointestinal tumours in regions with a poor or inconsistent supply of fresh vegetables. Many studies have confirmed a lower incidence of these cancers in vegetarians. It has been suggested that the decrease in gastrointestinal (GI) cancer in North America over the last five decades has been due to the increased intake of vitamin E in breakfast cereals, and more recently synthetic antioxidants in such agents as margarine and cooking oil (Shamberger *et al.*, 1972). Nitrosamines have been postulated as significant initiators of GI cancer. They have also been suggested as the ultimate carcinogens responsible for the increased lung cancer in tobacco smokers. Smokers, as a class, have lower vitamin C levels than non-smoking controls. Vitamin C has been shown to inhibit the conversion of amines to nitrosamines and to decrease the mutagenic and carcinogenic activity of amine/nitrite mixtures *in vitro* and in humans (Ohshima *et al.*, 1980).

In Ames tests it has been shown that vitamin C, vitamin E, sodium selenite, and the synthetic antioxidants butylated hydroxyanisole and butylated hydroxytoluene, will inhibit mutagenesis by substances requiring activation by microsomal oxidase enzymes (Coulter, 1982). Vitamin C is most effective as an inhibitor of water soluble promutagens; vitamin E and the two antioxidants which have been used in margarine and edible oils are more effective as inhibitors of fat soluble agents such as polycyclic hydrocarbons. While more work needs to be done in this area supplements of these two vitamins would seem to provide the possibility of cheap, safe, probably partial, protection for those exposed to amine drugs or drugs which become carcinogens after oxidative activation.

Non-patient Risks

Patients are not the only ones at risk from therapeutically used carcinogenic drugs. Anaesthetists and other operating room personnel have been shown to suffer a higher incidence of cancer and their children are more likely to be aborted or to be born with defects. Halogenated hydrocarbons such as trichlorethylene and chloroform have been used very extensively in the past and both are now considered to be carcinogens. Medical staff preparing carcinogenic drugs have been shown occasionally to ingest these agents for mutagenic tests on urine have revealed the presence of the drug or its active metabolites (Falck *et al.*, 1979). Mutagenicity tests on urine provide an extremely useful and sensitive way of confirming that an active or potentially active drug has indeed passed through the body exposing cells to the possibility of genetic damage. Agents used in hospital, other than drugs, also present a hazard. Radiation is well known and well controlled; less well known is ethylene oxide, a potent mutagen in many species with some evidence of human carcinogenicity, and formalin, which in the presence of hydrochloric acid can form bischloromethyl ether, an extremely active human carcinogen. Factory workers preparing and packaging carcinogenic drugs and other chemical carcinogens are also at risk unless good industrial hygiene is observed.

Conclusion

All DNA is built of the same four bases. Mutation arises when the sequence of these bases becomes modified through a process of damage followed by faulty repair. A substance which has been shown to cause genetic damage in one species will cause genetic damage in any other species provided it can reach the cellular DNA in a suitably active form. Whether this occurs or not depends on physiological factors such as absorption and metabolism rather than genetic factors peculiar to a particular species or cell. Mutation appears to be the initiating step in carcinogenesis. It is a necessary but in 'some' cases not a sufficient condition for the eventual appearance of a clinical cancer. The proportion of human cancers covered by the word 'some' is unknown. Animal species vary widely in their quantitative response to carcinogens. Some substances which appear to be very potent carcinogens in one or several species, including the human species, are non-carcinogenic in others, e.g. beta naphthylamine. Therefore extrapolations of quantitative dose response relationships from animals to humans are suspect. Nevertheless there are good data which allow a qualitative extrapolation from non-human tests to humans. If a substance is shown to be positive in an Ames mutagenicity or cell transformation test there is about an 85 per cent chance it will prove positive in an animal carcinogenicity test. If a substance is positive in one animal carcinogenicity test there is about an 85 per cent chance it will be positive in a second species, e.g. man. Thus, if a substance is positive in two animal species or one species and one of these short-term tests, then there is about a 98 per cent chance that it would prove carcinogenic in humans if the experiment could be carried out. In addition, genetic consequences other than cancer may follow administration of genetically toxic drugs (mutagens). These may include abortion or birth defect in the next or subsequent generations.

References

Ames, B.N. (1979). Identifying environmental chemicals causing mutations and cancer. *Science*, 204: 587-93
———— and Hooper, K. (1978). Does carcinogenic potency correlate with mutagenic potency in the Ames assay? *Nature*, 274: 19-20
Bartsch, H., Malaveille, C., Camus, A.M., Mantel-planche, G., Brun, G., Hautefeuille, A. *et al.* (1980). Bacterial and mammalian mutagenicity tests: validation and comparative studies on 180 chemicals. *International Agency for Research on Cancer Scientific Publications*, 27: 179-241
Bertell, R. (1977). X-ray exposure and premature ageing. *Journal of Surgical Oncology*, 9: 379-91
Boice, J.D. (1981). Cancer following medical irradiation. *Cancer*, 47: 1081-90
Bridges, B.A., Clemmeson, J. and Sugimura, T. (1979). Cigarette smoking – does it carry a genetic risk? *Mutation Research*, 65: 71-81
Burnet, M. (1974). *Intrinsic Mutagenesis: A Genetic Approach to Ageing*, Medical and Technical Publishing Co, Lancaster
Cohen, E.N., Brown, B.W., Bruce, D.L., Cascorbi, H.F., Corbett, T.H., Jones, T.W. *et al.* (1974). Occupational disease among operating room personnel: A national study. *Anaesthiology*, 41: 4: 321-40
Coulter, J.R. (1982). Unpublished data

Falck, K., Grohn, P., Sorsa, H., Vainio, H., Heinonen, E. and Holsti, L.R. (1979). Mutagenicity in urine of nurses handling cytostatic drugs. *Lancet*, 1: 1250-1

Forsberg, J.-G. (1979). Developmental mechanism of oestrogen-induced irreversible changes in the mouse cervicovaginal epithelium. *National Cancer Institute Monographs*, 51: 41-56

Green, M.H.L. (1980). The scientific basis for short-term tests for carcinogenecity: Non-mammalian systems. *International Agency for Research on Cancer Scientific Publications*, 27: 155-67

Herbst, A.L., Ulfelder, H. and Polkanzer, D.C. (1971). Adenocarcinoma of the vagina: Association of maternal stilboestrol therapy with tumour appearance in young women. *New England Journal of Medicine*, 284: 878-81

―――― Scully, R.E. and Robboy, S.J. (1979). Prenatal diethylstilboestrol exposure and human genital tract abnormalities. *National Cancer Institute Monographs*, 51: 25-35

Hicks, R.M., Wakefield, J. St. J. and Chowaniec, J. (1975). Evaluation of a new model to detect bladder carcinogens or co-carcinogens: Results obtained with saccharin, cyclamate and cyclophosphamide. *Chemico-Biological Interactions*, 11: 225-33

Hoover, R. and Fraumeni, J.F., Jr. (1981). Drug-induced cancer. *Cancer*, 47: 1071-80

Infante, P.F., Wagoner, J.K., McMichael, A.J., Waxweiler, R.J. and Falk, H. (1976). Genetic risks of vinyl chloride. *Lancet*, 1: 734-5

International Agency for Research on Cancer Monographs (1980a). Clofibrate. 24: 51

International Agency for Research on Cancer Monographs (1980b). General considerations on N-nitrosatable drugs. 24: 297-307

Kakunaga, T. (1975). The role of cell division in the malignant transformation of mouse cells treated with 3-methylcholanthrene. *Cancer Research*, 35: 1637-42

McCoy, E.C., Hankel, R., Rosenkranz, H.S., Giuffrida, J.G. and Bizzari, D.V. (1977). Detection of mutagenic activity in the urine of anaesthesiologists: a preliminary report. *Environmental Health Perspectives*, 21: 221-3

Metzler, M. (1975). Metabolic activation of diethylstilboestrol: Indirect evidence of a stilbene oxide in hamster and rat. *Biochemical Pharmacology*, 24: 1449-53

Michael, R.O. and Williams, G.M. (1974). Chloroquin inhibition of repair of DNA damage induced in mammalian cells by methyl methanesulphonate. *Mutation Research*, 25: 391-6

Miller, E.C. and Miller, J.A. (1981). Mechanisms of chemical carcinogenesis. *Cancer*, 47: 1055-64

Neubert, D. (1980). Teratogenicity: Any relationship with carcinogenicity? *International Agency for Research on Cancer Scientific Publications*, 27: 169-78

Ohshima, H., Béréziat, J.C. and Bourgade, M.C. (1980). Methods of monitoring nitrosation reactions in vivo. *International Agency for Research on Cancer Annual Report*, pp. 112-13

Purchase, I.F.H. (1980). Inter-species comparisons of carcinogenicity. *British Journal of Cancer*, 41: 454-68

―――― Longstaff, E., Ashby, J., Styles, J.A., Anderson, D., LeFevre, P.A. *et al.* (1978). An evaluation of 6 short-term tests for detecting organic chemical carcinogens. *British Journal of Cancer*, 37: 873-936

Reddy, E.P., Reynolds, R.K., Santos, E. and Barbacid, M. (1982). A point mutation is responsible for the acquisition of transforming properties by the T24 human bladder carcinoma oncogene. *Nature*, 300: 149-52

Reimer, R.R., Hoover, R., Fraumeni, J.F. and Young, R.C. (1977). Acute leukemia after alkylating agent therapy of ovarian cancer. *New England Journal of Medicine*, 297: 177-81

Rice, J.M. (1979). Problems and perpectives in perinatal carcinogenesis: A summary of the conference. *National Cancer Institute Monographs*, 51: 271-8

Shamberger, R.J., Tytko, S.A. and Willis, C.E. (1972). Antioxidants in cereals and food preservatives and the declining cancer death rate. *Cleveland Clinic Quarterly*, 39: 119-24

Sieber, S.M. (1977). The action of antitumor agents: a double-edged sword? *Medical and Pediatric Oncology*, 3(2): 123-31

Stewart, A.M. and Kneale, G.W. (1970). Age distribution of cancers caused by obstetric X-rays and their relevance to cancer latent periods. *Lancet*, 2: 4-8

Tabin, C.J., Bradley, S.M., Bargmann, C.I., Weinberg, R.A., Papageorge, A.G., Scolnick, E.M. *et al.* (1982). Mechanisms of activation of a human oncogene. *Nature*, 300: 143-9

Timson, J. (1977). Caffeine. *Mutation Research*, 47: 1-52

Tomatis, L. (1979). Prenatal exposure to chemical carcinogens and its effect on subsequent generations. *National Cancer Institute Monographs*, 51: 159-84

Weisburger, J.H., Marquardt, H., Hirota, N., Mori, H. and Williams, G.M. (1980). Induction of cancer of the glandular stomach in rats by an extract of nitrite-treated fish. *Journal of the National Cancer Institute*, 64: 163-7

World Health Organization, Technical Report Series 619 (1978). *Steroid Contraception and the Risk of Neoplasia*. World Health Organization, Geneva

Yamasaki, E. and Ames, B.N. (1977). Concentration of mutagens from urine by absorption with nonpolar resin XAD-2: Cigarette smokers have mutagenic urine. *Proceedings of the National Academy of Science USA*, 74: 3555-9

18 THE PREVENTION OF CANCER

C. Muir and D.M. Parkin

Hee is a better physician that keepes diseases off us than hee that cures them being on us. Prevention is so much better than healing because it saves the labour of being sick.

T. Adams (1612-1653)

Introduction

In the natural history of a chronic disease such as cancer there is a stage *before* any pathological change can be detected during which the individual is exposed to risk factors for the disease. The term 'prevention' should logically be reserved for action taken during this period to remove such factors and hence reduce the likelihood of disease occurrence. However, the concept has been extended to include the notion of improving outcome for the patient by commencing therapy at the soonest possible moment. Corresponding levels of prevention are accordingly recognised.

Primary prevention aims to reduce occurrence of disease by altering exposure to, or susceptibility to, risk factors. Prerequisites for primary prevention are:

(1) Risk factors are known for a particular cancer.
(2a) Reduction in level of risk factor is practicable *and*
(2b) reduction in level of risk factor is known (following a pilot study) to reduce the occurrence of disease. *or*
(3) Susceptibility to the risk factor can be reduced.

Some risk factors may be defined by lack of exposure — a possible example being vitamin A in the diet; in this instance risk factor reduction would be to add vitamin A to the diet.

Secondary prevention includes the improvement in outcome for patients (i.e. lower rates of complications or sequelae — including death) which results from diagnosis and treatment at an early stage. In general, secondary prevention is likely to be less effective than primary prevention since treatment of established disease (albeit less advanced than following conventional diagnosis) is involved. Secondary prevention would be the strategy of choice only when the criteria for primary prevention cannot be met — for example, no well-defined risk factors are known, or, if they are, they are not amenable to change.

Primary Prevention

The evidence for the attribution of a high proportion of human cancers to the environment, has been reviewed elsewhere (Higginson and Muir, 1979; Doll and Peto, 1981). These writers use environment in a very broad sense, including not only discrete chemical carcinogens in air, food and water and at work, but also the less well-defined life style factors such as dietary, social and cultural habits which impinge on the human organism.

If precise environmental causes can be identified for a particular cancer, then, in theory at least, prevention should be possible. In practice, two categories of cancer might be considered.

(i) Cancers caused by well-defined risk factors: Such cancers generally occur in adults, are usually epithelial, and arise in the skin, respiratory organs and upper digestive tract. Most have been shown to be associated with such personal habits as tobacco smoking, with or without excess alcohol consumption, betel quid chewing and exposure to solar radiation. A relatively small proportion can be related to specific occupational or iatrogenic exposures. In general, the aetiology of such tumours is clear, and it appears that disease would be prevented by removal or reduction of risk factors. The political and personal will to effect such change is, however, more difficult to ensure.

(ii) Cancers of suspected but unproved environmental aetiology: This group comprises cancers, largely of the gastrointestinal and genital tract, for which it seems rational to suspect environmental rather than genetic causes. This view is based on examination of geographical differences, time trends, changes in risk in migrants, case-control and cohort studies. However, the precise nature of the factors and mechanisms involved is usually unclear. When identified by case-control or other studies they are frequently in the nature of 'carcinogenic risk factors' such as age at first full-term pregnancy (breast cancer), age at first coitus (cervix uteri), low intake of dietary fibre or vitamin A (large bowel and lung, respectively). Many such factors may confound the

'true' cause or are likely to exert their effect indirectly by alteration of the body metabolism. Although almost certainly of environmental aetiology, preventing the occurrence of the tumours associated with such carcinogenic risk factors is probably currently not possible, for reasons discussed below.

Cancer Risk Factors

The Union Internationale Contre le Cancer (UICC) has published a summary of cancer risk factors (host and environmental) by site (Hirayama *et al.*, 1980). The examples given below are illustrative of the current state of knowledge on the potential for prevention in relation to some of these risk factors and cancer sites.

Diet. Although there is good circumstantial evidence that 30 per cent of cancers in males and perhaps 60 per cent of those in females are in some way influenced by diet (Higginson and Muir, 1979; Doll and Peto, 1981), at present this knowledge is not sufficient to advocate preventive measures other than in rather general terms. Cancer levels of Seventh-Day Adventists in the United States of America (USA) differ quite substantially from the national average, and not only for tobacco- and alcohol-related cancers; breast and colon cancer risk is significantly lower in this group of ovo-lacto-vegetarians, a difference ascribed to low animal fat intake following abstinence from meat (Phillips *et al.*, 1980). However, Mormons, another strict USA religious group of comparable socioeconomic background, who also eschew coffee, tea, alcohol and tobacco, eat considerable amounts of meat and have comparatively low incidence rates for these cancers (Lyon *et al.*, 1980). At this stage it would be unwise to draw too many conclusions.

A rather surprising finding to emerge from cohorts of males assembled for studies of cardiovascular disease has been the demonstration that high cholesterol levels in cohort members seem to be associated with a lower subsequent risk of colon cancer (Stemmermann *et al.*, 1981). This finding, which, although not entirely consistent from study to study, persists even when colon cancers appearing in the first few years after the estimation was made are discounted. The demonstration that raised vitamin A levels seem to protect smokers against lung cancer and possibly against other sites of cancer as well seems to open up immense possibilities for chemoprevention, although caution is needed until the whole problem has been thoroughly explored (Peto *et al.*, 1981).

Stomach. A series of case-control and prospective studies have shown in several populations that consumption of fresh fruit and vegetables protects against stomach cancer (Hirayama, 1971; Bjelke, 1974). The increased availability of these items throughout the world and over longer periods of the year may explain to a large measure the virtually universal fall in gastric cancer, a fall which began much earlier in the USA and Western Europe than in Japan and Eastern Europe. In a Japanese prospective study of over 250,000 persons followed for 13 years, the consumption of milk and milk products also resulted in lower risk. However, those households with a domestic refrigerator, which would be expected to lead to better food preservation and less fungal contamination and, in turn, a lesser need to pickle foods in salt, had fewer stomach cancer patients (Hirayama, 1977). The fall observed is thus likely to be due to a complex of factors and as yet no single one can be identified.

Large Bowel. Current hypotheses suggest that, whatever the initiating carcinogen may be for large bowel cancer, the risk is influenced by the promoting effect of bile acids or their metabolites. Bile acid production varies according to fat intake, hence the strong international correlation, shown by Armstrong and Doll (1975), for fat calorie intake and large bowel cancer. The concentration of bile acids is in turn influenced by the faecal bulk which can be modulated by the intake of dietary fibre. The results of a series of studies co-ordinated by the International Agency for Research on Cancer (IARC) in regions of Denmark and Finland where there is a three-fold difference in the incidence of large bowel cancer, are consistent with this hypothesis, but there are other differences in the foodstuffs consumed in these areas (Jensen *et al.*, 1982). Until the action and interaction of these has been thoroughly examined it would be unwise to suggest that the diet in rural Finland should be universally adopted, particularly when this region is known as 'a land of young widows' due to the very high mortality level from ischaemic heart disease (Table 18.1). It would hence appear premature at present to advocate an optimum or even a prudent diet other than in the most general terms – avoiding a high salt intake and over-eating.

If the evidence from animal experiments be considered, in which it has been consistently shown that caloric restriction in the equivalent of childhood leads to increased longevity and diminished levels of 'spontaneous' tumours, one wonders whether current attempts in many parts of the world, to 'improve' dietary intake of fat and protein are entirely without risk.

Diet does change over time, as McMichael *et al.* (1979) have shown

Table 18.1: Age-adjusted (World Standard) Mortality Rates (per 100,000) in Denmark and Finland, from Large Bowel Cancer (ICD 8th 153-154) and Cardiovascular Disease (ICD 8th 410-414) in 1978

	Large bowel		Cardiovascular	
	M	F	M	F
Finland	11	9	296	104
Denmark	25	19	235	106

for Australia and elsewhere, but present methods of estimation of past intake are imprecise and hamper progress in this important area. When the latent period is long, caution is more than ever necessary.

Sexual Intercourse. There is abundant evidence that the risk of cancer of the cervix uteri is raised in women who have first sexual intercourse at an early age and who have multiple sexual partners, hence the very high levels of risk in prostitutes. The pivotal variable seems to be age at first intercourse. A variety of explanations have been advanced which include susceptibility of the relatively young cervical epithelium to foreign DNA whether sperm, smegma or a virus. The relatively low social and economic status of many of the women with this disease is such that nutritional factors and lack of personal hygiene could also be involved. The role of contraception has been a controversial issue; oral contraceptive users have increased rates of disease, but this probably relates to increased sexual activity rather than any risk of the pill itself (WHO, 1978). The use of barrier methods of contraception seems to have a protective effect (Wright *et al.*, 1978).

To delay the age of first sexual intercourse and to discourage multiple partners would be difficult changes to introduce in many societies today. A consequence of doing so would be an increase in the age at first full-term pregnancy; this has been shown to augment the risk of breast cancer. Although the degree of protection conferred by an early first full-term pregnancy varies from country to country, any increased risk is not to be discounted at a time when the incidence of breast cancer is rising. Thus, on the face of it, measures to prevent cervical cancer are likely to increase breast cancer risk (and vice versa) and it is not until the mechanisms underlying both cancers are better understood that a more rational approach can be envisaged.

Although cancer of the penis is virtually never seen in men completely circumcised close to birth, it is likely that provision of an adequate water supply, avoidance of phimosis and good personal hygiene following retraction of the foreskin, would be sufficient to prevent this disease. Wives of males with penile cancer have been shown in some studies, but not others, to be at greater risk for cancer of the cervix. It is possible that the promiscuous male may harbour an oncogenic virus, a supposition rendered more plausible by the greatly increased risk of Kaposi's sarcoma — tentatively attributed to the cytomegalic virus — in promiscuous male homosexuals (*Lancet*, 1981). The candidate virus for cervical cancer has, however, been Herpes Type II.

Epidemiological research has been hampered by technical virological problems which possibly account for conflicting results in case-control and cohort studies.

Tobacco. The evidence for the carcinogenic effect of cigarette tobacco smoke on most organs of the body is overwhelming, as is that for other forms of serious damage to the respiratory and cardiovascular systems. It is probably true that in most occidental countries today few smokers are ignorant of the possible effects of this habit, yet many continue to smoke. Lung cancer risk 'freezes' on ceasing smoking and falls after several years towards that in non-smokers. In several countries of Europe and North America the proportion of males in the younger age groups and in the professional classes who smoke is diminishing, with corresponding falls in mortality rates. Young women, on the other hand, have chosen to continue to smoke, a choice reflected in the rapidly rising lung cancer mortality rates in this sex. Smokers of low tar and filter cigarettes have lower risk levels, but they still show rates considerably in excess of those in non-smokers.

While many governments have paid lip-service to the dangers of smoking, few have indexed taxation on tobacco to the overall cost of living, so that in real terms the habit has become cheaper. International organisations such as FAO, as well as national agricultural institutes, continue to advise governments and the individual farmer on methods of improving tobacco yield.

The tobacco industry continues without scruple to foster sales of its products aiming its advertising at the most vulnerable group, the adolescents. Advertising for cigarette and tobacco products is now banned from television and from newspapers and magazines in many countries, and has shifted to the support of sporting events, insidiously promoting the image, in a world where sport and sportsmen are adulated, of health rather than disease. The tobacco companies are energetically extending marketing efforts to the developing world, and promoting sales of non-filter, high tar brands of cigarette which they presumably recognise as too dangerous to the health of more affluent consumers!

The nature and extent of governmental policies are determined by a mixture of economic considerations and political philosophy, and range from direct curbs on the tobacco-related industries to attempts to counter their influence. In general, investment in anti-smoking propaganda is a tiny fraction of the tobacco industry's advertising budget. It has also proved far from easy to develop successful smoking cessation programmes, or to prevent the onset of smoking in adolescence (US Department of Health and Human Services, 1982). In particular, it is difficult to persuade the young that a habit of today may result in death 25 or more years hence, when they have before them governmental inertia and many living examples of those 'who got away with it', typified by 'Uncle Bill who has smoked for the past 50 years and is still fit and active'.

Substantially similar comments could be made about government attitudes to alcohol. The synergistic role of tobacco and alcohol has been shown for oesophagus and larynx cancer (Tuyns, 1979).

Breast. Miller (1978) has ascribed 20 per cent of breast cancer risk to dietary fat, 25 per cent to age at first pregnancy and 20 per cent to familial factors. Breast cancer risk has also been linked with age at the menarche. The fall in the age of onset of menstruation observed in the past 50 years in most occidental populations may be due to an increased fat intake resulting perhaps in the earlier existence of a critical mass of oestrogen producing fat cells. Early menarche seems to be associated with a late menopause. It is likely that these events, like pregnancy, entrain complex hormonal changes which may result in either endogenous carcinogen production or in increased level of promoting agents.

Rational prevention is unlikely until there is a better understanding of pathogenesis. In the interim, it has been repeatedly shown that removal of the ovaries before the age of 40 substantially reduces breast cancer risk. This one measure, probably socially and psychologically unacceptable, would fairly rapidly reduce breast cancer levels.

Bladder. In parts of Africa squamous cell cancer arising in the bilharzial bladder is very common. Current notions on pathogenesis are complex, involving the production of nitrosamines by bacteria in the infected organ. Prevention should be simple by breaking the life cycle of the parasite. This involves no more than persuading the population not to urinate into water but is very difficult to implement as cause and effect are by no means obvious. With rapidly increasing populations and extension of irrigation schemes schistosomiasis is likely to spread. For this cancer, prevention for the time being may have to be secondary and expensive by treatment of the schistosomal patient.

Viruses and Vaccines. In several parts of the world (Africa/Asia) the commonest cancer today is primary hepatocellular carcinoma. A series of what were essentially correlation studies showed that where incidence was high the average consumption of aflatoxin contaminated foods was also raised, evidence which, when taken in conjunction with animal experiments, seemed to explain the raised risk. However, the possible viral aetiology for primary liver cancer, advanced as long ago as 1940, has now been placed on a much stronger basis and very high relative risks, some in the order of 100-fold, for hepatitis B virus (HBV) carriers demonstrated in a series of populations and different countries (Beasley *et al.*, 1981). If this work is confirmed and if the vaccines currently under trial are effective and have no untoward effects, then it is possible that one of the current major tumours could be largely eliminated. Although the relative role of aflatoxin and the HBV has not yet been finally elucidated there are reasonable grounds for optimism. On the contrary, previous work suggesting a viral aetiology for breast cancer (and the possibility of production of a vaccine) has not been confirmed. While nasopharynx cancer is linked in some way to the Epstein-Barr virus and attempts are being made to produce a vaccine to this agent, it is premature even to speculate on the possible effect. It is worth noting that the evaluation of the efficacy of vaccines will not be easy for relatively rare diseases such as virus-induced cancer (Higginson *et al.*, 1971).

Occupational Exposures. Although the proportion of cancers due to occupational exposures is probably rather low, occupational cancers are by definition preventable. On the whole, the past record of industry, private or publicly owned, has not been good. The existence of a risk has been denied, efforts to investigate potential risks frequently frustrated and when risk is conclusively demonstrated the institution of adequate protection is claimed to be impossible on grounds of cost. This may be true for existing plants but modern engineering techniques seem to be able to control hazards when preventive measures are incorporated at the design stage. In several countries regulatory agencies have either been too lax or have lacked impartiality. The attitude of labour to protection has sometimes been ambivalent, 'danger money' being an acceptable alternative.

There are numerous examples of successful intervention for industrial occupational cancer. The measures taken in 1931 in England and Wales in relation to asbestos, measures which would be regarded as inadequate today, nonetheless resulted in a fall in mesothelioma risk and in the nickel industry the excess risk of nasal sinus cancers seems to have disappeared after changes in the manufacturing process were made (Doll, 1977).

When considering industrial risks in relation to other causes of cancer, it is easy to fall into the relative risk trap and forget that the extremely high relative risk for exposure to, say, vinylchloride monomer affects a relatively small number of people and that the 100-fold lower relative risks associated with moderate smoking but affecting a sizeable proportion of the population may in terms of numbers of cancers caused be vastly more important.

Prevention Strategies

Primary prevention has been most successful when individual susceptibility to disease can be easily reduced as by immunisation; the future potential for such protection in relation to oncogenic viruses has already been mentioned.

The other major preventive strategies involve alterations in exposure to potential carcinogens or risk factors. Control may involve regulatory or legislative activity to protect the *community* as a whole from potential carcinogens in food, air, water, the workplace, radiation and the like. The other broad category of preventive activity involves persuasion in an attempt to influence *personal* actions and habits, such as smoking or diet. Nonetheless there is considerable overlap. Legislation may reduce exposure to tobacco smoke by prohibiting smoking in public places; persuasion and financial incentives voted by law have influenced age of marriage and family size in, for example, China and Singapore.

Once a risk has been identified it has been suggested that if the truly high-risk groups could be identified and approached then it would be easier to induce these persons to alter their behaviour rather than exhorting all exposed individuals to do so. However, Salonen *et al.* (1981), after examining health behaviour in relation to estimated coronary heart disease risk during a community-based cardiovascular disease prevention programme in North Karelia, Finland, concluded that any changes observed were common to the community, bearing little relation to individual preintervention risk level, although the programme did nonetheless induce changes greater than those occurring in the reference population.

Face-to-face counselling of high-risk persons has been shown to be much more effective in changing behaviour and reducing risk. The problem is how to organise this for comparatively large numbers of people. The family physician has a central role. His most rewarding target is undoubtedly the smoker. His problem lies in a lack of access to the most vulnerable age group — from 9 to 14 years — and for this group other approaches will be needed.

While there is concern in many countries over the lack of availability or utilisation of medical services by the poorer sections of societies,

> the inequalities appear to be greatest (and most worrying) in the preventive services. Severe under-utilisation by the working classes is a complex resultant of under-provision, of costs (financial, psychological) of attendance, and perhaps of a lifestyle which profoundly inhibits any attempt at rational action in the interests of future well being. (Black, 1980)

If this conclusion is correct and can be generalised to more than one country, it is clear that the road for prevention goes through territories far removed from the simplistic 'removal-of-the-cause' approach, involves major changes in the fabric of society and has a timescale measured in generations.

Secondary Prevention

Secondary prevention of disease is a misnomer since there is no attempt to prevent pathological change occurring; here the objective is early detection so that treatment can be commenced at a stage at which medical aid would not normally have been sought. A rather arbitrary distinction is made between 'early diagnosis' — detection of disease which is symptomatic (but whose significance is not recognised by the patient), and 'screening' where the disease is detected whilst still asymptomatic. Most of the theoretical treatment of secondary prevention has been presented in terms of screening (Wilson and Junger, 1968; Cole and Morrison, 1978; Miller, 1982), but it is also applicable to early diagnosis.

Screening is usually defined in operational terms; it involves the use of relatively simple inexpensive tests or examinations which can be applied to subjects rapidly in order to distinguish a group with a high probability of having the disease in question who can then be subjected to full conventional diagnostic procedures. This process thus differs from usual medical practice where the clinical history and examination attempt to provide a definitive diagnosis upon which therapy can be based. In addition there is an important ethical difference since in screening programmes subjects who feel well are persuaded to take part with the implication that there will be a benefit from doing so. Such programmes thus have a special obligation to demonstrate their effectiveness, and for cancer screening this implies that they should reduce mortality and morbidity amongst those who agree to be screened.

Several sets of criteria have been suggested to help in the evaluation of proposed screening programmes (Wilson and Junger, 1968; Whitby, 1974; UICC, 1978). Although these are all rather differently formulated, the factors to be considered relate to the disease, the proposed screening test and to the treatment of detected cases.

Diseases for Screening

These should be significant public health problems either in terms of seriousness or frequency in the population. Most cancers are potentially serious, although for individual sites the prevalence of unrecognised disease is likely to be fairly low. Furthermore, if a screening programme is established in which the population is examined repeatedly the reservoir of undetected disease and hence the yield of screening will fall after the first or second cycles (Table 18.2). By confining examinations to population subgroups who are at increased risk of disease, prevalence of abnormality and hence yield of screening are increased. In practice all screening programmes are selective in some degree, at least on the basis of age group, and sometimes using other risk factors as well (e.g. smokers for chest X-ray screening). A good knowledge of the natural history of the disease is usually included in lists of criteria, and clearly it is desirable to understand the relationships between the preclinical stages of the condition which might be detected by screening, and the outcome of treatment in these stages. In general, however, there is a lack of precise quantitative knowledge concerning the behaviour of preclinical lesions in terms of their potential duration and rates of progression to established disease.

Table 18.2: Prevalence of Disease at First and Subsequent Screenings

Cancer	Survey	Prevalence (per 1,000 examined)	
		1st examination	Rescreening
Cervix (carcinoma *in situ only*)	Christopherson (1966): Females age 20+ in Louisville. Rescreen in under 3 years	3.9	1.3
Breast	Shapiro (1977): Females 40-64 in New York. Rescreen after 1 year	2.7	1.5
Lung	Brett (1968): Males 40-65 in S. England. Rescreen after 6 months	1.0	0.4

Screening Tests

Those which are intended to be applied to large numbers of individuals, should be simple, inexpensive, safe or free from side-effects, and acceptable to the population. Acceptability is, of course, partly related to safety and partly to cultural norms; for example routine regular proctoscopy may be acceptable to North Americans (American Cancer Society, 1980) but would not be so in many other cultures.

A distinction has been drawn between screening tests, which categorise subjects as 'probably ill' or probably well' and diagnostic tests which aim to reach a definitive decision. This difference is, however, only a question of the validity of the tests concerned, and the use of sensitivity and specificity as measures of validity is familiar in epidemiology. For screening tests there is a reciprocal relationship between the sensitivity and specificity which are usually determined by the 'cut-off point' or 'criterion of positivity' chosen for the test (Thorner and Remein, 1961). With the possible exception of the use of serum alphafoetoprotein as a screening test for hepatoma, cut-off points in cancer screening are not quantitatively defined. Instead, decisions are based upon subjective judgement of clinical findings, cytological or radiological patterns which are deemed to necessitate further investigation. In such instances choice is made more difficult if adequate quantitative knowledge of the precursor conditions is lacking.

Sensitivity and specificity of screening can also be altered by changing the number of different tests which can be applied at the same time (e.g. to screen for breast cancer) or the number of times the same test is applied (e.g. occult blood testing of faeces). Decisions on appropriate levels of sensitivity and specificity of screening procedures are not simple, and ultimately depend on considerations of costs and benefits, although such decisions are rarely explicitly expressed.

The validity of screening in terms of sensitivity and specificity can only be estimated if the true underlying presence or absence of disease is known, they cannot be deduced from the results of screening alone (Figure 18.1). Follow-up by further diagnostic procedures is usual for subjects screening positive, which allows the distinction between true and false positive tests (and hence the calculation of Predictive Value) but ascertainment of outcome for those screening negative is less often available. If the disease has a low prevalence, then reasonable estimates of specificity can be made (in nomenclature of Figure 18.1 since $b+d \doteq N$, specificity $\doteq 1-(b/N)$) but without follow-up of persons negative on screening (c+d) it is not possible to estimate sensitivity. Attempts to measure sensitivity by performing tests on patients with known disease are likely to be erroneous, since it is *unknown* cases that the screening test will try to detect in practice.

Figure 18.1: Possible Outcomes of Screening Examinations

Screening test result	Diagnosis		Total
	Diseased	Not diseased	
Positive	a (True positives)	b (False positives)	a + b
Negative	c (False negatives)	d (True negatives)	c + d
TOTAL	a + c	b + d	N = a + b + c + d

Sensitivity = $a/a+c$ Specificity = $d/b+d$
Predictive value of positive tests = $a/a+b$
Prevalence of disease = $a+c/N$

Treatment

Here the ethical issue raised earlier is of paramount consideration; for all diseases there is an obligation to provide accepted therapy whether this is efficacious or not; in screening programmes, however, it is essential to be certain that the treatment provides a better prognosis for patients detected by screening than if the disease had manifested itself later in its natural history. Improvement in prognosis may be measured simply as the increased survival or expectation of life following detection.

However, considerations of the improvement in quality of life are also important if earlier diagnosis leads to simpler or less traumatic methods of treatment. The difficulties in evaluating the results of screening are dealt with in the following section. It should be obvious that any treatment which is necessary for patients detected by screening should be acceptable to them and readily available. This means that health authorities should ensure that facilities for treating cases are provided before screening programmes are introduced into an area.

Evaluation of Prevention

Cochrane (1972) used the word 'effectiveness' to describe the degree of success of a programme in achieving its objective, and 'efficiency' to define the ratio between this observed outcome, and the input or expenditure required. The usefulness of prevention strategies can conveniently be discussed in these terms.

The Effectiveness of Prevention

Primary Prevention. Primary prevention has as its aim the reduction in exposure to risk factors (as already mentioned, this may take the form of an increased intake of a possible protective agent), and the prevention of disease *occurrence*. Thus, effectiveness of primary prevention can either be assessed by measuring the success in achieving the desired changes in exposure 'process measures' or in reducing the occurrence of disease 'outcome measures'.

Although the latter seems an inherently more sensible measure, because of the long latent period of most cancers it may be some time before the desired outcome could become manifest. Measuring of process allows immediate assessment of exposure reduction.

Measures of process may rely on routinely collected statistics, for example on production, or retail sales (of tobacco, alcohol), or regular surveys of the population for consumption patterns (for example government sponsored social and household expenditure surveys, or surveys undertaken by marketing organisations). Alternatively, and especially if a limited population is dealt with, the use of surveys of the behaviour of interest (e.g. dietary habits, sunlight exposure) can be made to see if prevention programmes seem to have had any impact.

Measures of outcome are concerned with reducing the occurrence of disease. The objectives of cancer prevention are to prevent or postpone the onset of disease, not to avoid the fact of death. The most appropriate statistics for judging whether or not these objectives are met are age-specific or age-standardised occurrence rates. Incidence rates (from cancer registration) are the preferred measure. In their absence mortality rates may be used as a proxy, although the relationship between the two depends upon survival; where this is relatively constant (which is probably true for the majority of cancers) changes in mortality rates are an adequate indicator of changes in cancer occurrence.

Secondary Prevention. Screening and early diagnosis will obviously not reduce cancer incidence. Apparent incidence may in fact rise, especially at the onset of screening programmes when many asymptomatic lesions are brought to light. It may be that some pre-cancers or early lesions detected by screening would have regressed or remained subclinical throughout the patient's lifespan and would never have appeared as incident cases of disease if a special search had not been undertaken.

Early detection aims to improve prognosis; usually this has been studied in terms of quantity of life gained. Quality of life may be an important consideration — unfortunately methods of measuring this are much more controversial. As far as quantity of life gained is concerned, data on case fatality rates (or duration of survival) would seem to be the most satisfactory method of assessment. Even in the ideal circumstances of a randomised controlled trial, however, there are two sources of difficulty in interpreting results of screening; lead time and length bias. Lead time is the interval between the time of detection by screening and the time at which the disease would otherwise have been diagnosed; any calculation of the real gain in survival following screening must therefore take into account this period by which diagnosis has been advanced (Hutchinson and Shapiro, 1968). Length bias can arise particularly at the beginning of a screening programme when the prevalent, undetected cases of disease in the population will comprise a disproportionate number with relatively slowly progressive disease, and hence better than average prognosis. Cases detected by screening will thus be a biased sample of diseased individuals, a sample with a relatively favourable prognosis (Feinleib and Zelen, 1969).

Proportionate distribution of cases by stage, a measure that can easily be derived from the results of a screening programme, is sometimes used as a proxy measure for prognosis (there is no need to wait months or years to calculate survival). It, too, will be subject to lead time and length biases but there are additional problems since it is difficult to make corrections using estimates of their magnitude.

The only valid measure of the effectiveness of screening is the change in the mortality rates that are achieved. If necessary this change can be presented as person-years of life saved, with weightings for 'quality of life' or life-years during different decades. Ideally such evaluation is by randomised controlled trial, but the logistics and ethical problems involved mean that relatively few have been performed. For lung cancer, regular screening by chest X-ray improves stage at diagnosis and duration of survival in cases found by screening, but mortality was no better in screened than control groups (Brett 1968; Taylor *et al.*, 1981). The Health Insurance Plan (HIP) trial of screening for breast cancer by mammography plus palpation resulted in improved mortality in the screened women over 50 years of age (Shapiro, 1977).

Two large-scale controlled trials to evaluate screening for colonic cancer by testing for faecal occult blood are in progress but so far results are not available (Winawer *et al.*, 1980; Gilbertson *et al.*, 1980). For the most widely practised cancer screening activity, cervical cytology, there have never been any trials; evidence of effectiveness is derived from observation and quasi-experimental situations. The observation that women who are screened have lower rates of invasive disease (Fidler *et al.*, 1968; McGregor, 1976) only confirms the well-known fact that subjects at lower risk of disease are the most frequent users of screening programmes. More convincing evidence comes from before–after comparisons, where mortality falls following population screening (Hakama, 1982) or intra-country comparisons of mortality in proportion to screening activity for different areas (Cramer, 1974; Miller *et al.*, 1976).

Efficiency of Prevention

Just as interest in cancer prevention has been stimulated by the relative ineffectiveness of therapy, so too the rapidly escalating cost of the latter has given rise to the hope that prevention may also cost less. Putting a value on the prevention of disease is conventionally done by reckoning which of the costs of a given illness might have been averted. The costing of disease is a controversial area, especially when the methods employed use monetary values, but no satisfactory or agreed alternative to financial costing has yet been developed.

The costs of illness are separated into direct costs, indirect costs, and social (or intangible) costs. Direct costs are those incurred in obtaining medical services (hospitalisation, physicians, transport, drugs, etc). The indirect costs of illness arise from the loss of normal working activity of the patient — either in conventional employment or in the home — and probably of the family too. The social or intangible costs of illness includes factors such as pain, suffering, anxiety and grief which are often very considerable in the case of cancer. The financial evaluation of the direct costs of illness is relatively easy, controversial for the indirect costs and exceedingly difficult for the social/intangible costs. Nevertheless, in the planning of health care services as in any other field of social policy, it is necessary to have some idea of the likely results of investment, not least because of ever-increasing pressure on budgets for health care. Moreover, some notion of the method of costing illness is necessary, or it may appear from a superficial viewpoint that prevention of disease is not worthwhile. For example, it is often asserted that if cancer is prevented, those who would have died from it will live to contract other chronic diseases of old age for which the necessary care and support may ultimately cost more. This may be true for direct costs, but since much prevention is concerned with postponement of illness and maintainance of a longer, healthy and active life, there are likely to be very large savings in indirect and social costs. In accounting terms also, the mere postponement of direct costs to a future date is valuable.

The question of whether prevention of disease is less expensive than cure involves using some form of analysis of costs versus outcome for the different possibilities. Cost-effectiveness analysis attempts to measure the relative expenses involved in achieving a given outcome — for example the saving of a 'life-year'. It is not always easy to use in health care since the outcomes of the different programmes being compared are often dissimilar, for instance the *quality* of a year of life gained by postponing the onset of cancer for one year may well be greater than a further year of life resulting from cancer therapy. For this reason it is often necessary to try to evaluate outcomes of intervention in some other units. In cost-benefit analysis financial costs are the most commonly used measures of outcome.

Formal cost-benefit analysis of a preventive programme requires that estimates of the following are made:

1. The financial (and other) costs of the preventive activities.
2. The results of the programme in preventing or postponing disease.

3. The evaluation of the benefits achieved in terms of financial cost of the disease which has been averted or delayed.

These are all hard to quantify in primary prevention programmes.

It is not easy to decide exactly who are the beneficiaries of legislative or persuasive efforts; furthermore, a single toxic factor may be involved in varying degrees in the causation of several diseases, and the link between preventive inputs and outcomes becomes obscure. It is not known, for example, how much bronchitis has been prevented or avoided by emission control regulations or anti-smoking campaigns. Furthermore, there may be complex considerations in evaluating the cost of the intervention — for example withdrawal of a carcinogenic chemical used in a manufacturing process may lead to a rise in the cost of the product to the consumer, or the control of a drug known to be carcinogenic involves costs in the use of a substitute, or inadequate treatment of the disease for which the drug was indicated. Other costs which result from primary prevention programmes may be borne at a national level, from the potential increase in unemployment or loss of export earnings.

The comparison of costs versus benefits is somewhat easier for programmes of screening (or early detection) which are largely confined to the field of health care services. Thus it is the high cost of achieving small *benefits* that inhibits the widespread introduction of such procedures as regular proctosigmoidoscopy for rectal carcinoma (Bolt, 1971) or screening for hepatocellular carcinoma by routine serum alphafoetoprotein estimation.

Within each screening programme, however, there are a number of variables which can be adjusted to alter the ratio between total expenditure and outcome.

The relationship between the sensitivity and specificity of the screening test and the 'criterion of positivity' that is chosen has already been discussed, and it has been pointed out that the variable which can easily be measured as a result of these changes is the predictive value of the test (the proportion of positive tests that are true positives). The predictive value of the test is also changed by alterations in the underlying prevalence of the disease sought (as, too, of course, is the total yield of cases from screening). The underlying prevalence can be increased if subgroups of the population are selected for screening on the basis of risk factors such as age, marital status, occupation, etc. In a sense this in itself is a form of screening, particularly if a history of some condition or symptom is used as the criterion for selection.

Prevalence of undetected disease can also be influenced by changing the frequency of examinations of the population.

Blumberg (1957) was the first to point out that there are different optimum levels for these variables in formulating a screening programme, depending on the relative values placed on the different outcomes of screening. His formula for the total value (Vt) to the community of a screening programme is expressed thus:

$$Vt = TP|x\ Vtp + TN \times Vtn + FP \times Vfp + FN \times Vfn$$

TP, TN, FP and FN are the numbers (or proportions) of true positives, true negatives, false positives and false negatives that are detected; they are determined by prevalence of disease and characteristics of the test, as already discussed. Vtp, Vtn, Vfp and Vfn are the 'health values' which can be imputed to a person in each of these states; the value may be positive or negative.

The value of a true positive test is related to the improved outcome (quantity and/or quality of life) following detection by screening rather than conventional diagnosis. The value of a true negative is related to the reassurance of a normal examination. The values of false results are clearly negative; false positive tests lead to unnecessary, time-consuming and possibly hazardous investigations (for example, breast cancer screening probably leads to more negative breast biopsies than would have taken place without screening), false negative tests may give misplaced reassurance, and lead to subsequent discovery of the tumour being delayed. The total value of a programme is, of course, debited by the costs of screening; these may be the direct costs of providing the examinations, but in addition the screening tests may be hazardous to the recipients. The precise magnitude of the risk of mammography depends on the assumptions made in the calculation; Bailar (1977) argued that risks outweigh any benefit from screening in women under 50 but the radiation dose from mammography is certainly much lower today.

The ability to explore these complex interrelationships between the variables in screening programmes has been enhanced by the development of models of the screening process based either on theoretical formulae (Eddy, 1980; Albert *et al.*, 1978) or using empirical data in computer simulation (Knox, 1973; Coppleson and Brown, 1975). At present perhaps their main limitation is inadequate data on the natural history of the cancers involved, but their undoubted value is the ability to examine outcomes of multiple variants of screening programmes in a way that would be quite impossible with real-life clinical trials.

The Future

It is not inconceivable that in years to come it may be possible to establish risk profiles comprising both measures of exposure and of susceptibility. The exposure indices could include not only those known today but also measurement of DNA adducts to known carcinogens: the indicators of susceptibility may go far beyond HLA profile, blood group and the like. It remains to be seen whether or not such refinements will influence attitudes to primary prevention. Although 'prevention is better than cure' has become an axiom for many human activities, if there were to be a survey to list the most desirable advances in knowledge, we venture to predict that in the developed world 'a cure for cancer' would be close to the top of the list and 'the prevention of cancer' would scarcely receive mention. In such a setting funding and acceptance of prevention will never be easy.

References

Albert, A., Gertman, P.M. and Louis, T.A. (1978). Screening for the early detection of cancer. *Mathematical Biosciences*, 40: 1-59

American Cancer Society (1980). Guidelines for the cancer-related checkup. *CA – A Cancer Journal for Clinicians*, 30: 194-240

Armstrong, B. and Doll, R. (1975). Environmental factors and cancer incidence and mortality in different countries with special reference to dietary practices. *International Journal of Cancer*, 15: 617-31

Bailar, J.C. (1977). Screening for early breast cancer: pros and cons. *Cancer*, 39: 2783-95

Beasley, R.P., Lin. C.-C., Hwang, L.-Y. and Chien, C.-S. (1981). Hepatocellular carcinoma and Hepatitis B virus. A prospective study of 22,707 men in Taiwan. *Lancet*, 2: 1129-33

Bjelke, E. (1974). Epidemiologic studies of cancer of the stomach, colon and rectum, with special emphasis on the role of diet. *Scandinavian Journal of Gastroenterology*, 9 (Suppl. 31): 42-53

Black, D. (Chairman) (1980). *Inequalities in Health*, Report of a Research Working Group. Department of Health and Social Security, London

Blumberg, M.S. (1957). Evaluating health screening procedures. *Operations Research*, 5: 351-60

Bolt, R.J. (1971). Sigmoidoscopy in detection and diagnosis in the asymptomatic individual. *Cancer*, 28: 121-2

Brett, G.Z. (1968). The value of lung cancer detection by six-monthly chest radiographs. *Thorax*, 23: 414-20

Christopherson, W.M. (1966). The control of cervix cancer. *Acta Cytologica*, 10: 6-10

Cochrane, A. (1972). *Effectiveness and Efficiency; Random reflections on the health service*, Nuffield Provincial Hospitals Trust, London

Cole, P. and Morrison, A.S. (1978). Basic issues in cancer screening. In: Miller, A.B. (ed.), *Screening in Cancer*, UICC Technical Report Series, 40, pp. 7-39

Copplesen, L.W. and Brown, B. (1975). Observations on a model of the biology of carcinoma of the cervix: a poor fit between observation and theory. *American Journal of Obstetrics and Gynecology*, 122: 127-36

Cramer, D.W. (1974). The role of cervical cytology in the declining morbidity and mortality of cervical cancer. *Cancer*, 34: 2018-27

Doll, R. (1977). Strategy for detection of cancer hazards to man. *Nature*, 265: 589-96

―――― and Peto, R. (1981). The causes of cancer: Quantitative estimates of avoidable risks of cancer in the United States today. *Journal of the National Cancer Institute*, 66: 1191-308

Eddy, D.M. (1980). *Screening for Cancer: Theory, Analysis and Design*, Prentice Hall, Englewood Cliffs, NJ

Feinleib, M. and Zelen, M. (1969). Some pitfalls in the evaluation of screening programs, *Archives of Environmental Health*, 19: 412-15

Fidler, H.K., Boyes, D.A. and Worth, A.J. (1968). Cervical cancer detection in British Columbia. *Journal of Obstetrics and Gynaecology of the British Commonwealth*, 75: 392-404

Gilbertson, V.A., Church, T., Grewe, F., Mandel, J., McHugh, R., Schuman, L. *et al.* (1980). The design of a study to assess occult blood screening for colon cancer. *Journal of Chronic Diseases*, 33: 107-14

Hakama, M. (1982). Trends in the incidence of cervical cancer in the Nordic countries. In: Magnus, K. (ed.), *Trends in Cancer Incidence*, Hemisphere Publishing, Washington

Higginson, J., de-Thé, G., Geser, A. and Day, N. (1971). An epidemiological analysis of cancer vaccines. *International Journal of Cancer*, 7: 565-74

―――― and Muir, C.S. (1979). Environmental carcinogenesis: misconceptions and limitations to cancer control. *Journal of the National Cancer Institute*, 63: 1291-8

Hirayama, T. (1971). Epidemiology of stomach cancer. *GANN Monograph on Cancer Research*, 11: 3-19

―――― (1977). Changing patterns of cancer in Japan with special reference to the decrease in stomach cancer mortality. In: Hiatt H.H., Watson, J.D. and Winston, J.A. (eds.), *Origins of Human Cancer*, New York, Cold Spring Harbor Laboratory, pp. 55-76

―――― Waterhouse, J.A.H. and Fraumeni, J.F. (eds.) (1980). *Cancer Risks by Site*, UICC Technical Report Series, 41, Geneva

Hutchinson, G.B. and Shapiro, S. (1968). Lead time gained by diagnostic screening for breast cancer. *Journal of the National Cancer Institute*, 41: 665-81

Jensen, O.M., MacLennan, R. and Wahrendorf, J. (1982). Diet, bowel function, fecal characteristics and large bowel cancer in Denmark and Finland. *Nutrition and Cancer*, 4 (1): 5-19

Knox, E.G. (1973). A simulation system for screening procedures. In: McLachlan, G. (ed.), *The Future, and Present Indicatives* (Problems & Progress in Medical Care, IX series), Nuffield Provincial Hospitals Trust, ch. 2, pp. 17-55

Lancet (editorial) (1981). Immunocompromised homosexuals, 2: 1325-6

Lyon, J.L., Gardner, J.W. and West, D.W. (1980). Cancer incidence in Mormons and non-Mormons in Utah during 1967-75. *Journal of the National Cancer Institute*, 65: 1055-61

McGregor, J.E. (1976). Evaluation of mass screening programmes for cervical cancer in N.E. Scotland. *Tumori*, 62: 287-95

McMichael, A., Potter, J.D. and Hetzel, B.S. (1979). Time-trends in colo-rectal cancer mortality in relation to food and alcohol consumption: United States, United Kingdom, Australia and New Zealand. *International Journal of Epidemiology*, 8: 295-303

Miller, A.B. (1978). An overview of hormone related cancers. *Cancer Research*, 38: 3985-90

—— (1982). Fundamental issues in screening. In: Schottenfeld, D. and Fraumeni, J.F. (eds.), *Cancer Epidemiology and Prevention*, Saunders, Philadelphia

—— Lindsay, J. and Hill, G.B. (1976). Mortality from cancer of the uterus in Canada and its relationship to screening for cancer of the cervix. *International Journal of Cancer*, 17: 602-12

Peto, R., Doll, R., Buckley, J.D. and Sporn, M.B. (1981). Can dietary beta-carotene materially reduce human cancer rates? *Nature*, 290: 201-8

Phillips, R.L., Garfinkel, L., Kuzma, J.W., Beeson, W.L., Lotz, T. and Brin, B. (1980). Mortality among California Seventh Day Adventists for selected cancer sites. *Journal of the National Cancer Institute*, 65: 1097-107

Salonen, J.K., Heinonen, O.P., Kottke, T.E. and Puska, P. (1981). Change in health behaviour in relation to estimated coronary heart disease risk during a community-based cardiovascular disease prevention programme. *International Journal of Epidemiology*, 10: 343-56

Shapiro, S. (1977). Evidence on screening for breast cancer from a randomised trial. *Cancer*, 39: 2772-82

Stemmermann, G.N., Nomura, A.M.Y., Heilbrun, L.K., Pollack, E.S. and Kagan, A. (1981). Serum cholesterol and colon cancer incidence in Hawaiian Japanese men. *Journal of the National Cancer Institute*, 67: 1179-82

Taylor, W.F., Fontana, R.S., Uhlerhopp, M.A. and Davis, C.S. (1981). Some results of screening for early lung cancer. *Cancer*, 47: 1114-20

Thorner, R.M. and Remein, Q.R. (1961). Principles and procedures in the evaluation of screening for disease. *Public Health Monograph No. 67*, US Government Printing Office, Washington

Tuyns, A. (1979). Epidemiology of alcohol and cancer. *Cancer Research*, 39: 2840-3

UICC (1978). Summary and recommendations. In: Miller, A.B. (ed.), *Screening in Cancer*, UICC Technical Report Series, 40: 334-8

US Department of Health and Human Services (1982). *The Health Consequences of Smoking; Cancer*, A report of the Surgeon General, US Government Printing Office, Washington, DC, Part V, p. 257

Whitby, L.G. (1974). Screening for disease: definitions and criteria. *Lancet*, 2: 819-21

WHO (1978). *Steroid Contraception and the Risk of Neoplasia*, WHO Technical Report Series, No 619

Wilson, J.M.G. and Junger, G. (1968). Principles and practice of screening for disease. *Public Health Papers*, No. 34, WHO, Geneva

Winawer, S.J., Andrewes, M., Flehinger, B., Sherlock, P., Schottenfeld, D. and Miller, D.G. (1980). Progress report on controlled trial of fecal occult blood testing for the detection of colorectal neoplasia. *Cancer*, 45: 2959-64

Wright, N.H., Vessey, M.P., Kenward, B., McPhersen, K. and Doll, R. (1978). Neoplasia and dysplasia of the cervix uteri and contraception: a possible protective effect of the diaphragm. *British Journal of Cancer*, 38: 273-9

INDEX